Body
Information
for Teens

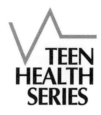

TEEN HEALTH SERIES

First Edition

Body Information for Teens

Health Tips about Maintaining Well-Being for a Lifetime

*Including Facts about the Development
and Functioning of the Body's Systems, Organs,
and Structures and the Health Impact
of Lifestyle Choices*

◆

Edited by Sandra Augustyn Lawton

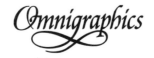

615 Griswold Street • Detroit, MI 48226

Bibliographic Note

Because this page cannot legibly accommodate all the copyright notices, the Bibliographic Note portion of the Preface constitutes an extension of the copyright notice.

Edited by Sandra Augustyn Lawton

Teen Health Series

Karen Bellenir, *Managing Editor*
David A. Cooke, M.D., *Medical Consultant*
Elizabeth Collins, *Research and Permissions Coordinator*
Cherry Stockdale, *Permissions Assistant*
Laura Pleva Nielsen, *Index Editor*
EdIndex, Services for Publishers, *Indexers*

* * *

Omnigraphics, Inc.

Matthew P. Barbour, *Senior Vice President*
Kay Gill, *Vice President—Directories*
Kevin Hayes, *Operations Manager*
David P. Bianco, *Marketing Director*

* * *

Peter E. Ruffner, *Publisher*

Frederick G. Ruffner, Jr., *Chairman*

Copyright © 2007 Omnigraphics, Inc.

ISBN 978-0-7808-0443-2

Library of Congress Cataloging-in-Publication Data

Body information for teens : health tips about maintaining well-being for a lifetime including facts about the development and functioning of the body's systems, organs, and structures and the health impact of lifestyle choices / edited by Sandra Augustyn Lawton.
    p. cm. -- (Teen health series)
    Summary: "Provides basic consumer health information for teens on understanding the body and and maintaining well-being. Includes index, resource information, and recommendations for further reading"--Provided by publisher.
    Includes bibliographical references and index.
    ISBN 978-0-7808-0443-2 (hardcover : alk. paper) 1. Teenagers--Health and hygiene. 2. Adolescent psychology. 3. Consumer information. I. Lawton, Sandra Augustyn.
    RJ140.B63 2007
    613'.0433--dc22
                                                                        2006101507

Printed in the United States

Table of Contents

Part Three: How Your Body Grows And Changes

Part Four: How To Keep Your Body Healthy

Part Five: How To Maintain Mental And Emotional Wellness

Part Six: How Lifestyle Choices Can Affect Your Health

Part Seven: How To Handle Illness And Injury

Part Eight: If You Need More Information

Preface

About This Book

The teen years are marked by changes—hormones stir, bodies transform, peer groups become more important, and independence calls. Parental influence decreases, and teens begin to assume more responsibility for the decisions they make about the foods they eat, the physical activities they pursue, the risks they take, and the lifestyles they adopt. Because all these decisions, and many more, have a direct impact on health, teens need to understand how their bodies work and how they can make choices that support life-long wellness.

Body Information for Teens explains how the body is shaped by heredity, how its various systems and organs work, and how it changes over time, beginning with the stages of fetal development and continuing through childhood, puberty, and the aging process. It describes the steps important to maintaining good health, including eating right, exercising, practicing good hygiene, and visiting healthcare providers for regular checkups. In addition, the importance of mental and emotional wellness is addressed, and a section about lifestyle choices explains how decisions regarding such matters as substance use, sexual activity, and body adornment can impact a person's health for a lifetime. Facts about how to handle common illness and injuries, safely use medications, and administer first aid are also included along with guidelines for understanding and evaluating medical information, a directory of health-related resources, and suggestions for additional reading.

How To Use This Book

This book is divided into parts and chapters. Parts focus on broad areas of interest; chapters are devoted to single topics within a part.

Part One: How Heredity Molds Your Body explains how genes govern not only a person's appearance but also his or her health risks. It describes the process of collecting a family's health history and discusses genetic testing.

Part Two: How Your Body Works provides facts about the major systems and organs of the body, including the skeletal, cardiovascular, respiratory, digestive, and lymphatic systems. It also describes hormones and sexual development. The part concludes with a chapter that addresses many common questions about seemingly mysterious body functions, such as why noses run or why people shiver or yawn.

Part Three: How Your Body Grows And Changes describes the stages by which a physical body grows and matures. It begins with a discussion of fetal development and describes the changes that occur throughout childhood and puberty and that continue even in adulthood.

Part Four: How To Keep Your Body Healthy discusses the care and maintenance of the human body. It describes the components of a healthy diet and talks about the importance of physical activity, good hygiene, and preventive health care.

Part Five: How To Maintain Mental And Emotional Wellness provides information about issues that often affect teens, including stress, depression, self-esteem, bullying, and dating violence. Dangerous behaviors such as eating disorders, self-injury, and suicide are also discussed.

Part Six: How Lifestyle Choices Can Affect Your Health presents information about alcohol, tobacco, and other drug use and other activities—including sexual practices, body piercing, tattooing, tanning, and cosmetic surgery—that can impact a person's wellbeing for a lifetime. Individual chapters discuss the specific risks involved and provide facts to support a well-informed decision-making process.

Part Seven: How To Handle Illness And Injury offers suggestions for improving communication with healthcare providers, an important aspect of maintaining good health but one many people find difficult. It also describes commonly used medicines and first aid techniques.

Part Eight: If You Need More Information provides tips on how to find medical information, how to evaluate health information on the internet, and how to interpret medical information in the news media. A directory of health resources and additional reading suggestions are also included.

Bibliographic Note

This volume contains documents and excerpts from publications issued by the following government agencies: Centers for Disease Control and Prevention (CDC), Health Resources and Services Administration (HRSA), Library of Congress, National Cancer Institute (NCI), National Guideline Clearinghouse, National Human Genome Research Institute, National Institute of Allergy and Infectious Diseases (NIAID), National Institute of Arthritis and Musculoskeletal and Skin Diseases (NIAMS), National Institute on Drug Abuse (NIDA), National Institute of Mental Health (NIMH), National Institutes of Health (NIH), National Library of Medicine (NLM), National Women's Health Information Center (NWHIC), President's Council on Physical Fitness and Sports (PCPFS), Substance Abuse and Mental Health Services Administration (SAMHSA), U.S. Department of Health and Human Services (HHS), and U.S. Food and Drug Administration (FDA).

In addition, this volume contains copyrighted documents and articles produced by the following organizations and individuals: American Academy of Family Physicians, American Board of Medical Specialties, American Geriatrics Society Foundation for Health in Aging, American Osteopathic Association, Child and Youth Health, FPWA Sexual Health Services, National Sleep Foundation, Nemours Foundation, *Science News for Kids*, University of Maine Cooperative Extension, University of Michigan Health System, and World Bank.

Full citation information is provided on the first page of each chapter. Every effort has been made to secure all necessary rights to reprint the copyrighted material. If any omissions have been made, please contact Omnigraphics to make corrections for future editions.

xii

The photograph on the front cover is from School Days/Digital Vision Photography.

Acknowledgements

In addition to the organizations listed above, special thanks are due to the *Teen Health Series* research and permissions coordinator, Elizabeth Collins, and to its managing editor, Karen Bellenir.

About the *Teen Health Series*

At the request of librarians serving today's young adults, the *Teen Health Series* was developed as a specially focused set of volumes within Omnigraphics' *Health Reference Series*. Each volume deals comprehensively with a topic selected according to the needs and interests of people in middle school and high school.

Teens seeking preventive guidance, information about disease warning signs, medical statistics, and risk factors for health problems will find answers to their questions in the *Teen Health Series*. The *Series*, however, is not intended to serve as a tool for diagnosing illness, in prescribing treatments, or as a substitute for the physician/patient relationship. All people concerned about medical symptoms or the possibility of disease are encouraged to seek professional care from an appropriate health care provider.

If there is a topic you would like to see addressed in a future volume of the *Teen Health Series*, please write to:

Editor
Teen Health Series
Omnigraphics, Inc.
615 Griswold Street
Detroit, MI 48226

Locating Information within the *Teen Health Series*

The *Teen Health Series* contains a wealth of information about a wide variety of medical topics. As the *Series* continues to grow in size and scope, locating the precise information needed by a specific student may become more challenging. To address this concern, information about books within the *Teen Health Series* is included in *A Contents Guide to the Health Reference Series*. The *Contents Guide* presents an extensive list of more than 13,000 diseases, treatments, and other topics of general interest compiled from the Tables of Contents and major index headings from the books of the *Teen Health Series* and *Health Reference Series*. To access *A Contents Guide to the Health Reference Series*, visit www.healthreferenceseries.com.

Our Advisory Board

We would like to thank the following advisory board members for providing guidance to the development of this *Series*:

Dr. Lynda Baker,
Associate Professor of Library and Information Science,
Wayne State University, Detroit, MI

Nancy Bulgarelli,
William Beaumont Hospital Library, Royal Oak, MI

Karen Imarisio,
Bloomfield Township Public Library, Bloomfield Township, MI

Karen Morgan,
Mardigian Library, University of Michigan-Dearborn,
Dearborn, MI

Rosemary Orlando,
St. Clair Shores Public Library, St. Clair Shores, MI

Medical Consultant

Medical consultation services are provided to the *Teen Health Series* editors by David A. Cooke, M.D. Dr. Cooke is a graduate of Brandeis University, and he received his M.D. degree from the University of Michigan. He completed residency training at the University of Wisconsin Hospital and Clinics. He is board-certified in internal medicine. Dr. Cooke currently works as part of the University of Michigan Health System and practices in Ann Arbor, MI. In his free time, he enjoys writing, science fiction, and spending time with his family.

Part One

How Heredity Molds Your Body

Chapter 1

Genes And How They Work

What is a cell?

Cells are the basic building blocks of all living things. The human body is composed of trillions of cells. They provide structure for the body, take in nutrients from food, convert those nutrients into energy, and carry out specialized functions. Cells also contain the body's hereditary material and can make copies of themselves.

Cells have many parts, each with a different function. Some of these parts, called organelles, are specialized structures that perform certain tasks within the cell. Human cells contain the following major parts, listed in alphabetical order:

- **Cytoplasm:** The cytoplasm is fluid inside the cell that surrounds the organelles.

- **Endoplasmic reticulum (ER):** This organelle helps process molecules created by the cell and transport them to their specific destinations either inside or outside the cell.

- **Golgi apparatus:** The Golgi apparatus packages molecules processed by the endoplasmic reticulum to be transported out of the cell.

About This Chapter: Information in this chapter is from "What is a cell?" "What is DNA?" "What is a gene?" "What is a chromosome?" "How many chromosomes do people have?" "How do cells divide?" and "What are proteins and what do they do?" Genetics Home Reference, a service of the U.S. National Library of Medicine, May 2006.

- **Lysosomes and peroxisomes:** These organelles are the recycling center of the cell. They digest foreign bacteria that invade the cell, rid the cell of toxic substances, and recycle worn-out cell components.

- **Mitochondria:** Mitochondria are complex organelles that convert energy from food into a form that the cell can use. They have their own genetic material, separate from the DNA (deoxyribonucleic acid) in the nucleus, and can make copies of themselves.

- **Nucleus:** The nucleus serves as the cell's command center, sending directions to the cell to grow, mature, divide, or die. It also houses DNA, the cell's hereditary material. A membrane called the nuclear envelope, which protects the DNA and separates the nucleus from the rest of the cell, surrounds the nucleus.

- **Plasma membrane:** The plasma membrane is the outer lining of the cell. It separates the cell from its environment and allows materials to enter and leave the cell.

- **Ribosomes:** Ribosomes are organelles that process the cell's genetic instructions to create proteins. These organelles can float freely in the cytoplasm or be connected to the endoplasmic reticulum.

What is DNA?

DNA, or deoxyribonucleic acid, is the hereditary material in humans and almost all other organisms. Nearly every cell in a person's body has the same DNA. Most DNA is located in the cell nucleus (where it is called nuclear DNA), but a small amount of DNA can also be found in the mitochondria (where it is called mitochondrial DNA or mtDNA).

The information in DNA is stored as a code made up of four chemical bases: adenine (A), guanine (G), cytosine (C), and thymine (T). Human DNA consists of about 3 billion bases, and more than 99 percent of those bases are the same in all people. The order, or sequence, of these bases determines the information available for building and maintaining an organism, similar to the way in which letters of the alphabet appear in a certain order to form words and sentences.

DNA bases pair up with each other, A with T and C with G, to form units called base pairs. Each base is also attached to a sugar molecule and a

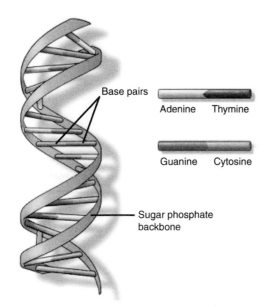

Figure 1.1. DNA is a double helix formed by base pairs attached to a sugar-phosphate backbone.

phosphate molecule. Together, a base, sugar, and phosphate are called a nucleotide. Nucleotides are arranged in two long strands that form a spiral called a double helix. The structure of the double helix is somewhat like a ladder, with the base pairs forming the ladder's rungs and the sugar and phosphate molecules forming the vertical side-pieces of the ladder.

An important property of DNA is that it can replicate, or make copies of itself. Each strand of DNA in the double helix can serve as a pattern for duplicating the sequence of bases. This is critical when cells divide because each new cell needs to have an exact copy of the DNA present in the old cell.

What is a gene?

A gene is the basic physical and functional unit of heredity. Genes, which are made up of DNA, act as instructions to make molecules called proteins. In humans, genes vary in size from a few hundred DNA bases to more than 2 million bases.

Every person has two copies of each gene, one inherited from each parent. Most genes are the same in all people, but a small number of genes (less than 1 percent of the total)

♣ It's A Fact!!

Humans have between 20,000 and 25,000 genes.

Source: "What is a gene?" Genetics Home Reference, National Library of Medicine.

are slightly different between people. Alleles are forms of the same gene with small differences in their sequence of DNA bases. These small differences contribute to each person's unique physical features.

What is a chromosome?

In the nucleus of each cell, the DNA molecule is packaged into thread-like structures called chromosomes. Each chromosome is made up of DNA tightly coiled many times around proteins, called histones that support its structure.

Chromosomes are not visible in the cell's nucleus—not even under a microscope—when the cell is not dividing. However, the DNA that makes up chromosomes becomes more tightly packed during cell division and is then visible under a microscope. Most of what researchers know about chromosomes was learned by observing chromosomes during cell division.

Each chromosome has a constriction point called the centromere, which divides the chromosome into two sections, or "arms." The short arm of the chromosome is labeled the "p arm." The long arm of the chromosome is labeled the "q arm." The location of the centromere on each chromosome gives the chromosome its characteristic shape and can be used to help describe the location of specific genes.

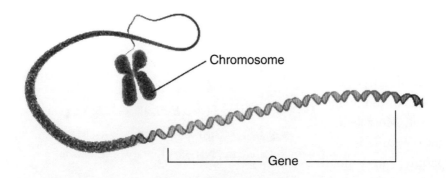

Figure 1.2. Genes are made up of DNA. Each chromosome contains many genes.

How many chromosomes do people have?

In humans, each cell normally contains 23 pairs of chromosomes, for a total of 46. Twenty-two of these pairs, called autosomes, look the same in both males and females. The 23rd pair, the sex chromosomes, differs between males and females. Females have two copies of the X chromosome, while males have one X and one Y chromosome.

How do cells divide?

There are two types of cell division: mitosis and meiosis. Most of the time when people refer to "cell division," they mean mitosis, the process of making new body cells. Meiosis is the type of cell division that creates egg and sperm cells.

Mitosis is a fundamental process for life. During mitosis, a cell duplicates all of its contents, including its chromosomes, and splits to form two identical daughter cells. Because this process is so critical, the steps of mitosis are carefully controlled by a number of genes. When mitosis is not regulated correctly, health problems, such as cancer, can result.

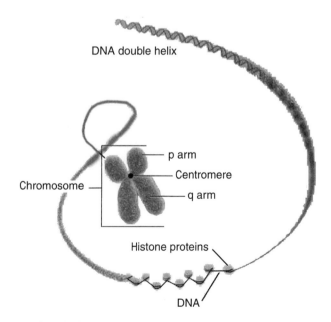

Figure 1.3. DNA and histone proteins are packaged into structures called chromosomes.

The other type of cell division, meiosis, ensures that humans have the same number of chromosomes in each generation. It is a two-step process that reduces the chromosome number by half—from 46 to 23—to form sperm and egg cells. When the sperm and egg cells unite at conception, each contributes 23 chromosomes so the resulting embryo will have the usual 46. Meiosis also allows genetic variation through a process of DNA shuffling while the cells are dividing.

What are proteins, and what do they do?

Proteins are large, complex molecules that play many critical roles in the body. They do most of the work in cells and are required for the structure, function, and regulation of the body's tissues and organs.

Proteins are made up of hundreds or thousands of smaller units called amino acids, which are attached to one another in long chains. There are 20 different types of amino acids that can be combined to make a protein. The sequence of amino acids determines each protein's unique 3-dimensional structure and its specific function.

Proteins can be described according to their large range of functions in the body. They are as follows, listed in alphabetical order:

- **Antibody:** Antibodies bind to specific foreign particles, such as viruses and bacteria, to help protect the body.

- **Enzyme:** Enzymes carry out almost all of the thousands of chemical reactions that take place in cells. They also assist with the formation of new molecules by reading the genetic information stored in DNA.

- **Messenger:** Messenger proteins, such as some types of hormones, transmit signals to coordinate biological processes between different cells, tissues, and organs.

- **Structural component:** These proteins provide structure and support for cells. On a larger scale, they also allow the body to move.

- **Transport/storage:** These proteins bind and carry atoms and small molecules within cells and throughout the body.

Chapter 2

Genetic Mutations And Health

What is a gene mutation, and how do mutations occur?

A gene mutation is a permanent change in the DNA sequence that makes up a gene. Mutations range in size from a single DNA building block (DNA base) to a large segment of a chromosome.

Gene mutations occur in two ways: they can be inherited from a parent or acquired during a person's lifetime. Mutations that are passed from parent to child are called hereditary mutations, or germline mutations (because they are present in the egg and sperm cells, which are also called germ cells). This type of mutation is present throughout a person's life in virtually every cell in the body.

Mutations that occur only in an egg or sperm cell, or those that occur just after fertilization, are called new (de novo) mutations. De novo mutations may explain genetic disorders in which an affected child has a mutation in every cell, but has no family history of the disorder.

Acquired (or somatic) mutations occur in the DNA of individual cells at some time during a person's life. These changes can be caused by environmental factors, such as ultraviolet radiation from the sun, or can occur if a

About This Chapter: Information in this chapter is from "Mutations and Health," Genetics Home Reference, a service of the U.S. National Library of Medicine, May 2006.

mistake is made as DNA copies itself during cell division. Acquired mutations in somatic cells (cells other than sperm and egg cells) cannot be passed on to the next generation.

Mutations may also occur in a single cell within an early embryo. As all the cells divide during growth and development, the individual will have some cells with the mutation and some cells without the genetic change. This situation is called mosaicism.

Some genetic changes are very rare; others are common in the population. Genetic changes that occur in more than 1 percent of the population are called polymorphisms. They are common enough to be considered a normal variation in the DNA. Polymorphisms are responsible for many of the normal differences between people, such as eye color, hair color, and blood type. Although many polymorphisms have no negative effects on a person's health, some of these variations may influence the risk of developing certain disorders.

How can gene mutations affect health and development?

> ✎ **What's It Mean?**
> A condition caused by mutations in one or more genes is called a genetic disorder.

To function correctly, each cell depends on thousands of proteins to do their jobs in the right places at the right times. Sometimes, gene mutations prevent one or more of these proteins from working properly. By changing a gene's instructions for making a protein, a mutation can cause the protein to malfunction or to be missing entirely. When a mutation alters a protein that plays a critical role in the body, it can disrupt normal development or cause a medical condition.

In some cases, gene mutations are so severe that they prevent an embryo from surviving until birth. These changes occur in genes that are essential for development and often disrupt the development of an embryo in its earliest stages. Because these mutations have very serious effects, they are incompatible with life.

It is important to note that genes themselves do not cause disease. Genetic disorders are caused by mutations that make a gene function improperly. For example, when people say that someone has "the cystic fibrosis gene," they are usually referring to a mutated version of the CFTR gene, which causes the disease. All people, including those without cystic fibrosis, have a version of the CFTR gene.

Do all gene mutations affect health and development?

No. Only a small percentage of mutations cause genetic disorders. Most have no impact on health or development. For example, some mutations alter a gene's DNA base sequence but do not change the function of the protein made by the gene.

Often, gene mutations that could cause a genetic disorder are repaired by certain enzymes before the gene is expressed (makes a protein). Each cell has a number of pathways through which enzymes recognize and repair mistakes in DNA. Because DNA can be damaged or mutated in many ways, DNA repair is an important process by which the body protects itself from disease.

A very small percentage of all mutations actually have a positive effect. These mutations lead to new versions of proteins that help an organism and its future generations better adapt to changes in their environment. For example, a beneficial mutation could result in a protein that protects the organism from a new strain of bacteria.

Can changes in chromosomes affect health and development?

Changes that affect entire chromosomes or segments of chromosomes can cause problems with growth, development, and function of the body's systems. These changes can affect many genes along the chromosome and alter the proteins made by those genes.

✎ **What's It Mean?**

Conditions caused by a change in the number, or structure of chromosomes, are known as chromosomal disorders.

Human cells normally contain 23 pairs of chromosomes, for a total of 46 chromosomes in each cell. A change in the number of chromosomes leads to a chromosomal disorder. These changes can occur during the formation of reproductive cells (eggs and sperm) or in early fetal development. A gain or loss of chromosomes from the normal 46 is called aneuploidy.

The most common form of aneuploidy is trisomy, or the presence of an extra chromosome in each cell. "Tri-" is Greek for "three"; people with trisomy have three copies of a particular chromosome in each cell instead of the normal two copies. Down syndrome is an example of a condition caused by trisomy. People with Down syndrome typically have three copies of chromosome 21 in each cell, for a total of 47 chromosomes per cell.

Monosomy, or the loss of one chromosome from each cell, is another kind of aneuploidy. "Mono-" is Greek for "one"; people with monosomy have one copy of a particular chromosome in each cell instead of the normal two copies. Turner syndrome is a condition caused by monosomy. Women with Turner syndrome are often missing one copy of the X chromosome in every cell, for a total of 45 chromosomes per cell.

Chromosomal disorders can also be caused by changes in chromosome structure. These changes are caused by the breakage and reunion of chromosome segments when an egg or sperm cell is formed or in early fetal development. Pieces of DNA can be rearranged within one chromosome or transferred between two or more chromosomes. The effects of structural changes depend on their size and location. Many different structural changes are possible; some cause medical problems, while others may have no effect on a person's health.

Many cancer cells also have changes in their chromosome number or structure. These changes most often occur in somatic cells (cells other than eggs and sperm) during a person's lifetime.

What are complex or multifactorial disorders?

Researchers are learning that nearly all conditions and diseases have a genetic component. Some disorders, such as sickle cell anemia and cystic fibrosis, are caused by mutations in a single gene. The causes of many other disorders, however, are much more complex. Common medical problems such as heart disease, diabetes, and obesity do not have a single genetic cause. They are likely associated with the effects of multiple genes in combination with lifestyle and environmental factors.

✎ What's It Mean?

Conditions caused by many contributing factors are called complex or multifactorial disorders.

Although complex disorders often cluster in families, they do not have a clear-cut pattern of inheritance. This makes it difficult to determine a person's risk of inheriting or passing on these disorders. Complex disorders are also difficult to study and treat because the specific factors that cause most of these disorders have not yet been identified. By 2010, however, researchers predict they will have found the major contributing genes for many common complex disorders.

What information about a genetic condition can statistics provide?

Statistical data can provide general information about how common a condition is, how many people have the condition, or how likely it is that a person will develop the condition. Statistics are not personalized; however, they offer estimates based on groups of people. By taking into account a person's family history, medical history, and other factors, a genetics professional can help interpret what statistics mean for a particular patient.

Some statistical terms are commonly used when describing genetic conditions and other disorders. These terms include the following:

- **Incidence:** The incidence of a gene mutation or a genetic disorder is the number of people who are born with the mutation or disorder in a specified group per year. Incidence is often written in the form "1 in [a number]" or as a total number of live births. Example: About 1 in 200,000 people in the United States are born with syndrome A each year. An estimated 15,000 infants with syndrome B were born last year worldwide.

- **Prevalence:** The prevalence of a gene mutation or a genetic disorder is the total number of people in a specified group at a given time who has the mutation or disorder. This term includes both newly diagnosed and pre-existing cases in people of any age. Prevalence is often written in the form "1 in [a number]" or as a total number of people who have a condition. Example: Approximately 1 in 100,000 people in the United States have syndrome A at the present time. About 100,000 children worldwide currently have syndrome B.

- **Mortality:** Mortality is the number of deaths from a particular disorder occurring in a specified group per year. Mortality is usually expressed as a total number of deaths. Example: An estimated 12,000 people worldwide died from syndrome C in 2002.

- **Lifetime risk:** Lifetime risk is the average risk of developing a particular disorder at some point during a lifetime. Lifetime risk is often written as a percentage or as "1 in [a number]." It is important to remember that the risk per year or per decade is much lower than the lifetime risk. In addition, other factors may increase or decrease a person's risk as compared with the average. Example: Approximately 1 percent of people in the United States develop disorder D during their lifetimes. The lifetime risk of developing disorder D is 1 in 100.

Chapter 3

Inheriting Genetic Conditions

What does it mean if a disorder seems to run in my family?

A particular disorder might be described as "running in a family" if more than one person in the family has the condition. Some disorders that affect multiple family members are caused by gene mutations, which can be inherited (passed down from parent to child). Other conditions that appear to run in families are not inherited. Instead, environmental factors such as dietary habits or a combination of genetic and environmental factors are responsible for these disorders.

It is not always easy to determine whether a condition in a family is inherited. A genetics professional can use a person's family history (a record of health information about a person's immediate and extended family) to help determine whether a disorder has a genetic component.

What are the different ways in which a genetic condition can be inherited?

Some genetic conditions are caused by mutations in a single gene. These conditions are usually inherited in one of several straightforward patterns, depending on the gene involved:

About This Chapter: Information in this chapter is excerpted from "Inheriting Genetic Conditions," Genetics Home Reference, a service of the U.S. National Library of Medicine, May 2006.

- **Autosomal dominant:** One mutated copy of the gene in each cell is sufficient for a person to be affected by an autosomal dominant disorder. Each affected person usually has one affected parent. Autosomal dominant disorders tend to occur in every generation of an affected family.

- **Autosomal recessive:** Two mutated copies of the gene are present in each cell when a person has an autosomal recessive disorder. An affected person usually has unaffected parents who each carry a single copy of the mutated gene (and are referred to as carriers). Autosomal recessive disorders are typically not seen in every generation of an affected family.

- **X-linked dominant:** X-linked dominant disorders are caused by mutations in genes on the X chromosome. Females are more frequently affected than males, and the chance of passing on an X-linked dominant disorder differs between men and women. Families with an X-linked dominant disorder often have both affected males and affected females in each generation. A striking characteristic of X-linked inheritance is that fathers cannot pass X-linked traits to their sons (no male-to-male transmission).

- **X-linked recessive:** X-linked recessive disorders are also caused by mutations in genes on the X chromosome. Males are more frequently affected than females, and the chance of passing on the disorder differs between men and women. Families with an X-linked recessive disorder often have affected males, but rarely affected females, in each generation. A striking characteristic of X-linked inheritance is that fathers cannot pass X-linked traits to their sons (no male-to-male transmission).

- **Codominant:** In codominant inheritance, two different versions (alleles) of a gene can be expressed, and each version makes a slightly different protein. Both alleles influence the genetic trait or determine the characteristics of the genetic condition.

- **Mitochondrial:** This type of inheritance, also known as maternal inheritance, applies to genes in mitochondrial DNA. Mitochondria, which are structures in each cell that convert molecules into energy, each contain a small amount of DNA. Because only egg cells contribute mitochondria to the developing embryo, only females can pass on mito-chondrial conditions to their children. Mitochondrial disorders can appear in every generation of a family and can affect both males and females, but fathers do not pass mitochondrial traits to their children.

Many other disorders are caused by a combination of the effects of multiple genes or by interactions between genes and the environment. Such disorders are more difficult to analyze because their genetic causes are often unclear, and they do not follow the patterns of inheritance described above. Examples of conditions caused by multiple genes or gene/environment interactions include heart disease, diabetes, schizophrenia, and certain types of cancer.

Disorders caused by changes in the number or structure of chromosomes do not follow the straightforward patterns of inheritance.

♣ It's A Fact!!
What are genetic disorders?

A genetic disorder is a disease caused in whole or in part by a "variation" (an unusual form) or "mutation" (alteration) of a gene. Genetic disorders can be passed on to family members who inherit the genetic abnormality. A small number of rare disorders are caused by a mistake in a single gene; but most disorders involving genetic factors, such as heart disease and most cancers, arise from a complex interplay of multiple genetic changes and environmental influences.

Geneticists group genetic disorders into the following three categories:

- **Single gene disorders** caused by a mistake in a single gene. The mutation may be present on one or both chromosomes of a pair. Sickle cell disease, cystic fibrosis and Tay-Sachs disease are examples of single gene disorders.

- **Chromosome disorders** caused by an excess or deficiency of the genes. An extra copy of a chromosome causes Down syndrome, but no individual gene on the chromosome is abnormal.

- **Multifactorial inheritance disorders** caused by a combination of small variations in genes, often in concert with environmental factors. Heart disease, most cancers, and Alzheimer's disease are examples of these disorders.

Source: Excerpted from "Genetics FAQ," National Human Genome Research Institute, National Institutes of Health, June 2006.

If a genetic disorder runs in my family, what are the chances that my children will have the condition?

When a genetic disorder is diagnosed in a family, family members often want to know the likelihood that they or their children will develop the condition. This can be difficult to predict in some cases because many factors influence a person's chances of developing a genetic condition. One important factor is how the condition is inherited. Here are some examples:

- **Autosomal dominant inheritance:** A person affected by an autosomal dominant disorder has a 50 percent chance of passing the mutated gene to each child. The chance that a child will not inherit the mutated gene is also 50 percent.

- **Autosomal recessive inheritance:** Two unaffected people who each carry one copy of the mutated gene for an autosomal recessive disorder (carriers) have a 25 percent chance with each pregnancy of having a child affected by the disorder. The chance with each pregnancy of having an unaffected child who is a carrier of the disorder is 50 percent, and the chance that a child will not have the disorder and will not be a carrier is 25 percent.

- **X-linked dominant inheritance:** The chance of passing on an X-linked dominant condition differs between men and women because men have one X chromosome and one Y chromosome, while women have two X chromosomes. A man passes on his Y chromosome to all of his sons and his X chromosome to all of his daughters. Therefore, the sons of a man with an X-linked dominant disorder will not be affected, but all of his daughters will inherit the condition. A woman passes on one or the other of her X chromosomes to each child. Therefore, a woman with an X-linked dominant disorder has a 50 percent chance of having an affected daughter or son with each pregnancy.

- **X-linked recessive inheritance:** Because of the difference in sex chromosomes, the probability of passing on an X-linked recessive disorder also differs between men and women. The sons of a man with an X-linked recessive disorder will not be affected, and his daughters will carry one copy of the mutated gene. With each pregnancy, a woman who carries an X-linked recessive disorder has a 50 percent chance of having sons who are affected and a 50 percent chance of having daughters who carry one copy of the mutated gene.

- **Codominant inheritance:** In codominant inheritance, each parent contributes a different version of a particular gene, and both versions influence the resulting genetic trait. The chance of developing a genetic condition with codominant inheritance, and the characteristic features of that condition, depend on which versions of the gene are passed from parents to their child.

- **Mitochondrial inheritance:** Mitochondria, which are the energy-producing centers inside cells, each contain a small amount of DNA. Disorders with mitochondrial inheritance result from mutations in mitochondrial DNA. Although mitochondrial disorders can affect both males and females, only females can pass mutations in mitochondrial DNA to their children. A woman with a disorder caused by changes in mitochondrial DNA will pass the mutation to all of her daughters and sons, but the children of a man with such a disorder will not inherit the mutation.

It is important to note that the chance of passing on a genetic condition applies equally to each pregnancy. For example, if a couple has a child with an autosomal recessive disorder, the chance of having another child with the disorder is still 25 percent (or 1 in 4). Having one child with a disorder does not "protect" future children from inheriting the condition. Conversely, having a child without the condition does not mean that future children will definitely be affected.

Although the chances of inheriting a genetic condition appear straightforward, factors such as a person's family history and the results of genetic testing can sometimes modify those chances. In addition, some people with a disease-causing mutation never develop any health problems or may experience only mild symptoms of the disorder. If a disease that runs in a family does not have a clear-cut inheritance pattern, predicting the likelihood that a person will develop the condition can be particularly difficult.

Estimating the chance of developing or passing on a genetic disorder can be complex. Genetics professionals can help people understand these chances and help them make informed decisions about their health.

Are chromosomal disorders inherited?

Although it is possible to inherit some types of chromosomal abnormalities, most chromosomal disorders (such as Down syndrome and Turner syndrome) are not passed from one generation to the next.

Some chromosomal conditions are caused by changes in the number of chromosomes. These changes are not inherited, but occur as random events during the formation of reproductive cells (eggs and sperm). An error in cell division called nondisjunction results in reproductive cells with an abnormal number of chromosomes. For example, a reproductive cell may accidentally gain or lose one copy of a chromosome. If one of these atypical reproductive cells contributes to the genetic makeup of a child, the child will have an extra or missing chromosome in each of the body's cells.

Changes in chromosome structure can also cause chromosomal disorders. Some changes in chromosome structure can be inherited, while others occur as random accidents during the formation of reproductive cells or in early fetal development. Because the inheritance of these changes can be complex, people concerned about this type of chromosomal abnormality may want to talk with a genetics professional.

Some cancer cells also have changes in the number or structure of their chromosomes. Because these changes occur in somatic cells (cells other than eggs and sperm), they cannot be passed from one generation to the next.

Why are some genetic conditions more common in particular ethnic groups?

People in an ethnic group often share certain versions of their genes, which have been passed down from common ancestors. If one of these shared genes contains a disease-causing mutation, a particular genetic disorder may be more frequently seen in the group.

Examples of genetic conditions that are more common in particular ethnic groups are sickle cell anemia, which is more common in people of African, African-American, or Mediterranean heritage; and Tay-Sachs disease, which is more likely to occur among people of Ashkenazi (eastern and central European) Jewish or French Canadian ancestry. It is important to note, however, that these disorders can occur in any ethnic group.

Chapter 4

Your Family's Health History

Questions And Answers About Your Family's Health History

What diseases in my family health history should I be concerned about?

Genetic factors contribute to the cause, natural history, and response to therapy of nearly every type of illness. Genetic disorders are influenced by abnormalities in your DNA. Some of these abnormalities cause more commonly recognized genetic conditions such as sickle cell disease or cystic fibrosis. As research continues, we all learn more about the role of genes in chronic diseases experienced throughout a lifetime.

Chronic diseases that have been associated with an increased family history include breast cancer, colon cancer, heart disease, stroke, diabetes, depression, and other psychiatric illnesses. Hearing loss and vision loss have also been found to have a genetic contribution. Sometimes a family history can even suggest variation in how useful certain drugs are in treating conditions

About This Chapter: Information in this chapter under the heading "Questions And Answers About Your Family's Health History" is excerpted from "Questions and Answers, Diseases and Conditions, Family History," U.S. Department of Health and Human Services, March 2006. Text under the heading "Your Family Health Portrait is from "My Family Health Portrait: The Surgeon General's Family History Initiative," U.S. Department of Health and Human Services, 2005.

experienced by family members. Side effects or responses to treatments can be influenced by genetic factors and may be cause for concern.

What if I can't find out my family health history?

Not everyone has access or knowledge to detail every member of their family's health history, so there may be blank areas. Seeking out legal records through state and government offices requires effort, but may provide additional details. Genealogy resources may also provide some leads for consideration in your searching for hard to find information. If you are adopted, the challenge may also include accessing family medical information from birth parents. The National Adoption Clearinghouse at http://naic.acf.hhs.gov is a resource that may be utilized to learn more about this process. It offers information about searching for birth parents that may be helpful at http://naic.acf.hhs.gov/adopted/search/index.cfm.

What aspects of family health history affect disease risk?

Everyone's family health history of disease is different. It is important to talk with other family members to gather information. Talking may help you and your family members identify key features in your family history that may point to increase risk for disease. These key features include the following:

- Diseases that occur at an earlier age than expected (10 to 20 years before most people get the disease)

- Disease in more than one close relative

- Disease that does not usually affect a certain gender (for example, breast cancer in a male)

- Certain combinations of diseases within a family (for example, breast and ovarian cancer, or heart disease and diabetes)

If a family has one or more of these features, there is an increased familial or family health risk. Sometimes, a family may have an inherited form of disease that is passed on from generation to generation. In these families, the risk for disease may be very high and disease may occur at young ages, and this is what your family history will help a health care professional to determine.

Is there anything I can do to protect myself if "bad" heart disease genes are in my family health history?

There are no "good" or "bad" genes. Most human diseases, especially common diseases such as heart disease, result from the interaction of genes with environmental and behavioral risk factors, both of which can be changed. The best disease prevention strategy for anyone, especially for people with an inherited risk, includes reducing risky behaviors (such as smoking), as well as increasing healthy behaviors (such as regular exercise).

How can knowing my family health history help lower my risk of disease?

You can't change your genes, but you can change behaviors that affect your health, such as smoking, inactivity, and poor eating habits. People with a family health history of chronic disease may have the most to gain from making lifestyle changes. In many cases, making these changes can reduce your risk of disease even if the disease runs in your family.

Another change you can make is to participate in screening tests, such as mammograms and colorectal cancer screening, for early detection of disease. People who have a family health history of a chronic disease may benefit the most from screening tests that look for risk factors or early signs of disease. Finding disease early, before symptoms appear, can mean better health in the long run. That is why it is important for your health care provider to know your family health history as well.

What does family health history have to do with genetics?

Your family health history reflects the combination of shared genes, environment, behavior, and culture. Traits like curly hair, dimples, leanness, and athletic ability are partly inherited. So are risks for health conditions like asthma, high blood pressure, diabetes, and heart disease. Knowing your family health history should be the first step in gathering information that may affect your health.

What will my healthcare professional do with family health history information?

Your healthcare provider will assess your risk of disease based on your family history and other risk factors. Your healthcare provider may also recommend things you can do to help prevent disease, such as exercising more, changing your diet, or using screening tests to detect disease early.

What if there is no family history of disease? Will I be healthy?

Even if you do not have a history of a disease in your family, you may still be at risk for that disease. This is true for the following reasons:

- Your lifestyle, personal health history, and other factors influence your chances of getting a disease.

- Your family could have a history of disease that you do not know about.

- You could have family members who died young, before they developed heart disease, diabetes, cancer, or other diseases.

♣ It's A Fact!!
U.S. Surgeon General's Family History Initiative

Healthcare professionals have known for a long time that common diseases such as heart disease, cancer, and diabetes—and even rare diseases like hemophilia, cystic fibrosis, and sickle cell anemia—can run in families. If one generation of a family has high blood pressure, it is not unusual for the next generation to have similarly high blood pressure. Tracing the illnesses suffered by your parents, grandparents, and other blood relatives can help your doctor predict the disorders to which you may be at risk and take action to keep you and your family healthy.

Americans know that family history is important to health. A recent survey found that 96 percent of Americans believe that knowing their family history is important. Yet, the same survey found that only one-third of Americans has ever tried to gather and write down their family's health history.

Because family health history is such a powerful screening tool, the Surgeon General has created a computerized tool to help make it fun and easy for anyone to create a sophisticated portrait of their family's health.

This tool, called "My Family Health Portrait," is a web-enabled program that runs on any computer that's connected to the web and running an up-to-date version of any major Internet browser.

Your Family Health Portrait

How To Create Your Family Health Portrait

To get the most accurate health history information, it is important to talk directly with your relatives. Explain to them that their health information can help improve prevention and screening of diseases for all family members.

Start by asking your relatives about any health conditions they have had including history of chronic illnesses, such as heart disease; pregnancy complications, such as miscarriage; and any developmental disabilities. Get as much specific information as possible.

It is most useful if you can list the formal name of any medical condition that has affected you or your relatives.

The web-based tool helps users organize family history information and then print it out for presentation to the family doctor. In addition, the tool helps users save their family history information to their own computer and even share family history information with other family members. The tool can be accessed at https://familyhistory.hhs.gov/.

The tool is available free to all users. No user information is saved on any computer of the U.S. federal government.

When you are finished organizing your family history information, the tool will create and print out a graphical representation of your family's generations and the health disorders that may have moved from one generation to the next. That is a powerful tool for predicting any illnesses for which you should be checked.

Whenever families gather, they should talk about, and write down, the health problems that seem to run in their family. Learning about their family's health history may help ensure a longer future together.

Source: Excerpted from "U.S. Surgeon General's Family History Initiative," U.S. Department of Health and Human Services, December 2005.

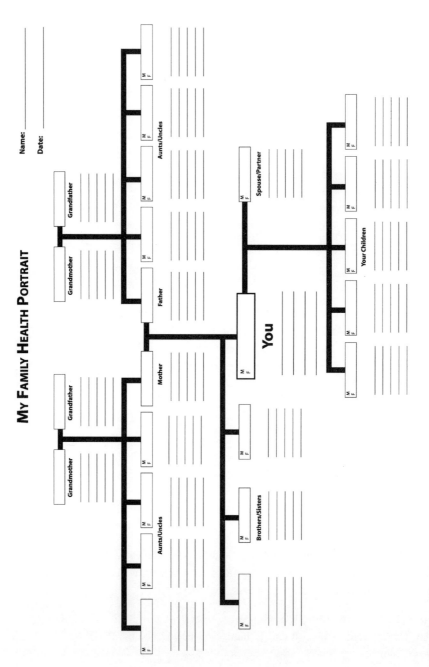

Figure 4.1. My Family Health Portrait

You can get help finding information about health conditions that have affected you or your family members, living or deceased, by asking relatives or healthcare professionals for information, or by getting copies of medical records.

If you are planning to have children, you and your partner should each create a family health portrait and show it to your healthcare professional.

Knowing your family health history is a powerful guide to understanding risk for disease. However, keep in mind that a family history of a particular illness may increase risk, but it almost never guarantees that other family members will develop the illness.

These are the people with whom you should talk:

- **Most important:** Parents, brothers, and sisters

- **Also important:** Grandparents, uncles and aunts, nieces and nephews, half brothers, and half sisters

- **Obtain information if you can:** Cousins, great uncles, and great aunts

How To Fill Out The Form

The "My Family Health Portrait" form will help you collect and organize your family information. No form can reflect every version of the American family, so use this chart as a starting point and adapt it to your family's needs.

First, write each of your relatives' names in the designated boxes and circle whether they are male (M) or female (F). On the next line, write the name of any health conditions they have had. If you know the age at which they were diagnosed with a condition, write that in parentheses after the condition. For example: "diabetes (diagnosed—age 37)."

If family members have died, write "deceased" and the age at which they died. For example: "heart attack (deceased—age 63)."

For twins, write "twin" on the first line for both individuals. If the twins are identical, write "identical twin" on the first line for both.

If your family includes half brothers or half sisters, write "half brother" or "half sister" on the first line and note "different father" or "different mother" on the next line.

Some conditions are more common in people with a shared background or ancestry. It is important to record the ancestry of your relatives and be as specific as possible. For example, if you know that your grandmother is Hispanic and her family comes from Mexico, write "Mexican" underneath her name. Likewise, if your family is from Africa, Asia, Europe, or South America, note the country they came from, if possible.

Once you complete "My Family Health Portrait," take it to your healthcare professional so that he or she can better individualize your health care. Be sure to make a copy for your records and update it as circumstances change or you learn more about your family's health history.

Congratulations on taking this step toward a longer, healthier life! "My Family Health Portrait" can be an effective way to improve your health today and in the future.

Chapter 5

Deciding About Genetic Testing

What is genetic testing?

Genetic tests look for abnormalities in a person's genes, or the presence/absence of key proteins whose production is directed by specific genes. Abnormalities in either could indicate an inherited disposition to a disorder. Genetic testing includes gene tests (DNA testing) and biochemical tests (protein testing).

In gene tests, DNA in cells taken from a person's blood, body fluids, or tissues is examined for an abnormality that flags a disease or disorder. The abnormality can be relatively large—a piece of a chromosome, or even an entire chromosome, missing or added. Sometimes the change is very small—as little as one extra, missing, or altered chemical base within the DNA strand. Genes can be amplified (too many copies), over-expressed (too active), inactivated, or lost altogether. Sometimes pieces of chromosomes become switched, transposed, or discovered in an incorrect location.

Gene tests use a variety of techniques to examine a person's DNA. Some tests involve using probes—short strings of DNA—with base sequences complementary to those of the mutated gene. These probes will seek their complements within an individual's genome. If the mutated sequence is present in the patient's genome, the probe will find it and bind to it, flagging the mutation.

About This Chapter: Information in this chapter is excerpted from "Genetics FAQ," National Human Genome Research Institute, National Institutes of Health, June 2006.

Another type of gene test involves comparing the sequence of DNA bases in a patient's gene to a normal version of the gene.

Biochemical tests look for the presence or absence of key proteins, which signal abnormal or malfunctioning genes.

What information can genetic testing provide?

Genetic testing can be predictive, discovering whether an individual has an inherited disposition to a certain disease, before symptoms appear. Genetic tests can also confirm a diagnosis if symptoms are present. Tests can determine whether a person is a carrier for the disease. Carriers won't get the disease, but can pass on the faulty gene to their children. Prenatal testing can help expectant parents know whether their unborn child will have a genetic disease or disorder. Newborn screening tests infants for abnormal or missing gene products.

Individuals in families at high risk for a disease live with troubling uncertainties about their own future as well as their children. A negative test, especially one that is strongly predictive, can provide an enormous sense of relief.

A positive test can also produce benefits. In the best circumstances, a positive test enables the person to take steps to reduce risk. These steps could include regular screening for the disease or lifestyle changes, such as a change in diet or regular exercise.

A positive test can relieve uncertainty, and can enable people to make informed decisions about their future.

Reasons For Genetic Testing:

- *Predictive testing* identifies people who are at risk of getting a disease before any symptoms appear. Predictive tests include those that screen for some inherited predispositions to certain forms of cancer, such as colon and breast cancer. Being predisposed does not mean that the individual will get the disease. It means the person has a certain risk of developing the disease.

- *Carrier testing* can tell individuals if they are carriers of an inherited disorder that they may pass on to their children. A person who has only one abnormal copy of a gene for a recessive condition is known as a carrier. Carriers won't get the disease, but can pass on the defective gene to their children. Cystic fibrosis and Tay-Sachs disease are examples of disorders for which parents can be carriers.

- *Prenatal testing* is available to people at risk for having children with a chromosomal abnormality or an inherited genetic condition. Two procedures are commonly used in prenatal testing. Amniocentesis involves analyzing a sample of amniotic fluid from the womb. CVS (chorionic villus sampling) involves taking a tiny tissue sample from outside the sac where the fetus develops. Prenatal testing is often used to look for disorders such as Down syndrome, spina bifida, cystic fibrosis, and Tay-Sachs disease.

- *Newborn screening*, the most widespread type of genetic testing, tests infant blood samples for abnormal or missing gene products. For example, infants are commonly screened for phenylketonuria (PKU), an enzyme deficiency that can lead to severe mental retardation if untreated.

How should I decide whether to be tested?

The decision to undergo testing is a very personal one. For many people, a pivotal consideration is whether there are preventive measures that can be taken if the test result is positive. For example, those who test positive for inherited forms of breast or colon cancer can benefit from preventive measures, screening for early detection, and early treatment.

In contrast, there are no preventive measures or cures for Huntington's disease; but a positive test for Huntington's disease might help an individual make lifestyle decisions, such as career choice, family planning, or insurance coverage.

Because the decision about whether to be tested for a genetic disease is complex, most people seek guidance from a genetic counselor trained to help individuals and families weigh the scientific, emotional, and ethical considerations that impact on this decision.

What are genetic counselors, and what do they do?

Genetic counselors work as members of healthcare teams providing information and support to individuals or families who have genetic disorders or may be at risk for inherited conditions. Genetic counselors will help with the following:

- Assess the risk of a genetic disorder by re-
  searching a family's history and evaluating medical records.

- Weigh the medical, social, and ethical
  decisions surrounding genetic testing.

- Provide support and information to help
  a person make a decision about testing.

> ♣ **It's A Fact!!**
> Genetics counselors are
> healthcare professionals with
> specialized graduate degrees
> and experience in medical
> genetics and counseling.

- Interpret the results of genetic tests and
  medical data.

- Provide counseling or refer individuals and families to support services.

- Serve as patient advocates.

- Explain possible treatments or preventive measures.

- Discuss reproductive options.

How do I find a genetic counselor?

Your doctor may refer you to a genetic counselor. Universities and medical centers also often have affiliated genetic counselors or can provide referrals to a counselor or genetics clinic.

As we've learned more about genetics, counselors have grown more specialized. For example, counselors may specialize in a particular disease (such as Parkinson's disease), an age group (such as adolescents), or a type of counseling (such as prenatal).

How do I decide whether I need to see a geneticist or other specialist?

A genetics counselor may refer you to a geneticist, a medical doctor or medical researcher, who specializes in your disease or disorder. A medical geneticist has completed a fellowship or has other advanced training in medical genetics. While a genetic counselor may help you with testing decisions and support issues, a medical geneticist will make the actual diagnosis of a disease or condition. Many genetic diseases are so rare that only a geneticist can provide the most complete and current information about your condition.

Part Two

How Your Body Works

Chapter 6

Your Bones: The Skeletal System

Functions Of The Skeletal System

Humans are vertebrates—animals having a vertebral column or backbone. They rely on a sturdy internal frame that is centered on a prominent spine.

The living bones in our bodies use oxygen and give off waste products in metabolism. They contain active tissues that consume nutrients, require a blood supply, and change shape or remodel in response to variations in mechanical stress. Bones provide a rigid framework, known as the skeleton, which support and protect the soft organs of the body.

The skeleton supports the body against the pull of gravity. The large bones of the lower limbs support the trunk when standing.

The skeleton also protects the soft body parts. The fused bones of the cranium surround the brain to make it less vulnerable to injury. Vertebrae surround and protect the spinal cord, and bones of the rib cage help protect the heart and lungs of the thorax.

Bones work together with muscles as simple mechanical lever systems to produce body movement.

About This Chapter: Information in this chapter is from "Skeletal System," at the National Cancer Institute's Surveillance, Epidemiology, and End Results (SEER)'s Training Website (http://training.seer.cancer.gov), 2000, accessed May 3, 2006. Note: Despite the older date of this document, the anatomical information it presents is still current.

Bones contain more calcium than any other organ. The intercellular matrix of bone contains large amounts of calcium salts, the most important being calcium phosphate.

When blood calcium levels decrease below normal, calcium is released from the bones so that there will be an adequate supply for metabolic needs. When blood calcium levels are increased, the excess calcium is stored in the bone matrix. The dynamic process of releasing and storing calcium goes on almost continuously.

Hematopoiesis, the formation of blood cells, mostly takes place in the red marrow of the bones.

In infants, red marrow is found in the bone cavities. With age, it is largely replaced by yellow marrow for fat storage. In adults, red marrow is limited to the spongy bone in the skull, ribs, sternum, clavicles, vertebrae, and pelvis. Red marrow functions in the formation of red blood cells, white blood cells, and blood platelets.

Bone Development And Growth

The terms osteogenesis and ossification are often used synonymously to indicate the process of bone formation. Parts of the skeleton form during the first few weeks after conception. By the end of the eighth week after conception, the skeletal pattern is formed in cartilage and connective tissue membranes and ossification begins.

♣ It's A Fact!!

Bone development continues throughout adulthood. Even after adult stature is attained, bone development continues for repair of fractures and for remodeling to meet changing lifestyles.

Osteoblasts, osteocytes, and osteoclasts are the three cell types involved in the development, growth, and remodeling of bones. Osteoblasts are bone-forming cells, osteocytes are mature bone cells, and osteoclasts break down and reabsorb bone.

There are two types of ossification: intramembranous and endochondral.

Intramembranous

Intramembranous ossification involves the replacement of sheet-like connective tissue membranes with bony tissue. Bones formed in this manner are called intramembranous bones. They include certain flat bones of the skull and some of the irregular bones. The future bones are first formed as connective tissue membranes. Osteoblasts migrate to the membranes and deposit bony matrix around themselves. When the osteoblasts are surrounded by matrix they are called osteocytes.

Endochondral Ossification

Endochondral ossification involves the replacement of hyaline cartilage with bony tissue. Most of the bones of the skeleton are formed in this manner. These bones are called endochondral bones. In this process, the future bones are first formed as hyaline cartilage models. During the third month after conception, the perichondrium that surrounds the hyaline cartilage "models" becomes infiltrated with blood vessels and osteoblasts and changes into a periosteum. The osteoblasts form a collar of compact bone around the diaphysis. At the same time, the cartilage in the center of the diaphysis begins to disintegrate. Osteoblasts penetrate the disintegrating cartilage and replace it with spongy bone. This forms a primary ossification center. Ossification continues from this center toward the ends of the bones. After spongy bone is formed in the diaphysis, osteoclasts break down the newly formed bone to open up the medullary cavity.

The cartilage in the epiphyses continues to grow so the developing bone increases in length. Later, usually after birth, secondary ossification centers form in the epiphyses. Ossification in the epiphyses is similar to that in the diaphysis except that the spongy bone is retained instead of being broken down to form a medullary cavity. When secondary ossification is complete, the hyaline cartilage is totally replaced by bone except in two areas. A region of hyaline cartilage remains over the surface of the epiphysis as the articular cartilage and another area of cartilage remains between the epiphysis and diaphysis. This is the epiphyseal plate or growth region.

Bone Growth

Bones grow in length at the epiphyseal plate by a process that is similar to endochondral ossification. The cartilage in the region of the epiphyseal plate, next to the epiphysis, continues to grow by mitosis. The chondrocytes, in the region next to the diaphysis, age and degenerate. Osteoblasts move in and ossify the matrix to form bone. This process continues throughout childhood and the adolescent years until the cartilage growth slows and finally stops. When cartilage growth ceases, usually in the early twenties, the epiphyseal plate completely ossifies so that only a thin epiphyseal line remains, and the bones can no longer grow in length. Bone growth is under the influence of growth hormone from the anterior pituitary gland and sex hormones from the ovaries and testes.

Even though bones stop growing in length in early adulthood, they can continue to increase in thickness or diameter throughout life in response to stress from increased muscle activity or to weight. The increase in diameter is called appositional growth. Osteoblasts in the periosteum form compact bone around the external bone surface. At the same time, osteoclasts in the endosteum break down bone on the internal bone surface, around the medullary cavity. These two processes together increase the diameter of the bone and, at the same time, keep the bone from becoming excessively heavy and bulky.

Classification Of Bones

- **Long Bones:** The bones of the body come in a variety of sizes and shapes. The four principal types of bones are long, short, flat, and irregular. Bones that are longer than they are wide are called long bones. They consist of a long shaft with two bulky ends or extremities. They are primarily compact bone but may have a large amount of spongy bone at the ends or extremities. Long bones include bones of the thigh, leg, arm, and forearm.

- **Short Bones:** Short bones are roughly cube shaped with vertical and horizontal dimensions approximately equal. They consist primarily of spongy bone, which is covered by a thin layer of compact bone. Short bones include the bones of the wrist and ankle.

- **Flat Bones:** Flat bones are thin, flattened, and usually curved. Most of the bones of the cranium are flat bones.

- **Irregular Bones:** Bones that are not in any of the above three categories are classified as irregular bones. They are primarily spongy bone that is covered with a thin layer of compact bone. The vertebrae and some of the bones in the skull are irregular bones.

All bones have surface markings and characteristics that make a specific bone unique. There are holes, depressions, smooth facets, lines, projections, and other markings. These usually represent passageways for vessels and nerves, points of articulation with other bones, or points of attachment for tendons and ligaments.

Divisions Of The Skeleton

The adult human skeleton usually consists of 206 named bones. These bones can be grouped in two divisions: axial skeleton and appendicular skeleton. The 80 bones of the axial skeleton form the vertical axis of the body. They include the bones of the head, vertebral column, ribs, and breastbone or sternum. The appendicular skeleton consists of 126 bones and includes the free appendages and their attachments to the axial skeleton. The free appendages are the upper and lower extremities, or limbs, and their attachments, which are called girdle.

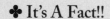

♣ It's A Fact!!

The adult human skeleton usually consists of 206 bones.

Articulations

An articulation, or joint, is where two bones come together. In terms of the amount of movement they allow, there are three types of joints: immovable, slightly movable, and freely movable.

Synarthroses

Synarthroses are immovable joints. The singular form is synarthrosis. In these joints, the bones come in very close contact and are separated only by a thin layer of fibrous connective tissue. The sutures in the skull are examples of immovable joints.

Amphiarthroses

Slightly movable joints are called amphiarthroses. The singular form is amphiarthrosis. In this type of joint, the bones are connected by hyaline cartilage or fibrocartilage. The ribs connected to the sternum by costal cartilages are slightly movable joints connected by hyaline cartilage. The symphysis pubis is a slightly movable joint in which there is a fibrocartilage pad between the two bones. The joints between the vertebrae and the intervertebral disks are also of this type.

Diarthroses

Most joints in the adult body are diarthroses, or freely movable joints. The singular form is diarthrosis. In this type of joint, the ends of the opposing bones are covered with hyaline cartilage, the articular cartilage, and they are separated by a space called the joint cavity. The components of the joints are enclosed in a dense fibrous joint capsule. The outer layer of the capsule consists of the ligaments that hold the bones together. The inner layer is the synovial membrane that secretes synovial fluid into the joint cavity for lubrication.

Because all of these joints have a synovial membrane, they are sometimes called synovial joints.

Chapter 7

The Muscular System

Functions Of The Muscular System

The muscular system is composed of specialized cells called muscle fibers. Their predominant function is contractibility. Muscles, where attached to bones or internal organs and blood vessels, are responsible for movement. Nearly all movement in the body is the result of muscle contraction. Exceptions to this are the action of cilia, the flagellum on sperm cells, and amoeboid movement of some white blood cells.

The integrated action of joints, bones, and skeletal muscles produces obvious movements such as walking and running. Skeletal muscles also produce more subtle movements that result in various facial expressions, eye movements, and respiration.

In addition to movement, muscle contraction also fulfills some other important functions in the body, such as posture, joint stability, and heat production. Posture, such as sitting and standing, is maintained as a result of muscle contraction. The skeletal muscles are continually making fine adjustments that hold the body in stationary positions. The tendons of many muscles extend over joints, and in this way, contribute to joint stability. This is particularly

About This Chapter: Information in this chapter is from "Muscular System," at the National Cancer Institute's Surveillance, Epidemiology, and End Results (SEER)'s Training Website (http://training.seer.cancer.gov), 2000, accessed May 3, 2006. Note: Despite the older date of this document, the anatomical information it presents is still current.

evident in the knee and shoulder joints, where
muscle tendons are a major factor in stabi-
lizing the joint. Heat production, to maintain body temperature, is an important
by-product of muscle metabolism.

> ♣ **It's A Fact!!**
> Nearly 85 percent of the
> heat produced in the body
> is the result of muscle
> contraction.

Structure Of Skeletal Muscle

A whole skeletal muscle is considered an organ of the muscular system. Each organ or muscle consists of skeletal muscle tissue, connective tissue, nerve tissue, and blood or vascular tissue.

Skeletal muscles vary considerably in size, shape, and arrangement of fibers. They range from extremely tiny strands, such as the stapedium muscle of the middle ear, to large masses, such as the muscles of the thigh. Some skeletal muscles are broad in shape and some narrow. In some muscles, the fibers are parallel to the long axis of the muscle, in some they converge to a narrow attachment, and in some they are oblique.

Each skeletal muscle fiber is a single cylindrical muscle cell. An individual skeletal muscle may be made up of hundreds, or even thousands, of muscle fibers bundled together and wrapped in a connective tissue covering. A connective tissue sheath, called the epimysium, surrounds each muscle. Fascia, connective tissue outside the epimysium, surrounds and separates the muscles. Portions of the epimysium project inward to divide the muscle into compartments. Each compartment contains a bundle of muscle fibers. Each bundle of muscle fiber is called a fasciculus and is surrounded by a layer of connective tissue called the perimysium. Within the fasciculus, each individual muscle cell, called a muscle fiber, is surrounded by connective tissue called the endomysium.

Skeletal muscle cells (fibers), like other body cells, are soft and fragile. The connective tissue covering furnishes support and protection for the delicate cells and allow them to withstand the forces of contraction. The coverings also provide pathways for the passage of blood vessels and nerves.

Commonly, the epimysium, perimysium, and endomysium extend beyond the fleshy part of the muscle, the belly or gaster, to form a thick rope-like tendon or a broad, flat sheet-like aponeurosis. The tendon and aponeurosis form indirect attachments from muscles to the periosteum of bones or to the connective tissue of other muscles. Typically a muscle spans a joint and is attached to bones by tendons at both ends. One of the bones remains relatively fixed or stable while the other end moves as a result of muscle contraction.

Skeletal muscles have an abundant supply of blood vessels and nerves. This is directly related to the primary function of skeletal muscle, which is contraction. Before a skeletal muscle fiber can contract, it has to receive an impulse from a nerve cell. Generally, an artery and at least one vein, accompany each nerve that penetrates the epimysium of a skeletal muscle. Branches of the nerve and blood vessels follow the connective tissue components of the muscle of a nerve cell, and with one or more minute blood vessels, called capillaries.

Muscle Types

In the body, there are three types of muscle: skeletal (striated), smooth, and cardiac.

Skeletal Muscle

Skeletal muscle, attached to bones, is responsible for skeletal movements. The peripheral portion of the central nervous system (CNS) controls the skeletal muscles. Thus, these muscles are under conscious, or voluntary, control. The basic unit is the muscle fiber with many nuclei. These muscle fibers are striated (having transverse streaks), and each acts independently of neighboring muscle fibers.

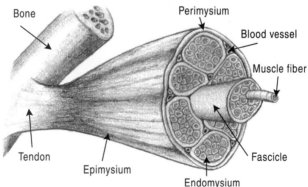

Figure 7.1. Structure of a Skeletal Muscle (SEER image redrawn by Alison DeKleine).

Smooth Muscle

Smooth muscle, found in the walls of the hollow internal organs, such as blood vessels, the gastrointestinal tract, bladder, and uterus, is under control of the autonomic nervous system. Smooth muscle cannot be controlled consciously, and thus acts involuntarily. The non-striated (smooth) muscle cell is spindle-shaped and has one central nucleus. Smooth muscle contracts slowly and rhythmically.

Cardiac Muscle

Cardiac muscle, found in the walls of the heart, is also under control of the autonomic nervous system. The cardiac muscle cell has one central nucleus, like smooth muscle, but it also is striated, like skeletal muscle. The cardiac muscle cell is rectangular in shape. The contraction of cardiac muscle is involuntary, strong, and rhythmical.

Muscle Groups

Most skeletal muscles have names that describe some feature of the muscle. Often several criteria are combined into one name. Associating the muscle's characteristics with its name will help you learn and remember them. The following are some terms relating to muscle features that are used in naming muscles:

- **Size:** vastus (huge); maximus (large); longus (long); minimus (small); brevis (short)

- **Shape:** deltoid (triangular); rhomboid (like a rhombus with equal and parallel sides); latissimus (wide); teres (round); trapezius (like a trapezoid, a four-sided figure with two sides parallel)

- **Direction of fibers:** rectus (straight); transverse (across); oblique (diagonally); orbicularis (circular)

- **Location:** pectoralis (chest); gluteus (buttock or rump); brachii (arm); supra- (above); infra- (below); sub- (under or beneath); lateralis (lateral)

- **Number of origins:** biceps (two heads); triceps (three heads); quadriceps (four heads)

Muscles Of The Head And Neck

Humans have well developed muscles in the face that permit a large variety of facial expressions. Because the muscles are used to show surprise, disgust, anger, fear, and other emotions, they are an important means of nonverbal communication. Muscles of facial expression include frontalis, orbicularis oris, laris oculi, buccinator, and zygomaticus.

There are four pairs of muscles that are responsible for chewing movements or mastication. All of these muscles connect to the mandible, and they are some of the strongest muscles in the body.

There are numerous muscles associated with the throat, the hyoid bone, and the vertebral column. Two of the more obvious and superficial neck muscles are the sternocleidomastoid and trapezius.

Muscles Of The Trunk

The muscles of the trunk include those that move the vertebral column, the muscles that form the thoracic and abdominal walls, and those that cover the pelvic outlet.

♣ **It's A Fact!!**
There are more than 600 muscles in the body, which together account for about 40 percent of a person's weight.

The erector spinae group of muscles on each side of the vertebral column is a large muscle mass that extends from the sacrum to the skull. These muscles are primarily responsible for extending the vertebral column to maintain erect posture. The deep back muscles occupy the space between the spinous and transverse processes of adjacent vertebrae.

The muscles of the thoracic wall are involved primarily in the process of breathing. The intercostal muscles are located in spaces between the ribs. They contract during forced expiration. External intercostal muscles contract to elevate the ribs during the inspiration phase of breathing. The diaphragm is a dome-shaped muscle that forms a partition between the thorax and the abdomen. It has three openings in it for structures that have to pass from the thorax to the abdomen.

The abdomen, unlike the thorax and pelvis, has no bony reinforcements or protection. The wall consists entirely of four muscle pairs, arranged in layers, and the fascia that envelops them.

Two muscular sheets, and their associated fascia, form the pelvic outlet.

Muscles Of The Upper Extremity

The muscles of the upper extremity include those that attach the scapula to the thorax and generally move the scapula, those that attach the humerus to the scapula and generally move the arm, and those that are located in the arm or forearm that move the forearm, wrist, and hand.

Muscles that move the shoulder and arm include the trapezius and serratus anterior. The pectoralis major, latissimus dorsi, deltoid, and rotator cuff muscles connect to the humerus and move the arm.

The muscles that move the forearm are located along the humerus, which include the triceps brachii, biceps brachii, brachialis, and brachioradialis. The 20 or more muscles that cause most wrist, hand, and finger movements are located along the forearm.

Muscles Of The Lower Extremity

The muscles that move the thigh have their origins on some part of the pelvic girdle and their insertions on the femur. The largest muscle mass belongs to the posterior group, the gluteal muscles, which, as a group, abduct the thigh. The iliopsoas, an anterior muscle, flexes the thigh. The muscles in the medial compartment adduct the thigh.

Muscles that move the legs are located in the thigh region. The quadriceps femoris muscle group straightens the leg at the knee. The hamstrings are antagonists to the quadriceps femoris muscle group, which are used to flex the leg at the knee.

The muscles located in the leg that move the ankle and foot are divided into anterior, posterior, and lateral compartments. The tibialis anterior, which dorsiflexes the foot, is antagonistic to the gastrocnemius and soleus muscles, which plantar flex the foot.

Chapter 8

The Heart And Cardiovascular System

Introduction To The Cardiovascular System

The cardiovascular system is sometimes called the blood-vascular, or simply the circulatory system. It consists of the heart, which is a muscular pumping device, and a closed system of vessels called arteries, veins, and capillaries. As the name implies, blood contained in the circulatory system is pumped by the heart around a closed circle, or circuit of vessels, as it passes again and again through the various "circulations" of the body.

As in the adult, survival of the developing embryo depends on the circulation of blood to maintain homeostasis and a favorable cellular environment. In response to this need, the cardiovascular system makes its appearance early in development and reaches a functional state long before any other major organ system.

The vital role of the cardiovascular system in maintaining homeostasis depends on the continuous and controlled movement of blood through the thousands of miles of capillaries that permeate every tissue and reach every cell in the body. It is in the microscopic capillaries that blood performs its

About This Chapter: Information in this chapter is from "Cardiovascular System," at the National Cancer Institute's Surveillance, Epidemiology, and End Results (SEER)'s Training Website (http://training.seer.cancer.gov), 2000, accessed May 3, 2006. Note: Despite the older date of this document, the anatomical information it presents is still current.

ultimate transport function. Nutrients and
other essential materials pass from capillary blood into fluids surrounding the
cells as waste products are removed.

Numerous control mechanisms help
to regulate and integrate the diverse functions and component parts of the cardiovascular
system in order to supply blood to specific body areas according to need. These
mechanisms ensure a constant internal environment surrounding each body cell
regardless of differing demands for nutrients or production of waste products.

Heart

The heart is a muscular pump that provides the force necessary to circulate
the blood to all the tissues in the body. Its function is vital because, to survive,
the tissues need a continuous supply of oxygen and nutrients, and metabolic
waste products have to be removed. Deprived of these necessities, cells soon

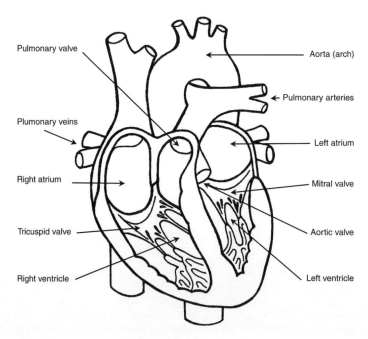

Figure 8.1. Internal View of the Heart

undergo irreversible changes that lead to death. While blood is the transport medium, the heart is the organ that keeps the blood moving through the vessels.

Structure Of The Heart

The human heart is a four-chambered muscular organ, shaped and sized roughly like a man's closed fist with two-thirds of the mass to the left of midline.

> ### ♣ It's A Fact!!
> The normal adult heart pumps about 5 liters of blood every minute throughout life. If it loses its pumping effectiveness for even a few minutes, the individual's life is jeopardized.

Chambers Of The Heart

The internal cavity of the heart is divided into four chambers. They are as follows:

• Right atrium

• Right ventricle

• Left atrium

• Left ventricle

The two atria are thin-walled chambers that receive blood from the veins. The two ventricles are thick-walled chambers that forcefully pump blood out of the heart. Differences in thickness of the heart chamber walls are due to variations in the amount of myocardium present, which reflect the amount of force each chamber is required to generate.

The right atrium receives deoxygenated blood from systemic veins; the left atrium receives oxygenated blood from the pulmonary veins.

Valves Of The Heart

Pumps need a set of valves to keep the fluid flowing in one direction and the heart is no exception. The heart has two types of valves that keep the blood flowing in the correct direction. The valves between the atria and ventricles are called atrioventricular valves (also called cuspid valves), while those at the bases of the large vessels leaving the ventricles are called semilunar valves.

The right atrioventricular valve is the tricuspid valve. The left atrioventricular valve is the bicuspid, or mitral, valve. The valve between the right ventricle and pulmonary trunk is the pulmonary semilunar valve. The valve between the left ventricle and the aorta is the aortic semilunar valve.

When the ventricles contract, atrioventricular valves close to prevent blood from flowing back into the atria. When the ventricles relax, semilunar valves close to prevent blood from flowing back into the ventricles.

Blood

Blood is the fluid of life, transporting oxygen from the lungs to body tissue and carbon dioxide from body tissue to the lungs. Blood is the fluid of growth, transporting nourishment from digestion, and hormones from glands, throughout the body. Blood is the fluid of health, transporting disease-fighting substances to the tissue and waste to the kidneys. Because it contains living cells, blood is alive. Red blood cells and white blood cells are responsible for nourishing and cleansing the body.

Without blood, the human body would stop working.

Classification And Structure Of Blood Vessels

Blood vessels are the channels or conduits through which blood is distributed to body tissues. The vessels make up two closed systems of tubes that begin and end at the heart. One system, the pulmonary vessels, transports blood from the right ventricle to the lungs and back to the left atrium. The other system, the systemic vessels, carries blood from the left ventricle to the tissues in all parts of the body and then returns the blood to the right atrium. Based on their structure and function, blood vessels are classified as arteries, capillaries, or veins.

Arteries

Arteries carry blood away from the heart. Pulmonary arteries transport blood that has low oxygen content from the right ventricle to the lungs. Systemic arteries transport oxygenated blood from the left ventricle to the body tissues. Blood is pumped from the ventricles into large elastic arteries that branch repeatedly into smaller and smaller arteries until the branching results in microscopic arteries called arterioles. The arterioles play a key role in regulating blood flow into the tissue capillaries. About 10 percent of the total blood volume is in the systemic arterial system at any given time. The wall of an artery consists of three layers. The innermost layer, the tunica intima (also called tunica interna), is simple squamous epithelium surrounded by a connective tissue basement membrane with elastic fibers. The middle layer, the tunica media, is primarily smooth muscle and is usually the thickest layer. It not only provides support for the vessel but also changes vessel diameter to regulate blood flow and blood pressure. The outermost layer, which attaches the vessel to the surrounding tissue, is the tunica externa or tunica adventitia. This layer is connective tissue with varying amounts of elastic and collagenous fibers. The connective tissue in this layer is quite dense where it is adjacent to the tunic media, but it changes to loose connective tissue near the periphery of the vessel.

Capillaries

Capillaries, the smallest and most numerous of the blood vessels, form the connection between the vessels that carry blood away from the heart (arteries) and the vessels that return blood to the heart (veins). The primary function of capillaries is the exchange of materials between the blood and tissue cells.

Capillary distribution varies with the metabolic activity of body tissues. Tissues such as skeletal muscle, liver, and kidney have extensive capillary networks because they are metabolically active and require an abundant supply of oxygen and nutrients. Other tissues, such as connective tissue, have a less abundant supply of capillaries. The epidermis of the skin and the lens and cornea of the eye completely lack a capillary network. About 5 percent of the total blood volume is in the systemic capillaries at any given time. Another 10 percent is in the lungs.

♣ It's A Fact!!

Blood pressure is measured with a sphygmomanometer and is recorded as the systolic pressure over the diastolic pressure.

Smooth muscle cells in the arterioles, where they branch to form capillaries, regulate blood flow from the arterioles into the capillaries.

Veins

Veins carry blood toward the heart. After blood passes through the capillaries, it enters the smallest veins, called venules. From the venules, it flows into progressively larger and larger veins until it reaches the heart. In the pulmonary circuit, the pulmonary veins transport blood from the lungs to the left atrium of the heart. This blood has high oxygen content because it has just been oxygenated in the lungs. Systemic veins transport blood from the body tissue to the right atrium of the heart. This blood has reduced oxygen content because the oxygen has been used for metabolic activities in the tissue cells.

The walls of veins have the same three layers as the arteries. Although all the layers are present, there is less smooth muscle and connective tissue. This makes the walls of veins thinner than those of arteries, which is related to the fact that blood in the veins has less pressure than in the arteries. Because the walls of the veins are thinner and less rigid than arteries, veins can hold more blood. Almost 70 percent of the total blood volume is in the veins at any given time. Medium and large veins have venous valves, similar to the semilunar valves associated with the heart that help keep the blood flowing toward the heart. Venous valves are especially important in the arms and legs, where they prevent the backflow of blood in response to the pull of gravity.

Physiology Of Circulation

Role Of The Capillaries

In addition to forming the connection between the arteries and veins, capillaries have a vital role in the exchange of gases, nutrients, and metabolic waste products between the blood and the tissue cells. Substances pass through the capillaries wall by diffusion, filtration, and osmosis. Oxygen and carbon dioxide move across the capillary wall by diffusion. Fluid movement across a capillary wall is determined by a combination of hydrostatic and osmotic pressure. The net result of the capillary microcirculation created by hydrostatic and osmotic pressure is that substances leave the blood at one end of the capillary and return at the other end.

Blood Flow

Blood flow refers to the movement of blood through the vessels from arteries to the capillaries and then into the veins. Pressure is a measure of the force that the blood exerts against the vessel walls as it moves the blood through the vessels. Like all fluids, blood flows from a high-pressure area to a region with lower pressure. Blood flows in the same direction as the decreasing pressure gradient: arteries to capillaries to veins.

The rate, or velocity, of blood flow varies inversely with the total cross-sectional area of the blood vessels. As the total cross-sectional area of the vessels increases, the velocity of flow decreases. Blood flow is slowest in the capillaries, which allows time for exchange of gases and nutrients.

Resistance is a force that opposes the flow of a fluid. In blood vessels, most of the resistance is due to vessel diameter. As vessel diameter decreases, the resistance increases and blood flow decreases.

Very little pressure remains by the time blood leaves the capillaries and enters the venules. Blood flow through the veins is not the direct result of ventricular contraction. Instead, venous return depends on skeletal muscle action, respiratory movements, and constriction of smooth muscle in venous walls.

Pulse And Blood Pressure

Pulse refers to the rhythmic expansion of an artery that is caused by ejection of blood from the ventricle. It can be felt where an artery is close to the surface and rests on something firm.

In common usage, the term blood pressure refers to arterial blood pressure, the pressure in the aorta and its branches. Systolic pressure is due to ventricular contraction. Diastolic pressure occurs during cardiac relaxation. Pulse pressure is the difference between systolic pressure and diastolic pressure.

Four major factors interact to affect blood pressure: cardiac output, blood volume, peripheral resistance, and viscosity. When these factors increase, blood pressure also increases.

Arterial blood pressure is maintained within normal ranges by changes in cardiac output and peripheral resistance. Pressure receptors (baroreceptors), located in the walls of the large arteries in the thorax and neck, are important for short-term blood pressure regulation.

Circulatory Pathways

The blood vessels of the body are functionally divided into two distinctive circuits: pulmonary circuit and systemic circuit. The pump for the pulmonary circuit, which circulates blood through the lungs, is the right ventricle. The left ventricle is the pump for the systemic circuit, which provides the blood supply for the tissue cells of the body.

Pulmonary Circuit

Pulmonary circulation transports oxygen-poor blood from the right ventricle to the lungs where blood picks up a new blood supply. Then it returns the oxygen-rich blood to the left atrium.

Systemic Circuit

The systemic circulation provides the functional blood supply to all body tissue. It carries oxygen and nutrients to the cells and picks up carbon dioxide and waste products. Systemic circulation carries oxygenated blood from the left ventricle, through the arteries, to the capillaries in the tissues of the body. From the tissue capillaries, the deoxygenated blood returns through a system of veins to the right atrium of the heart.

Major Systemic Arteries

All systemic arteries are branches, either directly or indirectly, from the aorta. The aorta ascends from the left ventricle, curves posteriorly and to the left, and then descends through the thorax and abdomen. This geography divides the aorta into three portions: ascending aorta, aortic arch, and descending aorta. The descending aorta is further subdivided into the thoracic aorta and abdominal aorta.

Major Systemic Veins

After blood delivers oxygen to the tissues and picks up carbon dioxide, it returns to the heart through a system of veins. The capillaries, where the gaseous exchange occurs, merge into venules, and these converge to form larger and larger veins until the blood reaches either the superior vena cava or inferior vena cava, which drain into the right atrium.

Chapter 9

Breathing And The Respiratory System

When the respiratory system is mentioned, people generally think of breathing, but breathing is only one of the activities of the respiratory system. The body cells need a continuous supply of oxygen for the metabolic processes that are necessary to maintain life. The respiratory system works with the circulatory system to provide this oxygen and to remove the waste products of metabolism. It also helps to regulate pH of the blood.

Every 3 to 5 seconds, nerve impulses stimulate the breathing process, or ventilation, which moves air through a series of passages into and out of the lungs. After this, there is an exchange of gases between the lungs and the blood. This is called external respiration. The blood transports the gases to and from the tissue cells. The exchange of gases between the blood and tissue cells is internal respiration. Finally, the cells utilize the oxygen for their specific activities. This is cellular metabolism, or cellular respiration. Together these activities constitute respiration.

Mechanics Of Ventilation

Ventilation, or breathing, is the movement of air through the conducting passages between the atmosphere and the lungs. The air moves through the

About This Chapter: Information in this chapter is from "Respiratory System," at the National Cancer Institute's Surveillance, Epidemiology, and End Results (SEER)'s Training Website (http://training.seer.cancer.gov), 2000, accessed May 3, 2006. Note: Despite the older date of this document, the anatomical information it presents is still current.

passages because of pressure gradients that are produced by contraction of the diaphragm and thoracic muscles.

Pulmonary Ventilation

Pulmonary ventilation is commonly referred to as breathing. It is the process of air flowing into the lungs during inspiration (inhalation) and out of the lungs during expiration (exhalation). Air flows because of pressure differences between the atmosphere and the gases inside the lungs.

Air, like other gases, flows from a region with higher pressure to a region with lower pressure. Muscular breathing movements and recoil of elastic tissues create the changes in pressure that result in ventilation. Pulmonary ventilation involves three different pressures, which are as follows:

- Atmospheric pressure

- Intraalveolar (intra-pulmonary) pressure

- Intrapleural pressure

> **♣ It's A Fact!!**
> Respiration is the sequence of events that results in the exchange of oxygen and carbon dioxide between the atmosphere and the body cells.

Atmospheric pressure is the pressure of the air outside the body. Intraalveolar pressure is the pressure inside the alveoli of the lungs. Intrapleural pressure is the pressure within the pleural cavity. These three pressures are responsible for pulmonary ventilation.

> **✎ What's It Mean?**
>
> Inspiration: Inspiration (inhalation) is the process of taking air into the lungs. It is the active phase of ventilation because it is the result of muscle contraction. During inspiration, the diaphragm contracts and the thoracic cavity increases in volume. This decreases the intraalveolar pressure so that air flows into the lungs. Inspiration draws air into the lungs.
>
> Expiration: Expiration (exhalation) is the process of letting air out of the lungs during the breathing cycle. During expiration, the relaxation of the diaphragm and elastic recoil of tissue decreases the thoracic volume and increases the intraalveolar pressure. Expiration pushes air out of the lungs.

Respiratory Volumes And Capacities

A breath is one complete respiratory cycle that consists of one inspiration and one expiration.

♣ It's A Fact!!
Under normal conditions, the average adult takes 12 to 15 breaths a minute.

An instrument called a spirometer is used to measure the volume of air that moves into and out of the lungs, and the process of taking the measurements is called spirometry. Respiratory (pulmonary) volumes are an important aspect of pulmonary function testing because they can provide information about the physical condition of the lungs.

Respiratory capacity (pulmonary capacity) is the sum of two or more volumes.

Factors such as age, sex, body build, and physical conditioning have an influence on lung volumes and capacities. Lungs usually reach their maximum capacity in early adulthood and decline with age after that.

Conducting Passages

The respiratory conducting passages are divided into the upper respiratory tract and the lower respiratory tract. The upper respiratory tract includes the nose, pharynx, and larynx. The lower respiratory tract consists of the trachea, bronchial tree, and lungs. These tracts open to the outside and are lined with mucous membranes. In some regions, the membrane has hairs that help filter the air. Other regions may have cilia to propel mucus.

Nose, Nasal Cavities, And Paranasal Sinuses

The framework of the nose consists of bone and cartilage. Two small nasal bones and extensions of the maxillae form the bridge of the nose, which is the bony portion. The remainder of the framework is cartilage and is the flexible portion. Connective tissue and skin cover the framework.

Air enters the nasal cavity from the outside through two openings, the nostrils, or external nares. The openings from the nasal cavity into the pharynx are the internal nares. Nose hairs at the entrance to the nose trap large inhaled particles.

Paranasal Sinuses

Paranasal sinuses are air-filled cavities in the frontal, maxillae, ethmoid, and sphenoid bones. These sinuses, which have the same names as the bones in which they are located, surround the nasal cavity and open into it. They function to reduce the weight of the skull, to produce mucus, and to influence voice quality by acting as resonating chambers.

Pharynx

The pharynx, commonly called the throat, is a passageway that extends from the base of the skull to the level of the sixth cervical vertebra. It serves both the respiratory and digestive systems by receiving air from the nasal cavity and air, food, and water from the oral cavity. Inferiorly, it opens into the larynx and esophagus. The pharynx is divided into three regions according to location: the nasopharynx, the oropharynx, and the laryngopharynx (hypopharynx).

The nasopharynx is the portion of the pharynx that is posterior to the nasal cavity and extends inferiorly to the uvula. The oropharynx is the portion of the pharynx that is posterior to the oral cavity. The most inferior portion of the pharynx is the laryngopharynx that extends from the hyoid bone down to the lower margin of the larynx.

The upper part of the pharynx (throat) lets only air pass through. Lower parts permit air, foods, and fluids to pass.

The pharyngeal, palatine, and lingual tonsils are located in the pharynx. They are also called Waldeyer's Ring.

The retromolar trigone is the small area behind the wisdom teeth.

Larynx And Trachea

Larynx

The larynx, commonly called the voice box or glottis, is the passageway for air between the pharynx above and the trachea below. It extends from the fourth to the sixth vertebral levels. The larynx is often divided into three sections: sublarynx, larynx, and supralarynx. It is formed by nine cartilages that are connected to each other by muscles and ligaments.

The larynx plays an essential role in human speech. During sound production, the vocal cords close together and vibrate as air expelled from the lungs passes between them. The false vocal cords have no role in sound production but help close off the larynx when food is swallowed.

The thyroid cartilage is the Adam's apple. The epiglottis acts like a trap door to keep food and other particles from entering the larynx.

Trachea

The trachea, commonly called the windpipe, is the main airway to the lungs. It divides into the right and left bronchi at the level of the fifth thoracic vertebra, channeling air to the right or left lung.

The hyaline cartilage in the tracheal wall provides support and keeps the trachea from collapsing. The posterior soft tissue allows for expansion of the esophagus, which is immediately posterior to the trachea.

The mucous membrane that lines the trachea is ciliated pseudostratified columnar epithelium, similar to that in the nasal cavity and nasopharynx. Goblet cells produce mucus that traps airborne particles and microorganisms, and the cilia propel the mucus upward, where it is either swallowed or expelled.

Bronchi, Bronchial Tree, And Lungs

Bronchi And Bronchial Tree

In the mediastinum, at the level of the fifth thoracic vertebra, the trachea divides into the right and left primary bronchi. The bronchi branch into smaller and smaller passageways until they terminate in tiny air sacs called alveoli.

The cartilage and mucous membrane of the primary bronchi are similar to that in the trachea. As the branching continues through the bronchial tree, the amount of hyaline cartilage in the walls decreases until it is absent in the smallest bronchioles. As the cartilage decreases, the amount of smooth muscle increases. The mucous membrane also undergoes a transition from ciliated pseudostratified columnar epithelium, to simple cuboidal epithelium, to simple squamous epithelium.

The alveolar ducts and alveoli consist primarily of simple squamous epithelium, which permits rapid diffusion of oxygen and carbon dioxide. Exchange of gases between the air in the lungs and the blood in the capillaries occurs across the walls of the alveolar ducts and alveoli.

Lungs

The two lungs, which contain all the components of the bronchial tree beyond the primary bronchi, occupy most of the space in the thoracic cavity. The lungs are soft and spongy because they are mostly air spaces surrounded by the alveolar cells and elastic connective tissue. They are separated from each other by the mediastinum, which contains the heart. The only point of attachment for each lung is at the hilum, or root, on the medial side. This is where the bronchi, blood vessels, lymphatics, and nerves enter the lungs.

The right lung is shorter, broader, and has a greater volume than the left lung. It is divided into three lobes and each lobe is supplied by one of the secondary bronchi. The left lung is longer and narrower than the right lung. It has an indentation, called the cardiac notch, on its medial surface for the apex of the heart. The left lung has two lobes.

Each lung is enclosed by a double-layered serous membrane, called the pleura. The visceral pleura is firmly attached to the surface of the lung. At the hilum, the visceral pleura is continuous with the parietal pleura that lines the wall of the thorax. The small space between the visceral and parietal pleurae is the pleural cavity. It contains a thin film of serous fluid that is produced by the pleura. The fluid acts as a lubricant to reduce friction as the two layers slide against each other, and it helps to hold the two layers together as the lungs inflate and deflate.

Chapter 10

The Digestive System

Functions Of The Digestive System

The digestive system includes the digestive tract and its accessory organs, which process food into molecules that can be absorbed and utilized by the cells of the body. Food is broken down, bit by bit, until the molecules are small enough to be absorbed, and the waste products are eliminated.

The digestive tract includes the mouth, pharynx, esophagus, stomach, small intestine, and large intestine. The tongue and teeth are accessory structures located in the mouth. The salivary glands, liver, gallbladder, and pancreas are major accessory organs that have a role in digestion. These organs secrete fluids into the digestive tract.

Food undergoes three types of processes in the body, which are as follows:

- Digestion
- Absorption
- Elimination

About This Chapter: Information in this chapter is from "Digestive System," at the National Cancer Institute's Surveillance, Epidemiology, and End Results (SEER)'s Training Website (http://training.seer.cancer.gov), 2000, accessed May 3, 2006. Note: Despite the older date of this document, the anatomical information it presents is still current.

Digestion and absorption occur in the digestive tract. After the nutrients are absorbed, they are available to all cells in the body and are utilized by the body cells in metabolism.

The digestive system prepares nutrients for utilization by body cells through six activities, or functions.

Ingestion

The first activity of the digestive system is to take in food through the mouth. This process, called ingestion, has to take place before anything else can happen.

> **♣ It's A Fact!!**
> The digestive tract, also called the alimentary canal or gastrointestinal (GI) tract, consists of a long continuous tube that extends from the mouth to the anus.

Mechanical Digestion

The large pieces of food that are ingested have to be broken into smaller particles that can be acted upon by various enzymes. This is mechanical digestion, which begins in the mouth with chewing, or mastication, and continues with churning and mixing actions in the stomach.

Chemical Digestion

The complex molecules of carbohydrates, proteins, and fats are transformed by chemical digestion into smaller molecules that can be absorbed and utilized by the cells. Chemical digestion, through a process called hydrolysis, uses water and digestive enzymes to break down the complex molecules. Digestive enzymes speed up the hydrolysis process, which is otherwise very slow.

Movements

After ingestion and mastication, the food particles move from the mouth into the pharynx, and then into the esophagus. This movement is deglutition, or swallowing. Mixing movements occur in the stomach as a result of smooth muscle contraction. These repetitive contractions usually occur in small segments of the digestive tract and mix the food particles with enzymes and other fluids. The movements that propel the food particles through the digestive tract are called peristalsis. These are rhythmic waves of contractions that move the food particles through the various regions in which mechanical and chemical digestion takes place.

Absorption

The simple molecules that result from chemical digestion pass through cell membranes of the lining in the small intestine into the blood or lymph capillaries. This process is called absorption.

Elimination

The food molecules that cannot be digested or absorbed need to be eliminated from the body. The removal of indigestible wastes through the anus, in the form of feces, is defecation or elimination.

Regions Of The Digestive System

At its simplest, the digestive system is a tube running from mouth to anus. Its chief goal is to break down huge macromolecules (proteins, fats, and starch), which cannot be absorbed intact, into smaller molecules (amino acids, fatty acids, and glucose) that can be absorbed across the wall of the tube and into the circulatory system for dissemination throughout the body.

Regions of the digestive system can be divided into two main parts: the alimentary tract and accessory organs. The alimentary tract of the digestive system is composed of the mouth, pharynx, esophagus, stomach, small and large intestines, rectum, and anus. Associated with the alimentary tract are the following accessory organs: salivary glands, liver, gallbladder, and pancreas.

Mouth

The mouth, or oral cavity, is the first part of the digestive tract. It is adapted to receive food by ingestion, break it into small particles by mastication, and mix it with saliva. The lips, cheeks, and palate form the boundaries. The oral cavity contains the teeth and tongue and receives the secretions from the salivary glands.

Lips And Cheeks

The lips and cheeks help hold food in the mouth and keep it in place for chewing. They are also used in the formation of words for speech. The lips contain numerous sensory receptors that are useful for judging the temperature and texture of foods.

Palate

The palate is the roof of the oral cavity. It separates the oral cavity from the nasal cavity. The anterior portion, the hard palate, is supported by bone. The posterior portion, the soft palate, is skeletal muscle and connective tissue. Posteriorly, the soft palate ends in a projection called the uvula. During swallowing, the soft palate and uvula move upward to direct food away from the nasal cavity and into the oropharynx.

Tongue

The tongue manipulates food in the mouth and is used in speech. The surface is covered with papillae that provide friction and contain the taste buds.

Teeth

A complete set of deciduous (primary) teeth contains 20 teeth. There are 32 teeth in a complete permanent (secondary) set. The shape of each tooth type corresponds to the way it handles food.

Pharynx And Esophagus

Pharynx

The pharynx is a fibromuscular passageway that connects the nasal and oral cavities to the larynx and esophagus. It serves both the respiratory and digestive systems as a channel for air and food. The upper region, the nasopharynx, is posterior to the nasal cavity. It contains the pharyngeal tonsils, or adenoids, functions as a passageway for air, and has no function in the digestive system. The middle region posterior to the oral cavity is the oropharynx. This is the first region food enters when it is swallowed. The opening from the oral cavity into the oropharynx is called the fauces. Masses of lymphoid tissue, the palatine tonsils, are near the fauces. The lower region, posterior to the larynx, is the laryngopharynx, or hypopharynx. The laryngopharynx opens into both the esophagus and the larynx.

Food is forced into the pharynx by the tongue. When food reaches the opening, sensory receptors around the fauces respond and initiate an involuntary swallowing reflex. This reflex action has several parts. The uvula is elevated to prevent food from entering the nasopharynx. The epiglottis drops downward to prevent food from entering the larynx and trachea in order to direct the food into the esophagus. Peristaltic movements propel the food from the pharynx into the esophagus.

Esophagus

The esophagus is a collapsible muscular tube that serves as a passageway between the pharynx and stomach. As it descends, it is posterior to the trachea and anterior to the vertebral column. It passes through an opening in the diaphragm, called the esophageal hiatus, and then empties into the stomach. The mucosa has glands that secrete mucus to keep the lining moist and well lubricated to ease the passage of food. Upper and lower esophageal sphincters control the

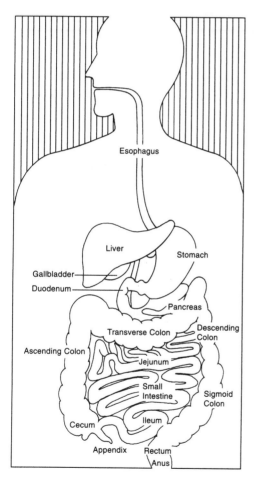

Figure 10.1. Organs Of The Digestive System (Source: National Institute of Diabetes and Digestive and Kidney Diseases (NIDDK), NIH Publication No. 04-2681)

movement of food into and out of the esophagus. The lower esophageal sphincter is sometimes called the cardiac sphincter and resides at the esophagogastric junction.

Stomach

The stomach, which receives food from the esophagus, is located in the upper left quadrant of the abdomen. The stomach is divided into the fundic, cardiac, body, and pyloric regions. The lesser and greater curvatures are on the right and left sides, respectively, of the stomach.

Gastric Secretions

The mucosal lining of the stomach is simple columnar epithelium with numerous tubular gastric glands. The gastric glands open to the surface of the mucosa through tiny holes called gastric pits. Four different types of cells make up the gastric glands and are as follows:

- Mucous cells
- Parietal cells
- Chief cells
- Endocrine cells

The secretions of the exocrine gastric glands, composed of the mucous, parietal, and chief cells, make up the gastric juice. The products of the endocrine cells are secreted directly into the bloodstream and are not a part of the gastric juice. The endocrine cells secrete the hormone gastrin, which functions in the regulation of gastric activity.

Regulation Of Gastric Secretions

The regulation of gastric secretion is accomplished through neural and hormonal mechanisms. Gastric juice is produced all the time, but the amount varies subject to the regulatory factors. Regulation of gastric secretions may be divided into cephalic, gastric, and intestinal phases. Thoughts and smells of food start the cephalic phase of gastric secretion; the presence of food in the stomach initiates the gastric phase; and the presence of acid chyme in the small intestine begins the intestinal phase.

Stomach Emptying

Relaxation of the pyloric sphincter allows chyme to pass from the stomach into the small intestine. The rate of which this occurs depends on the nature of the chyme and the receptivity of the small intestine.

Small And Large Intestine

Small Intestine

The small intestine extends from the pyloric sphincter to the ileocecal valve, where it empties into the large intestine. The small intestine finishes the process of digestion, absorbs the nutrients, and passes the residue on to the large intestine. The liver, gallbladder, and pancreas are accessory organs of the digestive system that are closely associated with the small intestine.

The small intestine is divided into the duodenum, jejunum, and ileum. The small intestine follows the general structure of the digestive tract in that the wall has a mucosa with simple columnar epithelium, submucosa, smooth muscle with inner circular and outer longitudinal layers, and serosa. The absorptive surface area of the small intestine is increased by plicae circulares, villi, and microvilli.

Exocrine cells in the mucosa of the small intestine secrete mucus, peptidase, sucrase, maltase, lactase, lipase, and enterokinase. Endocrine cells secrete cholecystokinin and secretin.

The most important factor for regulating secretions in the small intestine is the presence of chyme. This is largely a local reflex action in response to chemical and mechanical irritation from the chyme and in response to distention of the intestinal wall. This is a direct reflex action, thus the greater the amount of chyme, the greater the secretion.

Large Intestine

The large intestine is larger in diameter than the small intestine. It begins at the ileocecal junction, where the ileum enters the large intestine, and ends at the anus. The large intestine consists of the colon, rectum, and anal canal.

The wall of the large intestine has the same types of tissue that are found in other parts of the digestive tract, but there are some distinguishing characteristics. The mucosa has a large number of goblet cells but does not have any villi. The longitudinal muscle layer, although present, is incomplete. The longitudinal muscle is limited to three distinct bands, called teniae coli, that run the entire length of the colon. Contraction of the teniae coli exerts pressure on the wall and creates a series of pouches, called haustra, along the colon. Epiploic appendages, pieces of fat-filled connective tissue, are attached to the outer surface of the colon.

Unlike the small intestine, the large intestine produces no digestive enzymes. Chemical digestion is completed in the small intestine before the chyme reaches the large intestine. Functions of the large intestine include the absorption of water and electrolytes and the elimination of feces.

Rectum And Anus

The rectum continues from the sigmoid colon to the anal canal and has a thick muscular layer. It follows the curvature of the sacrum and is firmly attached to it by connective tissue. The rectum ends about 5 cm below the tip of the coccyx, at the beginning of the anal canal.

The last 2 to 3 cm of the digestive tract is the anal canal, which continues from the rectum and opens to the outside at the anus. The mucosa of the rectum is folded to form longitudinal anal columns. The smooth muscle layer is thick and forms the internal anal sphincter at the superior end of the anal canal. This sphincter is under involuntary control. There is an external anal sphincter at the inferior end of the anal canal. This sphincter is composed of skeletal muscle and is under voluntary control.

♣ It's A Fact!!
The salivary glands, liver, gallbladder, and pancreas are not part of the digestive tract, but they have a role in digestive activities and are considered accessory organs.

Salivary Glands

Three pairs of major salivary glands (parotid, submandibular, and sublingual glands), and numerous smaller ones, secrete saliva into the oral cavity, where it is mixed with food during mastication. Saliva contains water, mucus, and enzyme amylase. Functions of saliva include the following:

- It has a cleansing action on the teeth.

- It moistens and lubricates food during mastication and swallowing.

- It dissolves certain molecules so that food can be tasted.

- It begins the chemical digestion of starches through the action of amylase, which breaks down polysaccharides into disaccharides.

Liver

The liver is located primarily in the right hypochondriac and epigastric regions of the abdomen, just beneath the diaphragm. It is the largest gland in the body. On the surface, the liver is divided into two major lobes and two smaller lobes. The functional units of the liver are lobules with sinusoids that carry blood from the periphery to the central vein of the lobule.

The liver receives blood from two sources. Freshly oxygenated blood is brought to the liver by the common hepatic artery, a branch of the celiac trunk from the abdominal aorta. Blood that is rich in nutrients from the digestive tract is carried to the liver by the hepatic portal vein.

The liver has a wide variety of functions and many of these are vital to life. Hepatocytes perform most of the functions attributed to the liver, but the phagocytic Kupffer cells that line the sinusoids are responsible for cleansing the blood.

Liver functions include the following:

- Secretion

- Synthesis of bile salts

- Synthesis of plasma protein

- Storage

- Detoxification

- Excretion

- Carbohydrate metabolism

- Lipid metabolism

- Protein metabolism

- Filtering

Gallbladder

The gallbladder is a pear-shaped sac that is attached to the visceral surface of the liver by the cystic duct. The principal function of the gallbladder is to serve as a storage reservoir for bile. Bile is a yellowish-green fluid produced by liver cells. The main components of bile are water, bile salts, bile pigments, and cholesterol.

Bile salts act as emulsifying agents in the digestion and absorption of fats. Cholesterol and bile pigments from the breakdown of hemoglobin are excreted from the body in the bile.

Pancreas

The pancreas has both endocrine and exocrine functions. The endocrine portion consists of the scattered islets of Langerhans, which secrete the hormones insulin and glucagon into the blood. The exocrine portion is the major part of the gland. It consists of pancreatic acinar cells that secrete digestive enzymes into tiny ducts interwoven between the cells. Pancreatic enzymes include amylase, trypsin, peptidase, and lipase. Pancreatic secretions are controlled by the hormones secretin and cholecystokinin.

Chapter 11

Kidneys And The Urinary System

Functions Of The Urinary System

The principal function of the urinary system is to maintain the volume and composition of body fluids within normal limits. One aspect of this function is to rid the body of waste products that accumulate as a result of cellular metabolism, and because of this, it is sometimes referred to as the excretory system.

Although the urinary system has a major role in excretion, other organs contribute to the excretory function. The lungs in the respiratory system excrete some waste products, such as carbon dioxide and water. The skin is another excretory organ that rids the body of wastes through the sweat glands. The liver and intestines excrete bile pigments that result from the destruction of hemoglobin. The major task of excretion still belongs to the urinary system. If it fails, the other organs cannot take over and compensate adequately.

The urinary system maintains an appropriate fluid volume by regulating the amount of water that is excreted in the urine. Other aspects of its function include regulating the concentrations of various electrolytes in the body fluids and maintaining normal pH of the blood.

About This Chapter: Information in this chapter is from "Urinary System," at the National Cancer Institute's Surveillance, Epidemiology, and End Results (SEER)'s Training Website (http://training.seer.cancer.gov), 2000, accessed May 3, 2006. Note: Despite the older date of this document, the anatomical information it presents is still current.

In addition to maintaining fluid homeostasis in the body, the urinary system controls red blood cell production by secreting the hormone erythropoietin. The urinary system also plays a role in maintaining normal blood pressure by secreting the enzyme renin.

Components Of The Urinary System

The urinary system consists of the kidneys, ureters, urinary bladder, and urethra. The kidneys form the urine and account for the other functions attributed to the urinary system. The ureters carry the urine away from kidneys to the urinary bladder, which is a temporary reservoir for the urine. The urethra is a tubular structure that carries the urine from the urinary bladder to the outside.

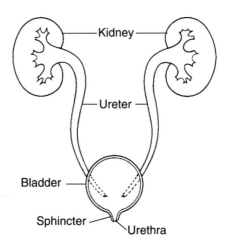

Figure 11.1. Components of the Urinary System (Source: National Kidney and Urologic Diseases Information Clearinghouse)

Kidneys

The kidneys are the organs that filter the blood, remove the wastes, and excrete the wastes in the urine. They are the organs that perform the functions of the urinary system. The other components are accessory structures to eliminate the urine from the body.

The paired kidneys are located between the twelfth thoracic and third lumbar vertebrae, one on each side of the vertebral column. The right kidney usually is slightly lower than the left because the liver displaces it downward. The kidneys protected by the lower ribs, lie in shallow depressions against the posterior abdominal wall and behind the parietal peritoneum. This means they are retroperitoneal. Each kidney is held in place by connective tissue, called renal fascia, and is surrounded by a thick layer of adipose tissue, called perirenal fat, which helps to protect it. A tough, fibrous, connective tissue renal capsule closely envelops each kidney and provides support for the soft tissue that is inside.

♣ **It's A Fact!!**

The kidneys are the primary organs of the urinary system.

In the adult, each kidney is approximately 3 cm thick, 6 cm wide, and 12 cm long. It is roughly bean-shaped with an indentation, called the hilum, on the medial side. The hilum leads to a large cavity, called the renal sinus, within the kidney. The ureter and renal vein leave the kidney, and the renal artery enters the kidney at the hilum.

The outer region is the renal cortex. This surrounds a region called the renal medulla. The renal medulla consists of a series of renal pyramids, which appear striated because they contain straight tubular structures and blood vessels. The wide bases of the pyramids are adjacent to the cortex and the pointed ends, called renal papillae, are directed toward the center of the kidney. Portions of the renal cortex extend into the spaces between adjacent pyramids to form renal columns. The cortex and medulla make up the parenchyma, or functional tissue, of the kidney.

The central region of the kidney contains the renal pelvis, which is located in the renal sinus and is continuous with the ureter. The renal pelvis is a large cavity that collects the urine as it is produced. The periphery of the renal pelvis is interrupted by cuplike projections called calyces. A minor calyx surrounds the renal papillae of each pyramid and collects urine from that pyramid. Several minor calyces converge to form a major calyx. From the major calyces the urine flows into the renal pelvis and from there into the ureter.

Each kidney contains over a million functional units, called nephrons, in the parenchyma (cortex and medulla). A nephron has two parts: a renal corpuscle and a renal tubule. The renal corpuscle consists of a cluster of capillaries, called the glomerulus, surrounded by a double-layered epithelial cup, called the glomerular capsule. An afferent arteriole leads into the renal corpuscle and an efferent arteriole leaves the renal corpuscle. Urine passes from the nephrons into collecting ducts then into the minor calyces.

The juxtaglomerular apparatus, which monitors blood pressure and secretes renin, is formed from modified cells in the afferent arteriole and the ascending limb of the nephron loop.

Ureters

Each ureter is a small tube, about 25 cm long, that carries urine from the renal pelvis to the urinary bladder. It descends from the renal pelvis, along the posterior abdominal wall, behind the parietal peritoneum, and enters the urinary bladder on the posterior inferior surface.

The wall of the ureter consists of three layers. The outer layer, the fibrous coat, is a supporting layer of fibrous connective tissue. The middle layer, the muscular coat, consists of inner circular and outer longitudinal smooth muscle. The main function of this layer is peristalsis to propel the urine. The inner layer, the mucosa, is transitional epithelium that is continuous with the lining of the renal pelvis and the urinary bladder. This layer secretes mucus, which coats and protects the surface of the cells.

Urinary Bladder

The urinary bladder is located in the pelvic cavity, posterior to the symphysis pubis, and below the parietal peritoneum. The size and shape of the urinary bladder varies with the amount of urine it contains and with the pressure it receives from surrounding organs.

The inner lining of the urinary bladder is a mucous membrane of transitional epithelium that is continuous with that in the ureters. When the bladder is empty, the mucosa has numerous folds called rugae. The rugae and transitional epithelium allow the bladder to expand as it fills.

The second layer in the walls is the submucosa that supports the mucous membrane. It is composed of connective tissue with elastic fibers.

The next layer is the muscularis, which is composed of smooth muscle. The smooth muscle fibers are interwoven in all directions and collectively these are called the detrusor muscle. Contraction of this muscle expels urine from the bladder. On the superior surface, the outer layer of the bladder wall is parietal peritoneum. In all other regions, the outer layer is fibrous connective tissue.

♣ It's A Fact!!

The urinary bladder is a temporary storage reservoir for urine.

There is a triangular area, called the trigone, formed by three openings in the floor of the urinary bladder. Two of the openings are from the ureters and form the base of the trigone. Small flaps of mucosa cover these openings and act as valves that allow urine to enter the bladder but prevent it from backing up from the bladder into the ureters. The third opening, at the apex of the trigone, is the opening into the urethra. A band of the detrusor muscle encircles this opening to form the internal urethral sphincter.

Urethra

The final passageway for the flow of urine is the urethra, a thin-walled tube that conveys urine from the floor of the urinary bladder to the outside. The opening to the outside is the external urethral orifice. The mucosal lining of the urethra is transitional epithelium. The wall also contains smooth muscle fibers and is supported by connective tissue.

The internal urethral sphincter surrounds the beginning of the urethra, where it leaves the urinary bladder. This sphincter is smooth (involuntary) muscle. Another sphincter, the external urethral sphincter, is skeletal (voluntary) muscle and encircles the urethra where it goes through the pelvic floor. These two sphincters control the flow of urine through the urethra.

In females, the urethra is short, only 3 to 4 cm (about 1.5 inches) long. The external urethral orifice opens to the outside just anterior to the opening for the vagina.

In males, the urethra is much longer, about 20 cm (7 to 8 inches) in length, and transports both urine and semen. The first part, next to the urinary bladder, passes through the prostate gland and is called the prostatic urethra. The second part, a short region that penetrates the pelvic floor and enters the penis, is called the membranous urethra. The third part, the spongy urethra, is the longest region. This portion of the urethra extends the entire length of the penis, and the external urethral orifice opens to the outside at the tip of the penis.

Chapter 12

The Immune System:
Your Body's First Line Of Defense

The immune system is a complex of organs—highly specialized cells and even a circulatory system separate from blood vessels—all of which work together to clear infection from the body.

The organs of the immune system, positioned throughout the body, are called lymphoid organs. The word "lymph" in Greek means a pure, clear stream—an appropriate description considering its appearance and purpose.

Lymphatic vessels and lymph nodes are the parts of the special circulatory system that carry lymph, a transparent fluid containing white blood cells, chiefly lymphocytes.

Lymph bathes the tissues of the body, and the lymphatic vessels collect and move it eventually back into the blood circulation. Lymph nodes dot the network of lymphatic vessels and provide meeting grounds for the immune system cells that defend against invaders. The spleen, at the upper left of the abdomen, is also a staging ground and a place where immune system cells confront foreign microbes.

About This Chapter: Information in this chapter is from "The Immune System," NIAID NetNews, National Institute of Allergy and Infectious Diseases (NIAID), September 2003.

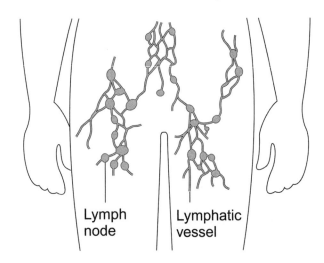

Lymph
node

Lymphatic
vessel

Figure 12.1. Immune cells and foreign particles enter the lymph nodes via incoming lymphatic vessels or the lymph nodes' tiny blood vessels (Source: NIAID, NIH Publication No. 03–5423)

Pockets of lymphoid tissue are in many other locations throughout the body, such as the bone marrow and thymus. Tonsils, adenoids, Peyer's patches, and the appendix are also lymphoid tissues.

Both immune cells and foreign molecules enter the lymph nodes via blood vessels or lymphatic vessels. All immune cells exit the lymphatic system and eventually return to the bloodstream. Once in the bloodstream, lymphocytes are transported to tissues throughout the body, where they act as sentries on the lookout for foreign antigens.

How The Immune System Works

Cells that will grow into the many types of more specialized cells that circulate throughout the immune system are produced in the bone marrow. This nutrient-rich, spongy tissue is found in the center shafts of certain long, flat bones of the body, such as the bones of the pelvis. The cells most relevant for understanding vaccines are the lymphocytes, numbering close to one trillion.

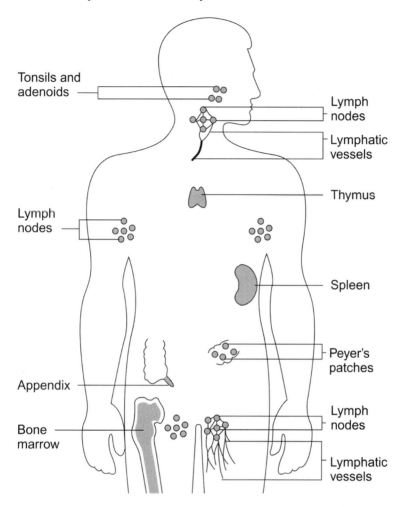

Tonsils and adenoids

Lymph nodes

Lymphatic vessels

Thymus

Lymph nodes

Spleen

Lymph nodes

Peyer's patches

Appendix

Bone marrow

Lymph nodes

Lymphatic vessels

Figure 12.2. Organs of the Immune System (Source: NIAID, NIH Publication No. 03–5423)

The two major classes of lymphocytes are B cells, which grow to maturity in the bone marrow, and T cells, which mature in the thymus, high in the chest behind the breastbone.

B cells produce antibodies that circulate in the blood and lymph streams and attach to foreign antigens to mark them for destruction by other immune cells.

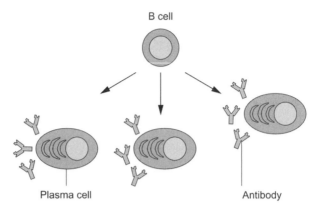

Figure 12.3. B cells mature into plasma cells that produce antibodies (Source: NIAID, NIH Publication No. 03–5423).

B cells are part of what is known as antibody-mediated or humoral immunity, so called because the antibodies circulate in blood and lymph, which the ancient Greeks called, the body's "humors."

Certain T cells, which also patrol the blood and lymph for foreign invaders, can do more than mark the antigens; they attack and destroy diseased cells they recognize as foreign. T lymphocytes are responsible for cell-mediated immunity (or cellular immunity). T cells also orchestrate, regulate, and coordinate the overall immune response. T cells depend on unique cell surface molecules, called the major histocompatibility complex (MHC), to help them recognize antigen fragments.

Antibodies

The antibodies that B cells produce are basic templates with a special region that is highly specific to target a given antigen. Much like a car coming off a production line, the antibody's frame remains constant, but through chemical and cellular messages, the immune system selects a green sedan, a red convertible, or a white truck to combat this particular invader.

However, in contrast to cars, the variety of antibodies is very large. Different antibodies are destined for different purposes. Some coat the foreign invaders to make them attractive to the circulating scavenger cells, called phagocytes, which will engulf an unwelcome microbe.

When some antibodies combine with antigens, they activate a cascade of nine proteins, known as complement, which have been circulating in inactive form in the blood. Complement forms a partnership with antibodies, once they have reacted with antigen, to help destroy foreign invaders and remove them from the body. Still other types of antibodies block viruses from entering cells.

T Cells

T cells have two major roles in immune defense. Regulatory T cells are essential for orchestrating the response of an elaborate system of different types of immune cells.

Helper T cells, for example, also known as CD4 positive T cells (CD4+ T cells), alert B cells to start making antibodies; they also can activate other T cells and immune system scavenger cells, called macrophages, and influence which type of antibody is produced.

Certain T cells, called CD8 positive T cells (CD8+ T cells), can become killer cells that attack and destroy infected cells. The killer T cells are also called cytotoxic T cells or CTLs (cytotoxic lymphocytes).

✎ What's It Mean?

Antibodies: Antibodies are special proteins that are part of the body's immune system. White blood cells make antibodies to neutralize harmful germs, or other foreign substances, called antigens. Antibodies are "good guys" that fight inside your body, protecting you from "bad guys" like bacteria and viruses.

B Cells: B cells play an important role in humoral immunity because they synthesize and secrete antibodies, which protect us from infection, viruses, etc.

T Cells: T cells are the major component of cell-mediated immunity. There are several types of T Cells: Cytotoxic T cells destroy cancer cells and foreign invaders; helper T cells that work in conjunction with white blood cells; and suppressor T cells that play a role in controlling white blood cell function.

Source: From the National Cancer Institute's Surveillance, Epidemiology, and End Results (SEER)'s Glossary, available at http://training.seer.cancer.gov/stws_glossary_a.html.

Immune System Process

Activation Of Helper T Cells

After it engulfs and processes an antigen, the macrophage displays the antigen fragments combined with a Class II MHC protein on the macrophage cell surface. The antigen-protein combination attracts a helper T cell, and promotes its activation.

Activation Of Cytotoxic T Cells

After a macrophage engulfs and processes an antigen, the macrophage displays the antigen fragments combined with a Class I MHC protein on the macrophage cell surface. A receptor on a circulating, resting cytotoxic T cell recognizes the antigen-protein complex and binds to it. The binding process and a helper T cell activate the cytotoxic T cell so that it can attack and destroy the diseased cell.

Activation Of B Cells To Make Antibody

A B cell uses one of its receptors to bind to its matching antigen, which the B cell engulfs and processes. The B cell then displays a piece of the antigen, bound to a Class II MHC protein, on the cell surface. This whole complex then binds to an activated helper T cell. This binding process stimulates the transformation of the B cell into an antibody-secreting plasma cell.

Chapter 13

The Lymphatic System: Your Body's Fluids

Functions Of The Lymphatic System

The lymphatic system has three primary functions. First of all, it returns excess interstitial fluid to the blood. Of the fluid that leaves the capillary, about 90 percent is returned. The 10 percent that does not return becomes part of the interstitial fluid that surrounds the tissue cells. Small protein molecules may "leak" through the capillary wall and increase the osmotic pressure of the interstitial fluid. This further inhibits the return of fluid into the capillaries, and fluid tends to accumulate in the tissue spaces. If this continues, blood volume and blood pressure decrease significantly and the volume of tissue fluid increases, which results in edema (swelling). Lymph capillaries pick up the excess interstitial fluid and proteins and returns them to the venous blood. After the fluid enters the lymph capillaries, it is called lymph.

The second function of the lymphatic system is the absorption of fats and fat-soluble vitamins from the digestive system and the subsequent transport of these substances to the venous circulation. The mucosa that lines the small intestine is covered with finger-like projections called villi. There are blood capillaries and special lymph capillaries, called lacteals, in the center of

About This Chapter: Information in this chapter is from "Lymphatic System," at the National Cancer Institute's Surveillance, Epidemiology, and End Results (SEER)'s Training Website (http://training.seer.cancer.gov), 2000, accessed May 3, 2006. Note: Despite the older date of this document, the anatomical information it presents is still current.

each villus. The blood capillaries absorb most nutrients, but the fats and fat-soluble vitamins are absorbed by the lacteals. The lymph in the lacteals has a milky appearance due to its high fat content and is called chyle.

The third, and probably most well known function of the lymphatic system, is defense against invading microorganisms and disease. Lymph nodes and other lymphatic organs filter the lymph to remove microorganisms and other foreign particles. Lymphatic organs contain lymphocytes that destroy invading organisms.

Components Of The Lymphatic System

Lymph

Lymph is a fluid similar in composition to blood plasma. It is derived from blood plasma as fluids pass through capillary walls at the arterial end. As the interstitial fluid begins to accumulate, it is picked up and removed by tiny lymphatic vessels and returned to the blood. As soon as the interstitial fluid enters the lymph capillaries, it is called lymph. Returning the fluid to the blood prevents edema and helps to maintain normal blood volume and pressure.

♣ **It's A Fact!!**
The lymphatic system consists of a fluid (lymph), vessels that transport the lymph, and organs that contain lymphoid tissue.

Lymphatic Vessels

Lymphatic vessels, unlike blood vessels, only carry fluid away from the tissues. The smallest lymphatic vessels are the lymph capillaries, which begin in the tissue spaces as blind-ended sacs. Lymph capillaries are found in all regions of the body except the bone marrow, central nervous system, and tissues, such as the epidermis, which lack blood vessels. The wall of the lymph capillary is composed of endothelium in which the simple squamous cells overlap to form a simple one-way valve. This arrangement permits fluid to enter the capillary but prevents lymph from leaving the vessel.

The microscopic lymph capillaries merge to form lymphatic vessels. Small lymphatic vessels join to form larger tributaries, called lymphatic trunks, which drain large regions. Lymphatic trunks merge until the lymph enters the two lymphatic ducts. The right lymphatic duct drains lymph from the upper right quadrant of the body. The thoracic duct drains all the rest.

Like veins, the lymphatic tributaries have thin walls and have valves to prevent backflow of blood. There is no pump in the lymphatic system like the heart in the cardiovascular system. The pressure gradients to move lymph through the vessels come from the skeletal muscle action, respiratory movement, and contraction of smooth muscle in vessel walls.

Lymphatic Organs

Lymphatic organs are characterized by clusters of lymphocytes and other cells, such as macrophages, enmeshed in a framework of short, branching connective tissue fibers. The lymphocytes originate in the red bone marrow with other types of blood cells and are carried in the blood from the bone marrow to the lymphatic organs. When the body is exposed to microorganisms and other foreign substances, the lymphocytes proliferate within the lymphatic organs and are sent in the blood to the site of the invasion. This is part of the immune response that attempts to destroy the invading agent.

Lymph Nodes

Lymph nodes are small bean-shaped structures that are usually less than 2.5 cm in length. They are widely distributed throughout the body along the lymphatic pathways where they filter the lymph before it is returned to the blood. Lymph nodes are not present in the central nervous system. There are three superficial regions on each side of the body where lymph nodes tend to cluster. These areas are the inguinal nodes in the groin, the axillary nodes in the armpit, and the cervical nodes in the neck.

The typical lymph node is surrounded by a connective tissue capsule and divided into compartments called lymph nodules. The lymph nodules are dense masses of lymphocytes and macrophages and are separated by spaces called lymph sinuses. Several afferent lymphatic vessels, which carry lymph into the node, enter the node on the convex side. The lymph moves through the lymph sinuses and enters an efferent lymphatic vessel, which carries the lymph away from the node. Because there are more afferent vessels than efferent vessels, the passage of lymph through the sinuses is slowed down, which allows time for the cleansing process. The efferent vessel leaves the node at an indented region called the hilum.

Tonsils

Tonsils are clusters of lymphatic tissue just under the mucous membranes that line the nose, mouth, and throat (pharynx).

Spleen

The spleen is located in the upper left abdominal cavity, just beneath the diaphragm, and posterior to the stomach. It is similar to a lymph node in shape and structure, but it is much larger. The spleen is the largest lymphatic organ in the body.

The spleen filters blood in much the same way that the lymph nodes filter lymph. Lymphocytes in the spleen react to pathogens in the blood and attempt to destroy them. Macrophages then engulf the resulting debris, the damaged cells, and the other large particles. The spleen, along with the liver, removes old and damaged erythrocytes from the circulating blood. Like other lymphatic tissue, it produces lymphocytes, especially in response to invading pathogens.

Thymus

The thymus is a soft organ with two lobes that is located anterior to the ascending aorta and posterior to the sternum. It is relatively large in infants and children, but after puberty, it begins to decrease in size so that in older adults it is quite small.

The primary function of the thymus is the processing and maturation of special lymphocytes called T-lymphocytes or T-cells. While in the thymus, the lymphocytes do not respond to pathogens and foreign agents. After the lymphocytes have matured, they enter the blood and go to other lymphatic organs where they help provide defense against disease. The thymus also produces a hormone, thymosin, which stimulates the maturation of lymphocytes in other lymphatic organs.

Chapter 14

Your Endocrine (Hormonal) System

Introduction To The Endocrine System

The endocrine system, along with the nervous system, functions in the regulation of body activities. The nervous system acts through electrical impulses and neurotransmitters to cause muscle contraction and glandular secretion. The effect is of short duration, measured in seconds, and localized. The endocrine system acts through chemical messengers, called hormones, which influence growth, development, and metabolic activities. The action of the endocrine system is measured in minutes, hours, or weeks and is more generalized than the action of the nervous system.

Exocrine Glands

Exocrine glands have ducts that carry their secretory product to a surface. These glands include the sweat, sebaceous, and mammary glands, and the glands that secrete digestive enzymes.

Endocrine Glands

The endocrine glands do not have ducts to carry their product to a surface. They are called ductless glands. The word endocrine is derived from the

About This Chapter: Information in this chapter is from "Endocrine System," at the National Cancer Institute's Surveillance, Epidemiology, and End Results (SEER)'s Training Website (http://training.seer.cancer.gov), 2000, accessed May 3, 2006. Note: Despite the older date of this document, the anatomical information it presents is still current.

Greek terms "endo," meaning within, and
"krine," meaning to separate or secrete.
The secretory products of endocrine
glands are called hormones and are secreted directly into the blood and then
carried throughout the body where they
influence only those cells that have receptor
sites for that hormone.

Endocrine Glands And Their Hormones

The endocrine system is made up of the endocrine glands that secrete
hormones. Although there are eight major endocrine glands scattered
throughout the body, they are still considered to be one system because they
have similar functions, similar mechanisms of influence, and many important interrelationships.

Some glands also have non-endocrine regions that have functions other
than hormone secretion. For example, the pancreas has a major exocrine
portion that secretes digestive enzymes and an endocrine portion that secretes hormones. The ovaries and testes secrete hormones and also produce
the ova and sperm. Some organs, such as the stomach, intestines, and heart,
produce hormones, but their primary function is not hormone secretion.

Pituitary And Pineal Glands

Pituitary Gland

The pituitary gland, or hypophysis, is a small gland about one centimeter in diameter, or the size of a pea. It is nearly surrounded by bone as it
rests in the sella turcica, a depression in the sphenoid bone. The gland is
connected to the hypothalamus of the brain by a slender stalk called the
infundibulum.

There are two distinct regions in the gland: the anterior lobe (adenohypophysis) and the posterior lobe (neurohypophysis). Releasing hormones from
the hypothalamus controls the activity of the adenohypophysis. The neurohypophysis is controlled by nerve stimulation.

Hormones Of The Anterior Lobe (Adenohypophysis): Growth hormone is a protein that stimulates the growth of bones, muscles, and other organs by promoting protein synthesis. This hormone drastically affects the appearance of an individual because it influences height. If there is too little growth hormone in a child, that person may become a pituitary dwarf of normal proportions but small stature. An excess of the hormone in a child results in an exaggerated bone growth, and the individual becomes exceptionally tall, or a giant.

Thyroid-stimulating hormone, or thyrotropin, causes the glandular cells of the thyroid to secrete thyroid hormone. When there is a hypersecretion of thyroid-stimulating hormone, the thyroid gland enlarges and secretes too much thyroid hormone.

Adrenocorticotropic hormone reacts with receptor sites in the cortex of the adrenal gland to stimulate the secretion of cortical hormones, particularly cortisol.

Gonadotropic hormones react with receptor sites in the gonads, or ovaries and testes, to regulate the development, growth, and function of these organs.

Prolactin hormone promotes the development of glandular tissue in the female breast during pregnancy and stimulates milk production after the birth of the infant.

Hormones Of The Posterior Lobe (Neurohypophysis): Antidiuretic hormone promotes the reabsorption of water by the kidney tubules, with the result that less water is lost as urine. This mechanism conserves water for the body. Insufficient amounts of antidiuretic hormone cause excessive water loss in the urine.

Oxytocin causes contraction of the smooth muscle in the wall of the uterus. It also stimulates the ejection of milk from the lactating breast.

Pineal Gland

The pineal gland, also called pineal body or epiphysis cerebri, is a small cone-shaped structure that extends posteriorly from the third ventricle of the brain. The pineal gland consists of portions of neurons, neuroglial cells, and specialized secretory cells, called pinealocytes. The pinealocytes synthesize the hormone melatonin and secrete it directly into the cerebrospinal fluid, which takes it into the blood. Melatonin affects reproductive development and daily physiologic cycles.

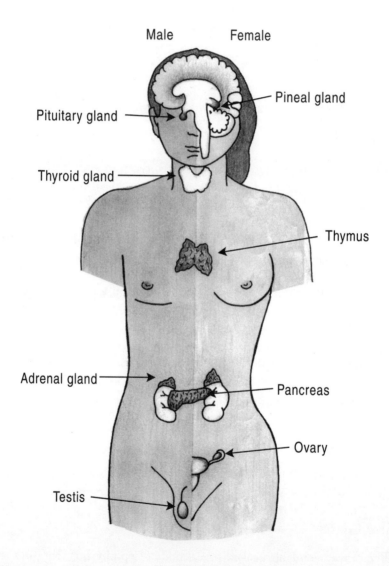

Figure 14.1. Major Endocrine Glands (SEER image redrawn by Alison DeKleine).

Thyroid And Parathyroid Glands

Thyroid Gland

The thyroid gland is a very vascular organ that is located in the neck. It consists of two lobes, one on each side of the trachea, just below the larynx or voice box. A narrow band of tissue, called the isthmus, connects the two lobes. Internally, the gland consists of follicles, which produce thyroxine and triiodothyronine hormones. These hormones contain iodine.

About 95 percent of the active thyroid hormone is thyroxine, and most of the remaining 5 percent is triiodothyronine. Both of these require iodine for their synthesis. Thyroid hormone secretion is regulated by a negative feedback mechanism that involves the amount of circulating hormone, hypothalamus, and adenohypophysis.

If there is an iodine deficiency, the thyroid cannot make sufficient hormone. This stimulates the anterior pituitary to secrete thyroid-stimulating hormone, which causes the thyroid gland to increase in size in a vain attempt to produce more hormones; but it cannot produce more hormones because it does not have the necessary raw material, iodine. This type of thyroid enlargement is called simple goiter, or iodine deficiency goiter.

The parafollicular cells of the thyroid gland secrete calcitonin. This hormone opposes the action of the parathyroid glands by reducing the calcium level in the blood. If blood calcium becomes too high, calcitonin is secreted until calcium ion levels decrease to normal.

Parathyroid Gland

Four small masses of epithelial tissue are embedded in the connective tissue capsule on the posterior surface of the thyroid glands. These are parathyroid glands, and they secrete parathyroid hormone or parathormone. Parathyroid hormone is the most important regulator of blood calcium levels. The hormone is secreted in response to low blood calcium levels, and its effect is to increase those levels.

Hypoparathyroidism, or insufficient secretion of parathyroid hormone, leads to increased nerve excitability. The low blood calcium levels trigger spontaneous and continuous nerve impulses, which then stimulate muscle contraction.

Adrenal Gland

The adrenal, or suprarenal, gland is paired with one gland located near the upper portion of each kidney. Each gland is divided into an outer cortex and an inner medulla. The cortex and medulla of the adrenal gland, like the anterior and posterior lobes of the pituitary, develop from different embryonic tissues and secrete different hormones. The adrenal cortex is essential to life, but the medulla may be removed with no life-threatening effects.

The hypothalamus of the brain influences both portions of the adrenal gland but by different mechanisms. The adrenal cortex is regulated by negative feedback involving the hypothalamus and adrenocorticotropic hormone; the medulla is regulated by nerve impulses from the hypothalamus.

Hormones Of The Adrenal Cortex

The adrenal cortex consists of three different regions, with each region producing a different group, or type, of hormones. Chemically, all the cortical hormones are steroid.

The outermost region of the adrenal cortex secretes mineralocorticoids. The principal mineralocorticoid is aldosterone, which acts to conserve sodium ions and water in the body. The middle region of the adrenal cortex secretes glucocorticoids. The principal glucocorticoid is cortisol, which increases blood glucose levels.

The third group of steroids secreted by the adrenal cortex is the gonadocorticoids, or sex hormones. The innermost region secretes these. Male hormones, androgens, and female hormones, estrogens, are secreted in minimal amounts in both sexes by the adrenal cortex, but their effect is usually masked by the hormones from the testes and ovaries. In females, the masculinization effect of androgen secretion may become evident after menopause, when estrogen levels from the ovaries decrease.

Hormones Of The Adrenal Medulla

The adrenal medulla develops from neural tissue and secretes two hormones, epinephrine and norepinephrine. These two hormones are secreted in response to stimulation by sympathetic nerve, particularly during stressful situations. A lack of hormones from the adrenal medulla produces no significant effects. Hypersecretion, usually from a tumor, causes prolonged or continual sympathetic responses.

Pancreas—Islets Of Langerhans

The pancreas is a long, soft organ that lies transversely along the posterior abdominal wall, posterior to the stomach, and extends from the region of the duodenum to the spleen. This gland has an exocrine portion that secretes digestive enzymes that are carried through a duct to the duodenum. The endocrine portion consists of the pancreatic islets, which secrete glucagons and insulin.

Alpha cells in the pancreatic islets secrete the hormone glucagons in response to a low concentration of glucose in the blood. Beta cells in the pancreatic islets secrete the hormone insulin in response to a high concentration of glucose in the blood.

> ### ♣ It's A Fact!!
> The gonads, the primary reproductive organs, are the testes in the male and the ovaries in the female.

Gonads

The gonads, the primary reproductive organs, are the testes in the male and the ovaries in the female. These organs are responsible for producing the sperm and ova, but they also secrete hormones and are considered to be endocrine glands.

Testes

Male sex hormones, as a group, are called androgens. The principal androgen is testosterone, which is secreted by the testes. A small amount is also produced by the adrenal cortex. Production of testosterone begins during fetal development, continues for a short time after birth, nearly ceases during childhood, and then resumes at puberty. This steroid hormone is responsible for the growth and development of the male reproductive structures, increased skeletal and muscular growth, enlargement of the larynx accompanied by voice changes, growth and distribution of body hair, and increased male sexual drive.

Testosterone secretion is regulated by a negative feedback system that involves releasing hormones from the hypothalamus and gonadotropins from the anterior pituitary.

Ovaries

Two groups of female sex hormones are produced in the ovaries, the estrogens and progesterone. These steroid hormones contribute to the development and function of the female reproductive organs and sex characteristics. At the onset of puberty, estrogens promote the development of the breasts, distribution of fat evidenced in the hips, legs, and breast, and maturation of reproductive organs such as the uterus and vagina.

Progesterone causes the uterine lining to thicken in preparation for pregnancy. Together, progesterone and estrogens are responsible for the changes that occur in the uterus during the female menstrual cycle.

Other Endocrine Glands

In addition to the major endocrine glands, other organs have some hormonal activity as part of their function. These include the thymus, stomach, small intestines, heart, and placenta.

✎ What's It Mean?

Goiter: Goiter is an enlargement of the thyroid gland. The resulting bulge on the neck may become extremely large, but most simple goiters are brought under control before this happens. Occasionally a simple goiter may cause some difficulty in breathing and swallowing.

Steroid: Any hormone affecting the development and growth of sex organs. Testosterone and estrogen are steroids.

Testosterone: A hormone that is produced especially by the testes or made synthetically and that is responsible for inducing and maintaining male secondary sex characters.

Source: National Cancer Institute's Surveillance, Epidemiology, and End Results (SEER)'s Glossary, available at http://training.seer.cancer.gov/stws_glossary_a.html.

Chapter 15

The Female Reproductive System

The organs of the female reproductive system produce and sustain the female sex cells (egg cells or ova), transport these cells to a site where they may be fertilized by sperm, provide a favorable environment for the developing fetus, move the fetus to the outside at the end of the development period, and produce the female sex hormones.

Ovaries

The primary female reproductive organs, or gonads, are the two ovaries. Each ovary is a solid, ovoid structure about the size and shape of an almond, about 3.5 cm in length, 2 cm wide, and 1 cm thick. The ovaries are located in shallow depressions, called ovarian fossae, one on each side of the uterus, in the lateral walls of the pelvic cavity. They are held loosely in place by peritoneal ligaments.

Structure

The ovaries are covered on the outside by a layer of simple cuboidal epithelium called germinal (ovarian) epithelium. This is actually the visceral peritoneum that envelops the ovaries. Underneath this layer there is a dense

About This Chapter: Information in this chapter is from "Reproductive System," at the National Cancer Institute's Surveillance, Epidemiology, and End Results (SEER)'s Training Website (http://training.seer.cancer.gov), 2000, accessed May 3, 2006. Note: Despite the older date of this document, the anatomical information it presents is still current.

connective tissue capsule, the tunica albuginea. The substance of the ovaries is distinctly divided into an outer cortex and an inner medulla. The cortex appears more dense and granular due to the presence of numerous ovarian follicles in various stages of development. Each of the follicles contains an oocyte, a female germ cell. The medulla is loose connective tissue with abundant blood vessels, lymphatic vessels, and nerve fibers.

> **♣ It's A Fact!!**
>
> The female reproductive system includes the ovaries, fallopian tubes, uterus, vagina, accessory glands, and external genital organs.

Oogenesis

Female sex cells, or gametes, develop in the ovaries by a form of meiosis called oogenesis. The sequence of events in oogenesis is similar to the sequence in spermatogenesis, but the timing and final result is different. Early in fetal development, primitive germ cells in the ovaries differentiate into oogonia. These divide rapidly to form thousands of cells, still called oogonia, which have a full complement of 46 (23 pairs) chromosomes. Oogonia then enter a growth phase, enlarge, and become primary oocytes. The diploid (46 chromosomes) primary oocytes replicate their DNA and begin the first meiotic division, but the process stops in prophase and the cells remain in this suspended

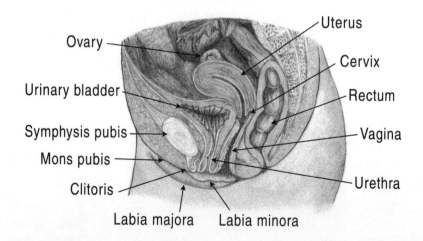

Figure 15.1. Organs of the Female Reproductive System (SEER image redrawn by Alison DeKleine).

state until puberty. Many of the primary oocytes degenerate before birth, but even with this decline, the two ovaries together contain approximately 700,000 oocytes at birth. This is the lifetime supply, and no more will develop. This is quite different than the male in which spermatogonia and primary spermatocytes continue to be produced throughout the reproductive lifetime. By puberty the number of primary oocytes has further declined to about 400,000.

Beginning at puberty, under the influence of follicle-stimulating hormone, several primary oocytes start to grow again each month. One of the primary oocytes seems to outgrow the others, and it resumes meiosis I. The other cells degenerate. The large cell undergoes an unequal division so that nearly all the cytoplasm, organelles, and half the chromosomes go to one cell, which becomes a secondary oocyte. The remaining half of the chromosomes goes to a smaller cell called the first polar body. The secondary oocyte begins the second meiotic division, but the process stops in metaphase. At this point ovulation occurs. If fertilization occurs, meiosis II continues. Again this is an unequal division with all of the cytoplasm going to the ovum, which has 23 single-stranded chromosomes. The smaller cell from this division is a second polar body. The first polar body also usually divides in meiosis I to produce two even smaller polar bodies. If fertilization does not occur, the second meiotic division is never completed and the secondary oocyte degenerates. Here again, there are obvious differences between the male and female. In spermatogenesis, four functional sperm develop from each primary spermatocyte. In oogenesis, only one functional fertilizable cell develops from a primary oocyte. The other three cells are polar bodies and they degenerate.

♣ It's A Fact!!
The primary female reproductive organs, or gonads, are the two ovaries.

Ovarian Follicle Development

An ovarian follicle consists of a developing oocyte surrounded by one or more layers of cells called follicular cells. At the same time that the oocyte is progressing through meiosis, corresponding changes are taking place in the follicular cells. Primordial follicles, which consist of a primary oocyte surrounded by a single layer of flattened cells, develop in the fetus and are the stage that is present in the ovaries at birth and throughout childhood.

Beginning at puberty follicle-stimulating hormone stimulates changes in the primordial follicles. The follicular cells become cuboidal, the primary oocyte enlarges, and it is now a primary follicle. The follicles continue to grow under the influence of follicle-stimulating hormone, and the follicular cells proliferate to form several layers of granulose cells around the primary oocyte. Most of these primary follicles degenerate along with the primary oocytes within them, but usually one continues to develop each month. The granulosa cells start secreting estrogen and a cavity, or antrum, forms within the follicle. When the antrum starts to develop, the follicle becomes a secondary follicle. The granulose cells also secrete a glycoprotein substance that forms a clear membrane, the zona pellucida, around the oocyte. After about 10 days of growth, the follicle is a mature vesicular (graafian) follicle, which forms a "blister" on the surface of the ovary and contains a secondary oocyte ready for ovulation.

Ovulation

Ovulation, prompted by luteinizing hormone from the anterior pituitary, occurs when the mature follicle at the surface of the ovary ruptures and releases the secondary oocyte into the peritoneal cavity. The ovulated secondary oocyte, ready for fertilization, is still surrounded by the zona pellucida and a few layers of cells called the corona radiata. If it is not fertilized, the secondary oocyte degenerates in a couple of days. If a sperm passes through the corona radiata and zona pellucida and enters the cytoplasm of the secondary oocyte, the second meiotic division resumes to form a polar body and a mature ovum.

After ovulation and in response to luteinizing hormone, the portion of the follicle that remains in the ovary enlarges and is transformed into a corpus luteum. The corpus luteum is a glandular structure that secretes progesterone and some estrogens. Its fate depends on whether fertilization occurs. If fertilization does not take place, the corpus luteum remains functional for about 10 days, and then it begins to degenerate into a corpus albicans, which is primarily scar tissue, and its hormone output ceases. If fertilization occurs, the corpus luteum persists and continues its hormone functions until the placenta develops sufficiently to secrete the necessary hormones. Again, the corpus luteum ultimately degenerates into corpus albicans, but it remains functional for a longer period of time.

Genital Tract

Fallopian Tubes

There are two uterine tubes, also called fallopian tubes or oviducts. There is one tube associated with each ovary. The end of the tube near the ovary expands to form a funnel-shaped infundibulum, which is surrounded by finger-like extensions called fimbriae. Because there is no direct connection between the infundibulum and the ovary, the oocyte enters the peritoneal cavity before it enters the fallopian tube. At the time of ovulation, the fimbriae increase their activity and create currents in the peritoneal fluid that help propel the oocyte into the fallopian tube. Once inside the fallopian tube, the oocyte is moved along by the rhythmic beating of cilia on the epithelial lining and by peristaltic action of the smooth muscle in the wall of the tube. The journey through the fallopian tube takes about 7 days. Because the oocyte is fertile for only 24 to 48 hours, fertilization usually occurs in the fallopian tube.

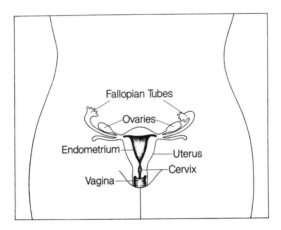

Figure 15.2. Uterus (Source: Cancer Visuals Online, National Cancer Institute)

Uterus

The uterus is a muscular organ that receives the fertilized oocyte and provides an appropriate environment for the developing fetus. Before the first pregnancy, the uterus is about the size and shape of a pear, with the narrow portion directed inferiorly. After childbirth, the uterus is usually larger, and then regresses after menopause.

The uterus is lined with the endometrium. The stratum functionale of the endometrium sloughs off during menstruation. The deeper stratum basale provides the foundation for rebuilding the stratum functionale.

Vagina

The vagina is a fibromuscular tube, about 10 cm long, that extends from the cervix of the uterus to the outside. It is located between the rectum and the urinary bladder. Because the vagina is tilted posteriorly as it ascends and the cervix is tilted anteriorly, the cervix projects into the vagina at nearly a right angle.

> ♣ **It's A Fact!!**
> The vagina serves as a passageway for menstrual flow, receives the erect penis during intercourse, and is the birth canal during childbirth.

External Genitalia

The external genitalia are the accessory structures of the female reproductive system that are external to the vagina. They are also referred to as the vulva or pudendum. The external genitalia include the labia majora, mons pubis, labia minora, clitoris, and glands within the vestibule.

The clitoris is an erectile organ, similar to the male penis, that responds to sexual stimulation. Posterior to the clitoris, the urethra, vagina, paraurethral glands, and greater vestibular glands open into the vestibule.

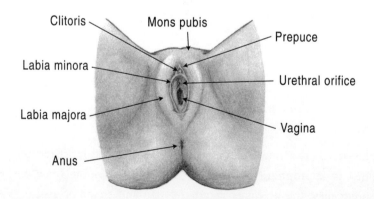

Figure 15.3. Female External Genitalia (SEER image redrawn by Alison DeKleine).

Female Sexual Response And Hormone Control

The female sexual response includes arousal and orgasm, but there is no ejaculation. A woman may become pregnant without having an orgasm.

Follicle-stimulating hormone, luteinizing hormone, estrogen, and progesterone have major roles in regulating the functions of the female reproductive system.

At puberty, when the ovaries and uterus are mature enough to respond to hormonal stimulation, certain stimuli cause the hypothalamus to start secreting gonadotropin-releasing hormone. This hormone enters the blood and goes to the anterior pituitary gland where it stimulates the secretion of follicle-stimulating hormone and luteinizing hormone. These hormones, in turn, affect the ovaries and uterus and the monthly cycles begin. A woman's reproductive cycles last from menarche to menopause.

The monthly ovarian cycle begins with the follicle development during the follicular phase, continues with ovulation during the ovulatory phase, and concludes with the development and regression of the corpus luteum during the luteal phase.

The uterine cycle takes place simultaneously with the ovarian cycle. The uterine cycle begins with menstruation during the menstrual phase, continues with repair of the endometrium during the proliferative phase, and ends with the growth of glands and blood vessels during the secretory phase.

Menopause occurs when a woman's reproductive cycles stop. Decreased levels of ovarian hormones and increased levels of pituitary follicle-stimulating hormone and luteinizing hormone mark this period. The changing hormone levels are responsible for the symptoms associated with menopause.

Mammary Glands

Functionally, the mammary glands produce milk; structurally, they are modified sweat glands. Mammary glands, which are located in the breast overlying the pectoralis major muscles, are present in both sexes, but usually are functional only in the female.

Externally, each breast has a raised nipple, which is surrounded by a circular pigmented area called the areola. The nipples are sensitive to touch, due to the fact that they contain smooth muscle that contracts and causes them to become erect in response to stimulation.

Internally, the adult female breast contains 15 to 20 lobes of glandular tissue that radiate around the nipple. The lobes are separated by connective tissue and adipose. The connective tissue helps support the breast. Some bands of connective tissue, called suspensory (Cooper's) ligaments extend through the breast from the skin to the underlying muscles. The amount and distribution of the adipose tissue determines the size and shape of the breast. Each lobe consists of lobules that contain the glandular units. A lactiferous duct collects the milk from the lobules within each lobe and carries it to the nipple. Just before the nipple, the lactiferous duct enlarges to form a lactiferous sinus (ampulla), which serves as a reservoir for milk. After the sinus, the duct again narrows and each duct opens independently on the surface of the nipple.

Hormones regulate mammary gland function. At puberty, increasing levels of estrogen stimulate the development of glandular tissue in the female breast. Estrogen also causes the breast to increase in size through the accumulation of adipose tissue. Progesterone stimulates the development of the duct system. During pregnancy these hormones enhance further development of the mammary glands. Prolactin from the anterior pituitary stimulates the production of milk within the glandular tissue, and oxytocin causes the ejection of milk from the glands.

✎ What's It Mean?

Chromosome: One of the linear, or sometimes circular DNA-containing bodies of viruses, prokaryotic organisms, and the cell nucleus of eukaryotic organisms, which contain most or all of the genes of the individual.

Estrogen: Any of various natural steroids that are secreted chiefly by the ovaries, placenta, adipose tissue, and testes, and that stimulate the development of female secondary sex characteristics and promote the growth and maintenance of the female reproductive system.

Fetus: A developing human from usually three months after conception to birth.

Source: National Cancer Institute's Surveillance, Epidemiology, and End Results (SEER)'s Glossary, available at http://training.seer.cancer.gov/stws_glossary_a.html.

Chapter 16

The Male Reproductive System

The male reproductive system, like that of the female, consists of those organs whose function is to produce a new individual, i.e., to accomplish reproduction. This system consists of a pair of testes and a network of excretory ducts (epididymis, ductus deferens (vas deferens), and ejaculatory ducts), seminal vesicles, the prostate, the bulbourethral glands, and the penis.

Testes

The male gonads, testes, or testicles, begin their development high in the abdominal cavity, near the kidneys. During the last two months before birth, or shortly after birth, they descend through the inguinal canal into the scrotum, a pouch that extends below the abdomen, posterior to the penis. Although this location of the testes, outside the abdominal cavity, may seem to make them vulnerable to injury, it provides a temperature about 3° C below normal body temperature. This lower temperature is necessary for the production of viable sperm. The scrotum consists of skin and subcutaneous tissue. A vertical septum, or partition, of subcutaneous tissue in the center divides it into two parts, each containing one testis. Smooth muscle fibers, called the dartos muscle, in the subcutaneous tissue contract to give the scrotum its wrinkled appearance. When these fibers are relaxed, the scrotum is smooth. Another muscle, the

About This Chapter: Information in this chapter is from "Reproductive System," at the National Cancer Institute's Surveillance, Epidemiology, and End Results (SEER)'s Training Website (http://training.seer.cancer.gov), 2000, accessed May 3, 2006. Note: Despite the older date of this document, the anatomical information it presents is still current.

cremaster muscle, consists of skeletal muscle fibers and controls the position of the scrotum and testes. When it is cold or a man is sexually aroused, this muscle contracts to pull the testes closer to the body for warmth.

Structure

Each testis is an oval structure about 5 cm long and 3 cm in diameter. A tough, white fibrous connective tissue capsule, the tunica albuginea, surrounds each testis and extends inward to form septa that partition the organ into lobules. There are about 250 lobules in each testis. Each lobule contains 1 to 4 highly coiled seminiferous tubules that converge to form a single straight tubule, which leads into the rete testis. Short efferent ducts exit the testes. Interstitial cells (cells of Leydig), which produce male sex hormones, are located between the seminiferous tubules within a lobule.

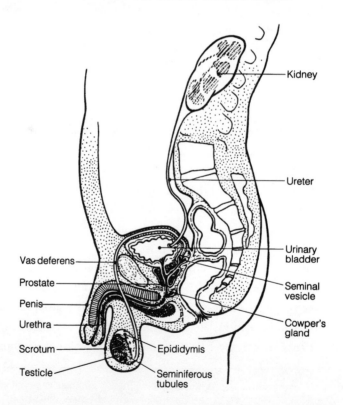

Figure 16.1. Male Reproductive System (Source: Cancer Visuals Online, National Cancer Institute)

Spermatogenesis

Sperm are produced by spermatogenesis within the seminiferous tubules. A transverse section of a seminiferous tubule shows that it is packed with cells in various stages of development. Interspersed with these cells, there are large cells that extend from the periphery of the tubule to the lumen. These large cells are the supporting, or sustentacular cells (Sertoli's cells), which support and nourish the other cells.

Early in embryonic development, primordial germ cells enter the testes and differentiate into spermatogonia, immature cells that remain dormant until puberty. Spermatogonia are diploid cells, each with 46 chromosomes (23 pairs) located around the periphery of the seminiferous tubules. At puberty, hormones stimulate these cells to begin dividing by mitosis. Some of the daughter cells produced by mitosis remain at the periphery as spermatogonia. Others are pushed toward the lumen, undergo some changes, and become primary spermatocytes. Because they are produced by mitosis, primary spermatocytes, like spermatogonia, are diploid and have 46 chromosomes.

Each primary spermatocyte goes through the first meiotic division, meiosis I, to produce two secondary spermatocytes, each with 23 chromosomes (haploid). Just prior to this division, the genetic material is replicated so that each chromosome consists of two strands, called chromatids, which are joined by a centromere. During meiosis I, one chromosome, consisting of two chromatids, goes to each secondary spermatocyte. In the second meiotic division, meiosis II, each secondary spermatocyte divides to produce two spermatids. There is no replication of genetic material in this division, but the centromere divides so that a single-stranded chromatid goes to each cell. As a result of the two meiotic divisions, each primary spermatocyte produces four spermatids. During spermatogenesis there are two cellular divisions, but only one replication of DNA so that each spermatid has 23 chromosomes (haploid), one from each pair in the original primary spermatocyte. Each successive stage in spermatogenesis is pushed toward the center of the tubule so that the more immature cells are at the periphery and the more differentiated cells are nearer the center.

Spermatogenesis (and oogenesis in the female) differs from mitosis because the resulting cells have only half the number of chromosomes as the original cell. When the sperm cell nucleus unites with an egg cell nucleus, the full number of chromosomes is restored. If sperm and egg cells were produced by mitosis, then each successive generation would have twice the number of chromosomes as the preceding one.

The final step in the development of sperm is called spermiogenesis. In this process, the spermatids formed from spermatogenesis become mature spermatozoa, or sperm. The mature sperm cell has a head, midpiece, and tail. The head, also called the nuclear region, contains the 23 chromosomes surrounded by a nuclear membrane. The tip of the head is covered by an acrosome, which contains enzymes that help the sperm penetrate the female gamete. The midpiece, metabolic region, contains mitochondria that provide adenosine triphosphate (ATP). The tail, locomotor region, uses a typical flagellum for locomotion. The sperm are released into the lumen of the seminiferous tubule and leave the testes. They then enter the epididymis where they undergo their final maturation and become capable of fertilizing a female gamete.

Sperm production begins at puberty and continues throughout the life of a male. The entire process, beginning with a primary spermatocyte, takes about 74 days. After ejaculation, the sperm can live for about 48 hours in the female reproductive tract.

Duct System

Sperm cells pass through a series of ducts to reach the outside of the body. After they leave the testes, the sperm passes through the epididymis, ductus deferens, ejaculatory duct, and urethra.

> ♣ **It's A Fact!!**
> Sperm production begins at puberty and continues throughout the life of a male.

Epididymis

Sperm leave the testes through a series of efferent ducts that enter the epididymis. Each epididymis is a long (about 6 meters) tube that is tightly coiled to form a comma-shaped organ located along the superior and posterior margins of the testes. When the sperm leave the testes, they are immature and incapable of fertilizing ova. They complete their maturation process and become fertile as they move through the epididymis. Mature sperm are stored in the lower portion, or tail, of the epididymis.

Ductus Deferens

The ductus deferens, also called vas deferens, is a fibromuscular tube that is continuous (or contiguous) with the epididymis. It begins at the bottom (tail) of the epididymis then turns sharply upward along the posterior margin of the testes. The ductus deferens enters the abdominopelvic cavity through the inguinal canal and passes along the lateral pelvic wall. It crosses over the ureter and posterior portion of the urinary bladder, and then descends along the posterior wall of the bladder toward the prostate gland. Just before it reaches the prostate gland, each ductus deferens enlarges to form an ampulla. Sperm are stored in the proximal portion of the ductus deferens, near the epididymis, and peristaltic movements propel the sperm through the tube.

The proximal portion of the ductus deferens is a component of the spermatic cord, which contains vascular and neural structures that supply the testes. The spermatic cord contains the ductus deferens, testicular artery and veins, lymph vessels, testicular nerve, cremaster muscle that elevates the testes for warmth and at times of sexual stimulation, and a connective tissue covering.

Ejaculatory Duct

Each ductus deferens, at the ampulla, joins the duct from the adjacent seminal vesicle (one of the accessory glands) to form a short ejaculatory duct. Each ejaculatory duct passes through the prostate gland and empties into the urethra.

Urethra

The male urethra is divided into three regions. The prostatic urethra is the proximal portion that passes through the prostate gland. It receives the ejaculatory duct, which contains sperm and secretions from the seminal vesicles, and numerous ducts from the prostate glands. The next portion, the

---

♣ It's A Fact!!

The urethra extends from the urinary bladder to the external urethral orifice at the tip of the penis. It is a passageway for sperm and fluids from the reproductive system and urine from the urinary system. While reproductive fluids are passing through the urethra, sphincters contract tightly to keep urine from entering the urethra.

membranous urethra, is a short region that passes through the pelvic floor. The longest portion is the penile urethra (also called spongy urethra or cavernous urethra), which extends the length of the penis and opens to the outside at the external urethral orifice. The ducts from the bulbourethral glands open into the penile urethra.

Accessory Glands

The accessory glands of the male reproductive system are the seminal vesicles, prostate gland, and the bulbourethral glands. These glands secrete fluids that enter the urethra.

Seminal Vesicles

The paired seminal vesicles are saccular glands posterior to the urinary bladder. Each gland has a short duct that joins with the ductus deferens at the ampulla to form an ejaculatory duct, which then empties into the urethra. The fluid from the seminal vesicles is viscous and contains fructose, which provides an energy source for the sperm; prostaglandins, which contribute to the mobility and viability of the sperm; and proteins that cause slight coagulation reactions in the semen after ejaculation.

Prostate

The prostate gland is a firm, dense structure that is located just inferior to the urinary bladder. It is about the size of a walnut and encircles the urethra as it leaves the urinary bladder. Numerous short ducts from the substance of the prostate gland empty into the prostatic urethra. The secretions of the prostate are thin, milky colored, and alkaline. They function to enhance the motility of the sperm.

Bulbourethral Glands

The paired bulbourethral (Cowper's) glands are small, about the size of a pea, and located near the base of the penis. A short duct from each gland enters the proximal end of the penile urethra. In response to sexual stimulation, the bulbourethral glands secrete an alkaline mucus-like fluid. This fluid neutralizes the acidity of the urine residue in the urethra, helps to neutralize the acidity of the vagina, and provides some lubrication for the tip of the penis during intercourse.

Seminal Fluid

Seminal fluid, or semen, is a slightly alkaline mixture of sperm cells and secretions from the accessory glands. Secretions from the seminal vesicles make up about 60 percent of the volume of the semen, with most of the remainder coming from the prostate gland. The sperm and secretions from the bulbourethral gland contribute only a small volume.

The volume of semen in a single ejaculation may vary from 1.5 to 6.0 ml. There are usually between 50 to 150 million sperm per milliliter of semen. Sperm counts below 10 to 20 million per milliliter usually present fertility problems.

Penis

The penis, the male copulatory organ, is a cylindrical pendant organ located anterior to the scrotum and functions to transfer sperm to the vagina. The penis consists of three columns of erectile tissue that are wrapped in connective tissue and covered with skin. The two dorsal columns are the corpora cavernosa. The single, midline ventral column surrounds the urethra and is called the corpus spongiosum.

♣ **It's A Fact!!**

Although only one sperm actually penetrates and fertilizes the ovum, it takes several million sperm in an ejaculation to ensure that fertilization will take place.

The penis has a root, body (shaft), and glans penis. The root of the penis attaches it to the pubic arch, and the body is the visible, pendant portion. The corpus spongiosum expands at the distal end to form the glans penis. The urethra, which extends throughout the length of the corpus spongiosum, opens through the external urethral orifice at the tip of the glans penis. A loose fold of skin, called the prepuce, or foreskin, covers the glans penis.

Male Sexual Response

The male sexual response includes erection and orgasm accompanied by ejaculation of semen. Orgasm is followed by a variable time period during which it is not possible to achieve another erection.

Three hormones are the principle regulators of the male reproductive system. Follicle-stimulating hormone (FSH) stimulates spermatogenesis; luteinizing hormone (LH) stimulates the production of testosterone; and testosterone stimulates the development of male secondary sex characteristics and spermatogenesis.

Chapter 17

The Nervous System: How Your Body Communicates With Itself And Its Environment

Functions Of The Nervous System

The nervous system is the major controlling, regulatory, and communicating system in the body. It is the center of all mental activity including thought, learning, and memory. Together with the endocrine system, the nervous system is responsible for regulating and maintaining homeostasis.

Like other systems in the body, the nervous system is composed of organs, principally the brain, spinal cord, nerves, and ganglia. These, in turn, consist of various tissues, including nerve, blood, and connective tissue. Together these carry out the complex activities of the nervous system.

The various activities of the nervous system can be grouped together as three general, overlapping functions, which are as follows: sensory; integrative; and motor.

About This Chapter: Information in this chapter is from "Nervous System," at the National Cancer Institute's Surveillance, Epidemiology, and End Results (SEER)'s Training Website (http://training.seer.cancer.gov), 2000, accessed May 3, 2006. Note: Despite the older date of this document, the anatomical information it presents is still current.

Millions of sensory receptors detect changes, called stimuli, which occur inside and outside the body. They monitor such things as temperature, light, and sound from the external environment. Inside the body, the internal environment, receptors detect variations in pressure, pH, carbon dioxide concentration, and the levels of various electrolytes. All of this gathered information is called sensory input.

♣ **It's A Fact!!**

Through its receptors, the nervous system keeps us in touch with our environment, both external and internal.

Sensory input is converted into electrical signals called nerve impulses that are transmitted to the brain. There the signals are brought together to create sensations, to produce thoughts, or to add to memory. Decisions are made each moment based on the sensory input. This is integration.

Based on the sensory input and integration, the nervous system responds by sending signals to muscles, causing them to contract, or to glands, causing them to produce secretions. Muscles and glands are called effectors because they cause an effect in response to directions from the nervous system. This is the motor output or motor function.

Nerve Tissue

Although the nervous system is very complex, there are only two main types of cells in nerve tissue. The actual nerve cell is the neuron. It is the "conducting" cell that transmits impulses and the structural unit of the nervous system. The other type of cell is neuroglia, or glial, cell. The word "neuroglia" means "nerve glue." These cells are nonconductive and provide a support system for the neurons. They are a special type of "connective tissue" for the nervous system.

Neurons

Neurons, or nerve cells, carry out the functions of the nervous system by conducting nerve impulses. They are highly specialized and amitotic. This means that if a neuron is destroyed, it cannot be replaced because neurons do not go through mitosis.

Each neuron has three basic parts: cell body (soma), one or more dendrites, and a single axon.

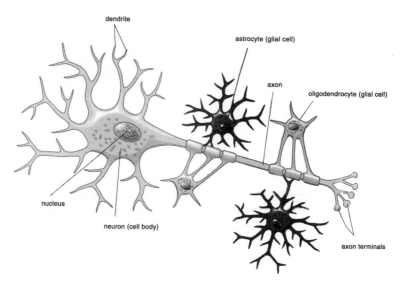

Figure 17.1. The archetiture of a neuron (Source: National Institute of Neurological Disorders and Stroke, NIH Publication No. 02-3440d).

Cell Body: In many ways, the cell body is similar to other types of cells. It has a nucleus with at least one nucleolus and contains many of the typical cytoplasmic organelles. It lacks centrioles, however. Because centrioles function in cell division, the fact that neurons lack these organelles is consistent with the amitotic nature of the cell.

Dendrites: Dendrites and axons are cytoplasmic extensions, or processes, that project from the cell body. They are sometimes referred to as fibers. Dendrites are usually, but not always, short and branching, which increases their surface area to receive signals from other neurons. The number of dendrites on a neuron varies. They are called afferent processes because they transmit impulses to the neuron cell body. There is only one axon that projects from each cell body. It is usually elongated, and because it carries impulses away from the cell body, it is called an efferent process.

Axon: An axon may have infrequent branches called axon collaterals. Axons and axon collaterals terminate in many short branches or telodendria. The distal ends of the telodendria are slightly enlarged to form synaptic bulbs. Many axons are surrounded by a segmented, white, fatty substance called myelin, or the myelin sheath. Myelinated fibers make up the white matter in the central nervous system (CNS), while cell bodies and unmyelinated fibers make the gray matter. The unmyelinated regions between the myelin segments are called the nodes of Ranvier.

In the peripheral nervous system, Schwann cells produce the myelin. The cytoplasm, nucleus, and outer cell membrane of the Schwann cell form a tight covering around the myelin and around the axon itself at the nodes of Ranvier. This covering is the neurilemma, which plays an important role in the regeneration of nerve fibers. In the CNS, oligodendrocytes produce myelin, but there is no neurilemma, which is why fibers within the CNS do not regenerate.

Functionally, neurons are classified as afferent, or interneurons (association neurons), according to the direction in which they transmit impulses relative to the central nervous system. Afferent, or sensory, neurons carry impulses from peripheral sense receptors to the CNS. They usually have long dendrites and relatively short axons. Efferent, or motor, neurons transmit impulses from the CNS to effector organs, such as muscles and glands. Efferent neurons usually have short dendrites and long axons. Interneurons, or association neurons, are located entirely within the CNS in which they form the connecting link between the afferent and efferent neurons. They have short dendrites and may have either a short or long axon.

Neuroglia

Neuroglia cells do not conduct nerve impulses, but instead, they support, nourish, and protect the neurons. They are far more numerous than neurons and, unlike neurons, are capable of mitosis.

Tumors

Schwannomas are benign tumors of the peripheral nervous system, which commonly occur in their sporadic, solitary form in otherwise normal individuals. Rarely, individuals develop multiple schwannomas arising from one or many elements of the peripheral nervous system.

Commonly called a Morton neuroma, this problem is fairly common benign nerve growth and begins when the outer coating of a nerve in your foot thickens. This thickening is caused by irritation of branches of the medial and lateral plantar nerves that results when two bones repeatedly rub together.

Organization Of The Nervous System

Although terminology seems to indicate otherwise, there is really only one nervous system in the body. Although each subdivision of the system is also called a "nervous system," all of these smaller systems belong to the single, highly integrated nervous system. Each subdivision has structural and functional characteristics that distinguish it from the others.

The Central Nervous System

✣ **It's A Fact!!**
The nervous system as a whole is divided into two subdivisions: the central nervous system (CNS) and the peripheral nervous system (PNS).

The brain and spinal cord are the organs of the central nervous system. Because they are so vitally important, the brain and spinal cord, located in the dorsal body cavity, are encased in bone for protection. The brain is in the cranial vault, and the spinal cord is in the vertebral canal of the vertebral column. Although considered to be two separate organs, the brain and spinal cord are continuous at the foramen magnum.

The Peripheral Nervous System

The organs of the peripheral nervous system are the nerves and ganglia. Nerves are bundles of nerve fibers, much like muscles are bundles of muscle fibers. Cranial nerves and spinal nerves extend from the CNS to peripheral organs such as muscles and glands. Ganglia are collections, or small knots, of nerve cell bodies outside the CNS.

The peripheral nervous system is further subdivided into an afferent (sensory) division and an efferent (motor) division. The afferent or sensory division transmits impulses from peripheral organs to the CNS. The efferent or motor division transmits impulses from the CNS out to the peripheral organs to cause an effect or action.

Finally, the efferent or motor division is again subdivided into the somatic nervous system and the autonomic nervous system. The somatic nervous system, also called the somatomotor, or somatic efferent nervous system, supplies motor impulses to the skeletal muscles. Because these nerves permit conscious control of the skeletal muscles, it is sometimes called the voluntary nervous system. The autonomic nervous system, also called the visceral efferent nervous system, supplies motor impulses to cardiac muscle, to smooth muscle, and to glandular epithelium. It is further subdivided into sympathetic and parasympathetic divisions. Because the autonomic nervous system regulates involuntary or automatic functions, it is called the involuntary nervous system.

Chapter 18

Why Does My Body Do That? Answers To Some Body Mysteries

Why Does My Nose Run?

You may have heard the old joke: If your nose is running and your feet smell, you must be upside down! But why does your nose run? Read on to find out the whole story.

What's Running?

To understand why your nose runs, you need to know what mucus (say: myoo-kus) is. This is the gooey, sticky, slimy material that is made inside your nose (also known as snot). Believe it or not, your nose makes a cup full of snot every day!

For something kind of gross, mucus does a lot of good. It keeps germs, dirt, pollen, and bacteria from getting into your lungs by stopping them in your nose; but sometimes mucus does not stay put.

About This Chapter: This chapter begins with "Why Does My Nose Run," 2004, "What Makes Me Sneeze," 2006, "Why Do I Yawn," 2005, "Why Do I Burp," 2006, "Why Do I Shiver," 2004, and "What's A Fart," 2003. This information was provided by KidsHealth, one of the largest resources online for medically reviewed health information written for parents, kids, and teens. For more articles like this one, visit www.KidsHealth.org, or www.TeensHealth.org. © The Nemours Foundation. Additional information under the questions "What Causes The Noise When You Crack A Joint," 2005, and "Why Do Fingers And Toes Wrinkle In The Bathtub," 2004, is from Everyday Mysteries, Library of Congress (http://www.loc.gov).

Reasons For Running

If your nose is running, here are several possible explanations:

• **You have a cold or the flu.** When you have either one of these, your nose goes into mucus-making overdrive to keep the germ invaders out of your lungs and the rest of your body where they might make you even sicker than you already are. You know what happens then. The mucus runs down your throat, out your nose, or into a tissue when you blow your nose; or it can fill your sinuses, which is why you get that stuffy feeling.

• **You have allergies.** Kids who have allergies get runny noses when they are around the thing they are allergic to (like pollen or animal hair). That is because their bodies react to these things like they are germs.

• **You are crying.** When you cry, tears come out of the tear glands under your eyelids and drain through the tear ducts that empty into your nose. Tears mix with mucus there, and your nose runs.

• **Baby, it's cold outside.** When you are outside on a cold day, the air in your nose is a lot warmer than the air around you. You know how the bathroom gets steamy when you take a shower? Something similar happens in your nose—water drops come together, or condense, then the drops mix with your mucus and run out your nose.

Stoppin' The Runnin'

If you have allergies or a bad cold, your parent or doctor might give you some medicine. A decongestant (say: dee-kun-jes-tunt) or antihistamine (say: an-tye-his-tuh-meen) could help you breathe easier and dry up some of that mucus; but sometimes the easiest thing to do is—you guessed it—blow your nose!

♣ It's A Fact!!

Sneezing, also called sternutation, is your body's way of removing an irritation from your nose.

Source: "What Makes Me Sneeze," © 2006 The Nemours Foundation.

What Makes Me Sneeze?

If you just sneezed, something was probably irritating or tickling the inside of your nose.

When the inside of your nose gets a tickle, a message is sent to a special part of your brain called the sneeze center. The sneeze center then sends a message to all the muscles that have to work together to create the amazingly complicated process that we call the sneeze.

Some of the muscles involved are the abdominal (belly) muscles, the chest muscles, the diaphragm (the large muscle beneath your lungs that makes you breathe), the muscles that control your vocal cords, and muscles in the back of your throat. Do not forget the eyelid muscles. Did you know that you always close your eyes when you sneeze?

It is the job of the sneeze center to make all these muscles work together, in just the right order, to send that irritation flying out of your nose.

Most anything that can irritate the inside of your nose can start a sneeze. Some common things include dust, cold air, or pepper. When you catch a cold in your nose, a virus has made a temporary home there and is causing lots of swelling and irritation. Some people have allergies, and they sneeze when they are exposed to certain things, such as animal dander (which comes from the skin of many common pets) or pollen (which comes from some plants).

Do you know anyone who sneezes when they step outside into the sunshine? About one out of every three people sneezes when exposed to bright light. They are called photic sneezers (photic means light). If you are a photic sneezer, you got it from one of your parents because it is an inherited trait. You could say that it runs in your family. Most people have some sensitivity to light that can trigger a sneeze.

Have you ever had the feeling that you are about to sneeze, but it just gets stuck? Next time that happens, try looking toward a bright light briefly (but do not look right into the sun). See if that doesn't unstick a stuck sneeze!

Why Do I Yawn?

Everybody yawns, from unborn babies to the oldest great-grandparent. Animals do it, too; but why, exactly, do people and animals yawn? No one knows for sure. But there are many theories (ideas) about why people yawn.

One is that when we are bored or tired, we just do not breathe as deeply as we usually do. As this theory goes, our bodies take in less oxygen because our breathing has slowed. Therefore, yawning helps us bring more oxygen into the blood and move more carbon dioxide out of the blood.

Yawning, then, would be an involuntary reflex (something we cannot really control) to help us control our oxygen and carbon dioxide levels. Sounds good, but other studies have shown that breathing more oxygen does not decrease yawning. Likewise, breathing more carbon dioxide does not increase yawning. Hmmm. Now what?

Another theory is that yawning stretches the lungs and lung tissue. Stretching and yawning may be a way to flex muscles and joints, increase heart rate, and feel more awake.

Other people believe that yawning is a protective reflex to redistribute the oil-like substance called surfactant (say: sur-fak-tunt) that helps keep lungs lubricated inside and keeps them from collapsing. So, if we did not yawn, according to this theory, taking a deep breath would become harder and harder; and that would not be good.

There is one idea about yawning that everyone knows to be true. It seems contagious. If you yawn in class, you will probably notice a few other people will start yawning, too. Even thinking about yawning can get you yawning. How many times have you yawned while reading this article? We hope not many!

Why Do I Burp?

"Burp!" You cover your mouth with your hand, but it is too late. The people at the next table in the lunchroom already heard. As you turn back to your soda, you think: Where did that burp come from?

A burp, sometimes called a belch, is nothing but gas. When you eat or drink, you do not just swallow food or liquid. You also swallow air at the same time. The air we breathe contains gases, like nitrogen (say: ny-truh-jen) and oxygen (say: ahk-sih-jen).

Sometimes when you swallow these gases, they need to get out. That is where burping comes in. Extra gas is forced out of the stomach, up through the esophagus (say: ih-sah-fuh-gus, the tube for food that connects the back of the throat to the stomach), and out of the mouth as a burp.

Some kids find that drinking soda or other carbonated beverages makes them burp more. Can you guess why? If you are thinking that it is because these drinks contain extra gas, you are right. The gas that makes the drinks fizzy is carbon dioxide (say: kar-bon dy-ahk-side), another gas that can bring on big burps. Sometimes eating or drinking too fast can make a person burp because this can send extra air into the stomach. The same thing happens when you drink through a straw—extra air in equals more burps out.

Burping is almost never anything to worry about. Everybody does it at least once in a while, and it is very unusual for burping to mean something is wrong in a kid's body.

What can you do if you are around people and you feel a burp coming on? It seems like the only people who can get away with really loud burps are little babies. Their parents cheer when they burp because it means that the babies will not feel the extra gas in their stomachs and cry. But unless you are tiny and bald, it is probably a good idea to be polite when it is time to burp. Try to burp quietly and cover your mouth. Of course, whether your burp is loud or quiet, saying, "excuse me" cannot hurt either.

Why Do I Shiver?

You have been floating along in the cool water of the lake for a while, and even though you were hot before you dove in, you feel your legs start to shake. You get out and wrap yourself in your towel, and your teeth start chattering. What is going on? You are probably shivering.

Nerves Know

Shivers are reflexes (say: ree-fleks-iz), which are things your body does automatically to keep you safe and healthy. Reflexes are controlled by your nervous system, which is made up of your brain, your spinal cord, and lots and lots of little nerves that stretch out all over your body. Nerves are like little strings or wires that carry information.

What kind of information? Well, your nerves sense that the cool water of the lake has lowered your body temperature. Your body needs to stay at a toasty 98.6 degrees Fahrenheit (37 degrees Celsius) for you to be safe and comfortable. The nerves send signals saying, "I'm cold! Warm me up!"

Muscles In Action

That is when things really start to get interesting. The signals go to your brain (telling you to wrap in the towel) and to your spinal cord, which sends a message to other nerves all over your body. What happens next? Your muscles tighten and loosen really fast. Why? They are trying to warm you up, just like taking a jog around the lake would do. Once you get all snug and cozy in your towel and your body warms back up, your brain and nerves tell your muscles to stop shivering.

There are other times when you might shiver, too. Sometimes you will shiver when you are excited or afraid. When you feel these things, your brain and nerves send out messages through your body that cause your muscles to get excited, so you shiver.

Great Goose Bumps!

You may notice that when you shiver, tiny bumps form all over your skin. Goose bumps happen because your skin is covered with hair. When the muscles that are attached to each hair get tight, they pull the hair and your skin up into the air.

We call them goose bumps because they look like the skin of a goose or a chicken. So do not be a silly goose the next time you get the goose bumps after swimming. Towel off and put on some dry clothes to warm yourself up.

What's A Fart?

P.U.! What is that smell? How can your body make something so stinky?

Farts, also called flatus (say: flay-tus) or intestinal (say: in-tes-tuh-null) gas, are made of, well, gas!

When you eat, you do not swallow just your food. You also swallow air, which contains gases like nitrogen (say: ny-truh-jen) and oxygen (say: ahk-sih-jen). Small amounts of these gases travel through your digestive system as you digest your food. Other gases like hydrogen (say: hy-droh-jen), carbon dioxide (say: kar-bon dy-ahk-side, the gas that makes soda fizzy), and methane (say: meth-ain) are made when food is broken down in the large intestine. All of these gases in the digestive system have to escape somehow, so they come out as farts.

Gases are also what can make farts smell bad. Tiny amounts of hydrogen, carbon dioxide, and methane combine with hydrogen sulfide (say: suhl-fide) and ammonia (say: uh-mow-nyuh) in the large intestine to give gas its smell. Phew!

All people fart sometimes, whether they live in France, the Fiji islands, or Fresno, California! If you have a dog, you may have even been unlucky enough to have heard (or smelled) Fido farting. Intestinal gas is totally normal, and it is very rare for farting to be a sign that something is wrong in the body.

The bathroom is also a good place to go if you are feeling particularly gassy because it is not polite to fart in social settings, like in class or at the dinner table. Do not worry if this happens accidentally. Just remember to say, "Excuse me!"

✔ Quick Tip

If you are feeling particularly farty and you want to get rid of some gas, try cutting back on foods like beans, onions, and fried foods. These can release larger amounts of gas as they break down in your body. If you have a lot of gas after you eat ice cream, yogurt, or milk, talk to your parent about it. Your body may have a difficult time digesting the natural sugar called lactose, which is found in dairy foods. Do not forget that farting can sometimes be your body's sign that it is time to take a trip to the bathroom.

Source: "What's A Fart," © 2003 The Nemours Foundation.

What Causes The Noise When You Crack A Joint?

The noise that is made when you crack a joint is made by escaping gases, movement, and rough surfaces.

Your joints can make a variety of sounds—popping, cracking, grinding, and snapping. The joints that crack are the knuckles, knees, ankles, back, and neck. The following are different reasons why these joints sound off:

- **Escaping gases:** Scientists explain that synovial fluid present in your joints acts as a lubricant. The fluid contains the gases oxygen, nitrogen, and carbon dioxide. When you pop or crack a joint, you stretch the joint capsule. Gas is rapidly released, which forms bubbles. In order to crack the same knuckle again, you have to wait until the gases return to the synovial fluid.

- **Movement of joints, tendons, and ligaments:** When a joint moves, the tendon's position changes and moves slightly out of place. You may hear a snapping sound as the tendon returns to its original position. In addition, your ligaments may tighten as you move your joints. This commonly occurs in your knee or ankle, and can make a cracking sound.

- **Rough surfaces:** Arthritic joints make sounds caused by the loss of smooth cartilage and the roughness of the joint surface.

Is joint cracking harmful? If you are feeling pain when your joints pop, then you should seek a health care professional. In terms of knuckle cracking, some studies show that knuckle cracking does not cause serious harm. Other studies show that repetitive knuckle cracking can do some damage to the soft tissue of the joint. It may also lead to a weak grip and a swelling hand.

Why Do Fingers And Toes Wrinkle In The Bathtub?

The outermost layer of the skin swells when it absorbs water. It is tightly attached to the skin underneath, so it compensates for the increased area by wrinkling.

There are various theories of why fingers and toes wrinkle in water. Most biologists suggest that the tough outer layer of skin made up of dead keratin

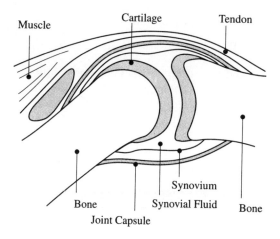

Figure 18.1. A Healthy Joint: In a healthy joint, the bones are encased in smooth cartilage. Together, they are protected by a joint capsule lined with a synovial membrane that produces synovial fluid. The capsule and fluid protect the cartilage, muscles, and connective tissues. (Source: National Institute of Arthritis and Musculoskeletal and Skin Diseases)

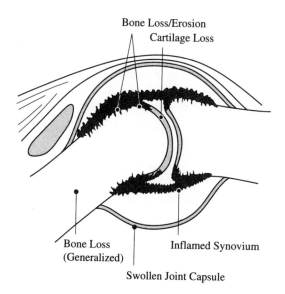

Figure 18.2. An Osteoarthritic Joint: With osteoarthritis, the cartilage becomes worn away. Spurs grow out from the edge of the bone, and synovial fluid increases. Altogether, the joint feels stiff and sore. (Source: National Institute of Arthritis and Musculoskeletal and Skin Diseases)

cells is responsible. Keratin is a protein found in hair, nails, and the outermost layer of our skin.

Our skin is made up of three layers. They are as follows:

- The subcutaneous tissue is the deepest layer. It contains fats and connective tissue, along with large blood vessels and nerves.

- The dermis is the middle layer. It contains the blood vessels, nerves, hair roots, and sweat glands.

- The epidermis is the topmost layer. It helps to prevent evaporation of water from the body and to protect the internal layers from harm.

The epidermis is made up of these four layers:

- The stratum corneum

- Granular layer

- Squamous cell layer

- Basal cell layer

The stratum corneum is the outer layer of our skin—the part that we can see and feel. This is the layer with the dead keratin cells.

While a person is in the pool or a bathtub for a long time, the dead keratin cells absorb water. This absorption causes the surface area of the skin to swell, but the outer layer is tightly attached to the living tissue. So, to compensate for the increased surface area, our skin wrinkles.

So why does this happen to hands and feet and not to other parts of the body? It is because the hands and feet have the thickest layer of dead keratin cells. Our hands and feet are subjected to a lot of wear and tear. Imagine if the palm of our hands had skin as thin as that on our backs. No fun playing basketball with skin that thin!

Part Three

How Your Body Grows And Changes

Chapter 19

Fetal Development

First Month

About five to seven days after a sperm fertilizes an egg, the egg attaches to the lining of the uterus. This process is called implantation. The fertilized egg then begins to grow in the uterus, doubling in size every day. At this stage of development, the baby is called an embryo.

Shortly after implantation, the placenta and umbilical cord begin to form. The placenta and umbilical cord provide nourishment and oxygen to the baby and carry away the baby's wastes. The baby is enclosed in a sac of fluid, called the amniotic sac, to protect the baby from bumps and pressure.

In another week, the baby has a spinal cord. A few days later, five to eight bones of the spinal column (vertebrae) are in place. Nerve development is beginning. By the end of the first six weeks of pregnancy, the baby has a head and trunk.

The embryo becomes three layers around the fifth week. The outer layer consists of the brain, nerves, and skin. The middle layer becomes the bones, muscles, blood vessels, heart, and sex organs. The inner layer holds the stomach, liver, intestines, lungs, and urinary tract. The eyes and other features

About This Chapter: Reprinted with permission. Excerpts from "Pregnancy Month by Month." University of Michigan Health System. © 2005. All rights reserved.

begin to form, as do tiny buds that will be the arms and legs. The heart also forms, and it begins to beat on the 25th day after conception (five to six weeks after the last menstrual period). However, it is impossible to hear the heart beating at this time.

By the end of six weeks, the baby is about ½ inch long and weighs a fraction of an ounce.

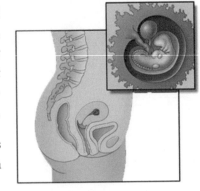

Figure 19.1. First Month Of Fetal Development

Second Month

This month is especially critical in the development of the baby. Any disturbance from drugs, viruses, or environmental factors, such as pesticides, may cause birth defects.

The baby's development is very rapid during the second month. By the end of the second month, all of the baby's major body organs and body systems, including the brain, lungs, liver, and stomach, have begun to develop. The first bone cells appear during this time. Eyelids form and grow but remain sealed shut. The inner ear is forming. Ankles, toes, wrists, fingers, and sexual organs are developing.

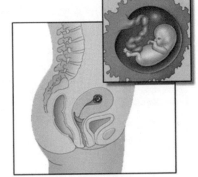

Figure 19.2. Second Month Of Fetal Development

At the end of the second month of pregnancy, the baby looks like a tiny human infant. If it is a boy, the penis will begin to appear. The baby is a little over one inch long and still weighs less than one ounce. From now on the baby is called a fetus.

Third Month

The baby will be completely formed by the end of the third month. The baby may have begun moving its hands, legs, and head, and opening and closing its mouth, but he or she is still too small for the mother to feel this movement.

The fingers and toes are now more distinct and have soft nails. The baby's hands are more developed than the feet, and the arms are longer than the legs. The baby's head is quite large compared to the rest of its body. Hair may have started to form on the head. Tooth buds have formed under the baby's gums. Vocal cords develop around the 13th week of pregnancy.

The baby's heart has four chambers and beats at 120 to 160 beats per minute. Kidneys are now developed and start draining urine into the bladder. Intestines have formed outside of the baby (on the umbilical cord) because they cannot fit inside the baby. By the end of this month, the umbilical cord, which carries nutrients to the baby and takes wastes away, will be fully formed.

At the end of the third month, the baby will weigh just over one ounce and will be about four inches long.

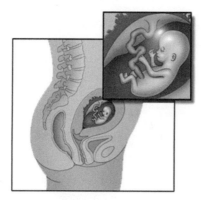

Figure 19.3. Third Month Of Fetal Development

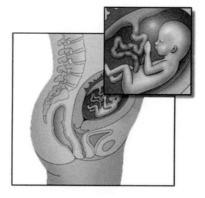

Figure 19.4. Fourth Month Of Fetal Development

Fourth Month

The baby's skin is pink and somewhat transparent. Eyebrows and eyelashes begin to appear in this month. Buds on the side of the head begin to form into the outer ear. The baby's face continues to develop. The tail has disappeared from the fetus and the head makes up about half of the baby's size. The baby's neck is long enough to lift the head from the body.

The baby moves, kicks, sleeps, wakes, swallows, and passes urine. The mother may start to feel a slight sensation in her lower abdomen (called quickening). This feels like bubbles or fluttering. When the mother feels the baby's movement, she should write down the date and tell her health care provider. This helps determine when the baby is due.

By the end of the fourth month, the baby will be eight to ten inches long and will weigh about six ounces.

✎ What's It Mean?

Ovaries: Part of a woman's reproductive system, the ovaries produce her eggs. Each month, through the process called ovulation, the ovaries release eggs into the fallopian tubes, where they travel to the uterus, or womb. If a man's sperm fertilizes an egg, a woman becomes pregnant and the egg grows and develops inside the uterus. If the egg is not fertilized, the egg and the lining of the uterus are shed during a woman's monthly menstrual period. [1]

Placenta: During pregnancy, a temporary organ joining the mother and fetus. The placenta transfers oxygen and nutrients from the mother to the fetus and permits the release of carbon dioxide and waste products from the fetus. The placenta is expelled during the birth process with the fetal membranes. [1]

Scrotum: In males, the external sac that contains the testicles. [2]

Sperm: The male reproductive cell, formed in the testicle. A sperm unites with an egg to form an embryo. [2]

Testicles (Testes): The male sex gland. There is a pair of testes behind the penis in a pouch of skin called the scrotum. The testes make and store sperm and make the male hormone testosterone. [1]

Umbilical Cord: Connected to the placenta and provides the transfer of nutrients and waste between the woman and the fetus. [1]

Uterus: A woman's womb, or the hollow, pear-shaped organ located in a woman's lower abdomen between the bladder and the rectum. [1]

Source: [1] "NWHIC Web Site Glossary," National Women's Health Information Center, U.S. Department of Health and Human Services, Office on Women's Health; cited August 2006. [2] "Dictionary of Cancer Terms," National Cancer Institute, U.S. National Institutes of Health; cited August 2006.

Fifth Month

This is a period of tremendous growth for the baby. The internal organs are maturing. The baby's fingernails have grown to the tips of the fingers. Fat is now being stored beneath the baby's skin. The baby is also growing muscle and is getting stronger every day. The blood cells take over for the liver the job of producing blood. The baby's gall bladder will become functional, producing bile that is necessary for digestion. Milk teeth will begin forming under the

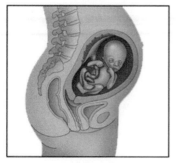

baby's gums. Body hair, including eyebrows and eyelashes, are starting to grow.

The baby sleeps and wakes at regular intervals. The mother will find that the baby is much more active now. He or she turns from side to side and head over heels. The baby may suck its thumb.

At the end of the fifth month, the baby will be about 10 to 12 inches long and will weigh about one pound.

Figure 19.5. Fifth Month Of Fetal Development

Sixth Month

This month continues to be a period of rapid growth. The baby's skin is wrinkled and red. It is covered with lanugo (fine, soft hair) and vernix (a substance consisting of oil, sloughed skin cells, and lanugo). Real hair and toenails are beginning to grow. The baby's brain is developing rapidly. Fatty sheaths, which transmit electrical impulses along nerves, are forming. Meconium, the baby's first stool, is developing. A special type of fat (brown fat),

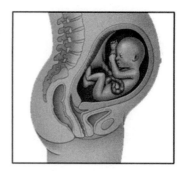

Figure 19.6. Sixth Month Of Fetal Development

which keeps the baby warm at birth, is forming. Baby girls will develop eggs in their ovaries during this month. The baby's bones are becoming solid.

The baby is almost fully formed and looks like a miniature human. However, because the lungs are not well developed and the baby is still very small, a baby cannot usually live outside the uterus at this stage without highly specialized care.

By the end of the sixth month, the baby will be around 11 to 14 inches long and will weigh about 1 to 1½ pounds.

Seventh Month

The baby is continuing to grow and develop. The baby's eyes can now open and close and can sense light changes. The lanugo is starting to disappear from the baby's face. The baby's hearing is getting better. He or she can now hear the outside world quite well over the sound of your heartbeat. The baby exercises by kicking and stretching. He or she can also make grasping motions and likes to suck its thumb.

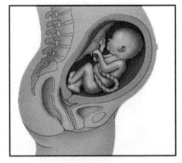

Figure 19.7. Seventh Month Of Fetal Development

By the end of this month, the baby will be approximately 15 inches long and weigh about 2 or 2½ pounds. If the baby was born now, its chances of survival are better than last month.

Eighth Month

The baby's body continues to grow quickly. The bones are getting stronger, limbs are fatter, and the skin has a healthy glow. The brain is now forming its different regions. The brain and nerves are directing bodily functions. Taste buds are developing. The baby may now hiccup, cry, taste sweet and sour, and respond to pain, light, and sound. If the baby is a boy, his testicles have dropped from his abdomen, where they will then descend into his scrotum.

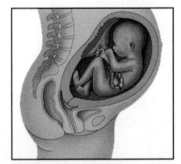

Figure 19.8. Eighth Month Of Fetal Development

The baby will be about 16 to 18 inches long and will weigh about 4 pounds at the end of this month.

Ninth Month

The baby is now gaining about a ½ pound each week. The baby is getting fatter and its skin is less rumpled. He or she is getting ready for birth and is settling into the fetal position with its head down against the birth canal, its legs tucked up to its chest, and its knees against its nose.

The mother's antibodies to disease are beginning to flow rapidly through the placenta. The rapid flow of blood through the umbilical cord keeps it taut, which prevents tangles.

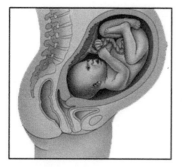

Figure 19.9. Ninth Month Of Fetal Development

The baby is beginning to develop sleeping patterns. The baby will continue to kick and punch, although it will move lower in the mother's abdomen to under her pelvis (this is a process called "lightening"). The mother will also feel the baby roll around as it gets too cramped inside the uterus for much movement. The baby's lungs are now mature and the baby will have a great chance of survival if born a little early. The bones of the baby's head are soft and flexible to ease the process of delivery through the birth canal.

The baby is now about 20 inches long and weighs approximately 6 to 9 pounds. The baby may be born anytime between the 37th and 42nd week of pregnancy. Only 5 percent of babies are born on their due date.

Chapter 20

Child Development Stages

Birth To 3 Months

From birth to 3 months, children do the following things:

- Learn about the world through all their senses
- Track people and objects with their eyes
- Respond to faces and bright colors
- Reach and discover hands and feet
- Lift their heads and turn toward sounds
- Cry, but are often soothed when held
- Begin to smile
- Begin to develop a sense of self

From birth to 3 months, children need the following:

- Protection from physical danger
- Adequate nutrition (exclusive breastfeeding is best)

About This Chapter: Information in this chapter is excerpted from *Early Childhood Counts: Programming Resources for Early Childhood Care and Development*, by the World Bank Institute. Copyright 2000 World Bank. Reproduced with permission of World Bank, via Copyright Clearance Center. Note: Despite the older date of this document, the developmental milestones described are still accurate.

- Adequate health care (immunization, oral re-hydration therapy as required, hygiene)
- An adult with whom to form an attachment
- An adult who can understand and respond to their signals
- Things to look at, touch, hear, smell, and taste
- Opportunity to be held, sung to, and rocked

4 To 6 Months

From 4 to 6 months, children do the following things:

- Smile often
- Prefer parents and older siblings
- Repeat actions with interesting results
- Listen intently
- Respond when spoken to
- Laugh, gurgle, and imitate sounds
- Explore their hands and feet
- Put objects in their mouths
- Sit when propped, roll over, scoot, and bounce
- Grasp objects without using their thumbs

From 4 to 6 months, children need the following:

- All of the previous needs, plus:
- Opportunities to explore the world
- Appropriate language stimulation
- Daily opportunities to play with a variety of objects

7 To 12 Months

From 7 to 12 months, children do the following things:

- Remember simple events
- Identify themselves, body parts, and familiar voices

- Understand their own name and other common words
- Say their first meaningful words
- Explore, bang, and shake objects
- Find hidden objects and put objects in containers
- Sit alone
- Creep, pull themselves up to stand, and walk
- May seem shy or upset with strangers

From 7 to 12 months, children need the following:

- All of the previous needs, plus:
- Introduction of supplementary foods
- Opportunities to hear stories and be read to
- A safe environment to explore

1 To 2 Years

From 1 to 2 years, children do the following things:

- Imitate adult actions
- Speak and understand words and ideas
- Enjoy stories and experimenting with objects
- Walk steadily, climb stairs, and run
- Assert their independence, but prefer familiar people
- Recognize ownership of objects
- Development friendships
- Solve problems
- Show pride in their accomplishments
- Like to help with tasks
- Begin pretend play

From 1 to 2 years, children need the following:

- All of the previous needs, plus:

- Support in acquiring new motor, language, and thinking skills
- A chance to develop some independence
- Help in learning how to control their behavior
- Opportunities to begin to learn to care for themselves
- Opportunities for play and exploration
- Play with other children
- Read to and tell stories daily
- Health care must also include de-worming if required

2 To 3½ Years

From 2 to 3½ years, children do the following things:

- Enjoy learning new skills
- Learn language rapidly
- Are always on the go
- Gain control of their hands and fingers
- Are easily frustrated
- Act more independent, but are still dependent
- Act out familiar scenes

From 2 to 3½ years, children need the following:

- All of the previous needs, plus opportunities to:
- Make choices
- Engage in dramatic play
- Sing favorite songs
- Work simple puzzles

3½ To 5 Years

From 3½ to 5 years, children do the following things:

- Have a longer attention span
- Act silly and boisterous

- Talk a lot and ask many questions
- Want real adult things
- Keep art projects
- Test physical skills and courage with caution
- Reveal feelings in dramatic play
- Like to play with friends and do not like to lose
- Share and take turns sometimes

From 3½ to 5 years, children need the following:

- All of the previous needs, plus:
- Opportunities to develop fine motor skills
- Encouragement of language through talking, reading, and singing
- Activities which will develop a positive sense of mastery
- Opportunities to learn cooperation, helping, and sharing
- Experimentation with pre-writing and pre-reading skills
- Hands-on exploration for learning through action
- Opportunities for taking responsibility and making choices
- Encouragement to develop self-control, cooperation, and persistence in completing projects
- Support for their sense of self-worth and pride in accomplishments
- Opportunities for self-expression (drawing, painting, working with clay or mud)
- Encouragement of creativity
- Rhythmic movement
- Listening to music of all kinds

5 To 8 Years

From 5 to 8 years, children do the following things:

- Grow curious about people and how the world works
- Show an increasing interest in numbers, letters, reading, and writing

- Read
- Become more and more interested in final products
- Gain more confidence in physical skills
- Use words to express feelings and to cope
- Like grown-up activities
- Become more outgoing and play cooperatively

From 5 to 8 years, children need the following:

- In addition to the previous needs:
- Support in acquiring additional motor, language, and thinking skills
- Additional opportunities to develop independence
- Opportunities to become self-reliant in terms of personal care
- Opportunities to develop a wide variety of skills
- Support for the further development of language through talking, reading, and singing
- Activities that will further develop a positive sense of mastery
- Opportunities to learn cooperation, helping, and teamwork
- Hands-on manipulation of objects to support learning
- Opportunities for taking responsibility and for making choices
- Support in the development of self-control and persistence in completing projects
- Support for their sense of self-worth and pride in accomplishments
- Motivation and reinforcement for academic achievement
- Opportunities to practice questioning and observing
- Opportunities to make music, accomplish art, and dance
- Attend basic education

Source: Adapted from National Association for the Education of Young Children. (1985, 1995); Donohue-Colletta. (1992); additions made by others.

Chapter 21

The Ins And Outs Of Puberty

What Is Puberty?

Puberty is the time when a person's body starts to change from being the body of a child to the body of an adult, and when their reproductive organs begin to develop. These changes can affect the way a person looks, feels, and thinks. Some people find the changes confusing, strange, and uncomfortable, while others think they feel great. Puberty feels different for everybody.

Puberty usually starts to happen between the ages of 9 and 16. Most girls will notice their bodies starting to change around the age of 10 or 11, while most boys begin puberty around the age of 12 or 13. Everybody is different, however; so do not be alarmed if you notice changes earlier or later than this. You might find it useful to know when your mom or dad went through puberty, as you may be similar to them in this way.

What Happens At Puberty?

Both boys and girls go through physical and emotional changes at puberty caused by hormones. This happens when the pituitary gland at the base of the brain triggers your reproductive organs (testes for boys, ovaries for girls) into producing hormones. The main male hormone is called testosterone, and the main female hormones are called estrogen and progesterone.

Changes boys may notice at puberty can include the following:

- Wet dreams (when semen is released during sleep)

- Penis and testes (testicles) get larger

- An increase in height

- Body hair starts to grow under the arms and in the pubic area, as well as facial hair

- More frequent (and sometimes unwanted) erections

- Voice changes, or "breaks," and eventually becomes deeper

- Skin changes, including pimples

Changes girls may notice at puberty can include the following:

- Hips get wider

- Breasts start to develop

- Periods (menstruation) begin

- An increase in height and sometimes a weight gain

- Skin changes, including pimples

- Body hair starts to grow under the arms and in the pubic area

It can be handy to know what is happening to girls at puberty if you are a boy, and to boys if you are a girl. Everyone experiences some changes; in fact, some changes happen to both boys and girls.

☞ **Remember!!**

Whether you like or dislike the changes that are happening to your body, puberty is a natural and healthy part of growing up. Puberty is a sign that your body is becoming physically ready to create a baby, even though being a parent is probably the last thing on your mind.

Source: Copyright © 2006 FPWA Sexual Health Services. Reprinted with permission. For additional information, visit http://www.fpwa.org.au.

Girl's Stuff

Periods Explained

Periods are part of the monthly menstrual cycle. They are caused by the changes in a girl's body that happen when an egg develops and the body prepares for a possible pregnancy. Part of this preparation happens each month when the lining of the uterus (womb) becomes thick with blood. If a pregnancy does not occur, the lining breaks down and is passed out of the body through the vagina. This is called a period.

The menstrual cycle starts when a girl has her period. Most menstrual cycles last for around 1 month (from the first day of one period to the first day of the next period), but this varies for each girl. Things such as stress, weight loss, exercise, and traveling can affect the length of the cycle. A period, or the time when bleeding occurs, usually lasts for 3 to 7 days, and the total amount of blood lost is usually around 1–2 tablespoons.

At first, periods can be very irregular, but after the first year or so they usually settle into a pattern. The pattern is different for each girl. A calendar can be useful to help work out when your period is due next.

Most girls start to have periods between the ages of 10 and 14 and will continue to have them until they are about 50 years old. Some girls feel fine when they have their period, while others feel a bit sick or sore in the stomach. Some gentle exercise, placing a hot water bottle over the stomach, or taking a mild painkiller like can help.

Many girls worry that other people will be able to tell when they have their period. The only way that other people can tell if you have your period is if you choose to tell them. They cannot tell just by looking at you.

Pads And Tampons

Pads and tampons are used to absorb period blood. They come in a variety of sizes and are available from supermarkets and pharmacies. Pads have a sticky strip on the back that attaches to the inside of your underpants, while tampons are inserted into the vagina. Tampons cannot slip out accidentally, nor can they get lost inside you. Some girls prefer to use tampons so they can continue to swim or wear a leotard during their period, but it is important to use what you feel comfortable with.

In case your period comes when you are at school or out with friends, it is a good idea to plan ahead and carry some pads or tampons in your school bag or purse. In an emergency situation, toilet paper or tissues can be used (wrap them around the crotch of your underpants). If you are at school, a teacher or nurse will be able to help you. They are used to dealing with these situations every day, so there is no need to be embarrassed.

It is important to wash your hands before and after changing pads or tampons and to change them about every 4 hours (or as necessary). Only wear pads overnight, as leaving tampons in the vagina for a long period of time can lead to infection. When disposing of pads and tampons, wrap them in toilet paper and place them in a sanitary or rubbish bin (do not flush them down the toilet, as it blocks up the pipes).

PMS

PMS, or premenstrual syndrome, affects some girls in the week leading up to their period. You may feel tired or irritable, or your breasts may be sore. A healthy diet and regular exercise can help with PMS.

Breasts

All girls develop breasts during puberty. Some girls feel embarrassed, while others cannot wait to buy a bra. Wearing a loose t-shirt can help if you feel anxious about your growing chest. Breasts come in all different sizes; so do not worry if yours seem larger or smaller than anyone else's. It is also quite normal for your own two breasts to be slightly different sizes.

My Vagina's Leaking!

At puberty, girls start to produce vaginal secretions (or discharge). Discharge is part of a normal, healthy vagina. For most girls, discharge looks different at different times between their periods, but it is usually thin and clear (though often dries a whitish-yellow on underpants). Healthy discharge has a slight smell that is unnoticeable to others. If you notice your discharge is different from usual, such as heavier or with a different or unpleasant smell, see a doctor, as this can indicate an infection.

Hair Everywhere

Some girls experience significant hair growth on their body at puberty, such as hair on their forearms, upper lip, around their nipples, or on their thighs. This is normal and usually settles down. If it does not, there are many safe ways of removing unwanted hair.

Boy's Stuff

Sperm

At puberty, a boy's testicles become larger and begin to produce sperm (the male reproductive cells), which is contained in a whitish fluid called semen. Ejaculation, or "coming", is when semen comes out of an erect penis. The amount of semen ejaculated is about 1 teaspoon.

Sweet Dreams

A wet dream is when a boy ejaculates (or "comes") while he is asleep. These types of dreams usually bring pleasurable feelings and are a normal part of growing up. Wet dreams happen because sometimes there is too much sperm made in the testes, and your body needs to release it.

For some boys they are a regular occurrence, while for others they may only happen occasionally. Your sheets and pajamas may be slightly sticky when you wake up. This can usually be cleaned up with a wet cloth or by putting things into the wash. While there is no need to be embarrassed, you may prefer to wash the items yourself.

Embarrassing Erections

When a boy reaches puberty he will experience more frequent erections (when the penis swells and gets hard). Sometimes erections happen for no obvious reason. Thinking about something really boring can help make erections go away. Some boys prefer to wear clothing that makes erections less noticeable, such as baggy shorts or pants.

Help! My Voice Has Broken!

At puberty, a boy's voice changes and becomes deeper. This is usually known as the voice breaking. This is a gradual process and means that a boy's voice may alternate between high and squeaky and deep and throaty while his voice box grows and vocal cords stretch. A boy's voice usually "breaks" between the ages of 13 and 16 before eventually settling down.

I Thought Only Girls Were Supposed To Get Breasts

Many boys develop some breast enlargement, or swelling in the chest area, during puberty. This is normal and nothing to worry about. The swelling usually lasts for 4–6 months. Wearing a loose t-shirt can help if you feel embarrassed.

Everyone's Changing

Not Another Pimple!

At puberty, the glands which cause pimples become more active, and many boys and girls develop pimples or acne on their face and other parts of their body, such as the back and chest.

Washing your face twice a day with an antibacterial face wash can help, as can a healthy diet and wearing less make-up. Medication is available for severe conditions. See your doctor for more information. Try not to touch your face too much, as this can make pimples worse.

The good news is that pimples are temporary for most people.

Is It Okay To Masturbate?

Touching or rubbing the genital area so that it feels good is called masturbation. Most people masturbate and it is not something to feel guilty about. As long as it is done in private, masturbation is a normal and healthy way of experiencing pleasure and learning about your body.

Eek…I've Put On Weight

Some boys and girls put on weight around the time of puberty, and this is completely normal. Girls' hips usually widen, and their thighs become more rounded, while boys' shoulders and chests get wider. Eating a well-balanced diet and exercising regularly will help prevent a large weight gain. Speak to your doctor for more details.

While many people want to be super slim, it is more important to be healthy.

I've Got The Puberty Blues

Not all changes at puberty are physical ones. Your hormones are also changing, which may cause you to feel happy and excited one moment, then sad or angry the next.

The changes that are happening to your body can also leave you feeling confused, frustrated, or anxious. You may feel easily irritated by friends and family (especially your parents), or that things are overwhelming. Remember you are not the only one feeling like this, and that it will not always be this way. In the meantime, it can help to talk to someone you trust about any feelings you are having.

A Sweaty Situation

The hormones developing at puberty can also affect sweat glands, and boys especially need to take extra care about their personal hygiene at this time. Shower regularly using plenty of soap and use antiperspirant deodorant, especially if playing a sport.

Feeling Sexy

For some people, puberty is a time of discovering new types of relationships. Sometimes these relationships can lead to sex. It is important, however, that when it comes to relationships and sex, not to feel pressured. It is okay to take your time deciding, and do not let yourself be pressured into something you do not want to do.

☞ Remember!!

Learning to like your new adult body will help you to be happy and healthy with who you are.

Source: Copyright © 2006 FPWA Sexual Health Services. Reprinted with permission. For additional information, visit http://www.fpwa.org.au.

If you do decide to have sex, remember to always use a condom to reduce the risk of getting, or passing on, a sexually transmissible infection and to protect against pregnancy.

Liking The New You

While everyone's experience at puberty is different, the most important thing to remember is that it does not last forever. Talking about any problems you are having can help, whether it be with a parent, teacher, school nurse, counselor, or friend. Remember you are not alone in having problems or feeling confused.

Finding ways of expressing yourself and doing things that make you happy can help make puberty easier. These may include playing a sport, being part of a social club, or going out with friends.

Chapter 22

The Teenage Brain: Still Under Construction

Even though adults were once teenagers, they often treat teens like they are from Mars. Many times, teens feel they would fit in better on another planet.

The feelings are so widespread that bookstores are full of titles such as *Now I Know Why Tigers Eat Their Young: Surviving a New Generation of Teenagers* and *Help! My Family Is Driving Me Crazy: A Survival Guide for Teenagers*.

Surging hormones are often blamed for adolescent anxieties. More and more, however, scientists are realizing that important changes occur in the brain during the teen years.

Spurts in brain development, not sudden bouts of madness, they say, may help explain why kids start caring about different things, acting in new ways, and taking risks as they make the transition to adulthood.

"We don't think [teenage brains are] damaged," says neuroscientist Jay Giedd. He is the chief of brain imaging at the National Institutes of Health (NIH) in Bethesda, Md. "They're under construction."

Brain Scans

Every two years since 1991, a group of kids (and now adults) has been coming to Giedd's lab. There, the participants have their brains scanned by magnetic

About This Chapter: Information in this chapter is from "Teen Brains, Under Construction." Reprinted with permission from *SCIENCE NEWS for Kids*, copyright © 2005.

resonance imaging (MRI) machines, which show details of brain structure. Study members also answer questions about their lives and mental health.

At first, Giedd looked only at the brains of healthy children to see if he could find evidence of physical brain changes in kids who later developed mental illnesses. Initial re-

> ♣ **It's A Fact!!**
>
> By the first grade, the brain is already about 90 percent of its adult size.

sults, he says, were disappointing. Brains seemed to develop early and quickly.

However, even though the size of the brain does not change much, a closer look shows that the size of its parts does change a lot.

In 1996, Giedd's team reported that the amount of gray matter (the type of brain tissue that processes information) increases until about age 11 in girls and 13 in boys. After that, gray matter decreases, while the amount of white matter goes up and up. White matter connects areas of gray matter and helps brain cells communicate with each other.

What these results mean, for one thing, is that girls' brains tend to mature more quickly than boys' brains do. The results also suggest that kids are best at learning how to play musical instruments or sports and developing other skills between ages 7 and 11. That is when their gray matter is increasing the fastest. Once gray matter starts to go down, skills can be perfected, but it is harder to learn new ones.

Learning Machine

The brain's frontal lobe seems to undergo a lot of development during the teen years. That is the part of the brain that controls social activity, and that is the time of life when kids start to care more about friends and what other people think of them.

"The bottom line is that the brain is very plastic," Giedd says. "It changes much more than we used to think."

Adolescence, in particular, appears to be a very busy time for that wrinkled lump behind your forehead. "During this time, there are so many changes, the potential to learn things is about as high as it will ever be," Giedd says.

Among the most surprising things that Giedd and his coworkers have found is that brains do not stop developing until people are in their mid-20s.

"Initially, we thought we'd study them until they were 16 or 18," Giedd says. "Only recently, we thought, 'Wow, we should follow them longer to find out when things stop maturing.'"

The scientists now have about 4,000 brain scans from 2,000 people. For some individuals, they have six or seven scans covering 15 years of development.

Taking Risks

It took ten years for the researchers to map the patterns and timing of brain development. Now, they are trying to figure out how changes in the brain contribute to changes in behavior. They also want to know whether school, music, sports, diet, video games, parenting, TV watching, medicine, or other factors influence those changes during adolescence.

One goal is to learn what teachers can do to take advantage of the time when their students' brains change the most.

If some parts of the brain develop sooner than others, for example, perhaps school subjects should be taught in a different order. "Maybe the parts of the brain doing geometry are different from the parts doing algebra," Giedd says. "We haven't had solid links like this, but that's what we're shooting for."

Knowing what their brains are going through might also motivate teenagers to change their own priorities. "What you do with your brain during that time," Giedd says, "could have a lot of good and bad implications for the rest of your life."

Eventually, brain studies might help resolve conflicts at home. Teenagers are capable of learning a lot, but the parts of their brains related to emotions and decision-making are still in the works. As their brains undergo rewiring, teenagers are particularly vulnerable to risky behavior, such as drinking and driving too fast.

Brain development is no excuse for breaking curfew or taking big risks. Understanding what is going on in there, however, can make the situation more manageable for everyone.

Chapter 23

Adults And Aging

Genetic And Environmental Factors

As we age, our bodies change in many ways that affect the function of both individual cells and organ systems. These changes occur little by little and progress inevitably over time. However, the rate of this progression can be very different from person to person. Research in aging is beginning to find out the reasons for these changes and the genetic and environmental factors that control them.

The aging process depends on a combination of both genetic and environmental factors. Recognizing that every individual has his or her own unique genetic makeup and environment, which interact with each other, helps us understand why the aging process can occur at such different rates in different people. Overall, genetic factors seem to be more powerful than environmental factors in determining the large differences among people in aging and lifespan. There are even some specific genetic disorders that speed up the aging process, such as Hutchinson-Gilford, Werner's, and Down syndromes. However, many environmental conditions, such as the quality of health care

About This Chapter: Information in this chapter is from "The Aging Process," reprinted with permission from the American Geriatrics Society Foundation for Health in Aging, http://www.healthinaging.org, from the Aging in the Know website, http://www.healthinaging.org/agingintheknow. For more information, visit the AGS online at www.americangeriatrics.org.

that you receive, have a substantial effect on aging. A healthy lifestyle is an especially important factor in healthy aging and longevity. Environmental factors can significantly extend lifespan.

Cellular Changes Associated With Aging

Aging causes functional changes in cells. For example, the rate at which cells multiply tends to slow down as we age. Certain cells that are important for our immune system to work properly (called T-cell lymphocytes) also decrease with age. In addition, age causes changes in our responses to environmental stresses or exposures, such as ultraviolet light, heat, not enough oxygen, poor nutrition, and toxins (poisons) among others.

Age also interferes with an important process called apoptosis, which programs cells to self-destruct or die at appropriate times. This process is necessary for tissues to remain healthy, and it is especially important in slowing down immune responses once an infection has been cleared from the body.

Different diseases that are common in elderly people can affect this process in different ways. For example, cancer results in a loss of apoptosis. The cancer cells continue to multiply and invade or take over surrounding tissue, instead of dying as originally programmed. Other diseases may cause cells to die too early. In Alzheimer's disease, a substance called amyloid builds up and causes the early death of brain cells, which results in a progressive loss of memory and other brain functions. Toxins produced as byproducts of nerve cell transmissions are also thought to be involved in the death of nerve cells in Parkinson's disease.

♣ It's A Fact!!
Behaviors Of A Healthy Lifestyle

- Not smoking

- Drinking alcohol in moderation

- Exercising

- Getting adequate rest

- Eating a diet high in fruits and vegetables

- Coping with stress

- Having a positive outlook

Bodily Changes Associated With Aging

Our bodies normally change in appearance as we age.

Changes In Height

We all lose height as we age, although when the height loss begins, and how quickly it progresses, vary quite a bit among different people. Generally, our height increases until our late forties and then decreases about two inches by age 80. The reasons for height loss include the following:

- Changes in posture
- Changes in the growth of vertebrae (the bones that make up the spine)
- A forward bending of the spine
- Compression of the discs between the vertebrae
- Increased curvature of the hips and knees
- Decreased joint space in the trunk and extremities
- Joint changes in the feet
- Flattening of the arches

The length of the bones in our legs does not change much.

Changes In Weight

In men, body weight generally increases until their mid-fifties; then it decreases, with weight being lost faster in their late sixties and seventies. In women, body weight increases until the late sixties and then decreases at a rate slower than that of men.

People that live in less technologically developed societies do not show this pattern of weight change. This suggests that reduced physical activity and changes in eating habits may be causes of the change in body weight rather than the aging process.

Changes In Body Composition

The proportion of the body that is made up of fat doubles between age 25 and age 75. Exercise programs may prevent or reverse much of the proportional decrease in muscle mass and increase in total body fat. This change in body composition is important to consider in nutritional planning and level of activity. The change in body composition also has an important effect on how the body handles various drugs. For example, when our body fat increases, drugs that are dissolved in fatty tissues remain in the body much longer than when our body was younger and more muscular.

Other Changes With Aging

Normal aging in the absence of disease is a remarkably benign process. In other words, our body can remain healthy as we age. Although our organs may gradually lose some function, we may not even notice these changes except during periods of great exertion or stress. We may also experience slower reaction times.

Normal Aging And Disease

Aging and disease are related in subtle and complex ways. Several conditions that were once thought to be part of normal aging have now been shown to be due to disease processes that can be influenced by lifestyle. For example, heart and blood vessel diseases are more common in people who eat a lot of meat and fat. Similarly, cataract formation in the eye largely depends on the amount of exposure to direct sunlight.

We should remember that there is a range of individual response to aging. Biologic and chronologic ages are not the same. In addition, body systems do not age at the same rate within any individual. For example, you might have severe arthritis or loss of vision while the function of your heart or kidneys is excellent. Even those aging changes that are considered "usual" or "normal" are not inevitable consequences of aging.

Changes In The Regulation Of Body Systems

The way our body regulates certain systems changes with age. Some examples are as follows:

- Progressive changes in the heart and blood vessels interfere with your body's ability to control blood pressure.

- Your body cannot regulate its temperature as it could when you were younger. This can result in dangerously low body temperature from prolonged exposure to the cold or in heat stroke if the outside temperature is too high.

- There may be aging-related changes in your body's ability to develop a fever in response to an infection.

- The regulation of the amount and makeup of body fluids is slowed down in healthy older persons. Usual (resting) levels of the hormones that control the amount of body fluids are unchanged, but problems in fluid regulation commonly develop during illness or other stress. Also, elderly people do not feel as thirsty after water deprivation as they did when younger.

What do these age-related changes in our body systems mean?

- First, with advancing age, we become less like each other biologically, so our health care needs to be more individualized.

- Body systems that can be minimally affected by age are often profoundly influenced by lifestyle behaviors such as cigarette smoking, physical activity, and nutritional intake, and by circumstances such as financial means.

- Finally, it is helpful to consider ahead of time our possible choices in case certain situations arise. For example, if you become less physically able to take part in an athletic activity you did before, is there a different activity you might enjoy? Are there things you might like to do to keep your mind active? More serious situations to consider might include death of a spouse, or if you find your abilities becoming more and more limited. Have you discussed how you would like to handle such situations and your wishes with your family?

It is important to remember that the ability to learn and adjust continues throughout life and is strongly influenced by interests, activities, and motivation. With years of rich experience and reflection, we can rise above our own circumstances. Old age, despite the physical limitations, can be a time of variety, creativity, and fulfillment.

Part Four

How To Keep Your Body Healthy

Chapter 24

A Guide To Healthy Eating

The typical American diet is low in fruits, vegetables, and whole grains, and high in saturated fat, salt, and sugar. As a result, more Americans than ever are overweight, obese, and at increased risk for chronic diseases such as heart disease, high blood pressure, diabetes, and certain cancers.

Of course old habits are hard to break, and the notion of change can seem overwhelming; but it can be done with planning and a gradual approach. Some people can improve eating habits on their own, while others need a registered dietitian to guide them through the process. You may need a dietitian if you are trying to lose weight or if you have a health condition.

Look At What You Eat Now

Write down what you eat for a few days to get a good picture of what you're taking in. By looking at what you eat and how much you're eating, you can figure out what adjustments you need to make.

Start With Small Changes

You don't have to go cold turkey. In the end, you want to achieve a long-term healthy lifestyle. Small changes over time are the most likely to stick. If you want to eat more vegetables, try to add one more serving by sneaking it

About This Chapter: Information in this chapter is excerpted from "A Guide To Healthier Eating," *FDA & You*, Issue #8, Fall 2005, U.S. Food and Drug Administration.

in by adding bits of broccoli to something you already eat like pizza or soup. If you need more whole grains, add barley, whole-wheat pasta, or brown rice to your soup.

When you think about what you need to get more of, the other things tend to fall into place. If you have a carrot with lunch or add a banana to your cereal in the morning, you're going to feel full longer and you won't need a food that's high in sugar or fat an hour later.

Look for healthier versions of what you like to eat. If you like luncheon meat sandwiches, try a reduced-fat version. If you like the convenience of frozen dinners, look for ones with lower sodium. If you love fast-food meals, try a salad with reduced-calorie dressing as your side dish instead of French fries.

Use The Nutrition Facts Label

To make smart food choices quickly and easily, compare the nutrition facts labels on products. Look at the percent daily value (%DV) column. The general rule of thumb is that 5 percent or less of the daily value is considered low, and 20 percent or more is high.

Keep saturated fat, trans fat, cholesterol, and sodium low, while keeping fiber, potassium, iron, calcium, and vitamins A and C high. Be sure to look at the serving size and the number of servings per package. The serving size affects calories, amounts of each nutrient, and the percentage of daily value.

The %DV is based on a 2,000-calorie diet, but recommended calorie intake differs for individuals based on age, gender, and activity level. Some people need less than 2,000 calories a day. You can use the %DV as a frame of reference whether or not you consume more or less than 2,000 calories. The %DV makes it easy to compare the nutrients in each food product to see which ones are higher or lower. When comparing products, just make sure the serving sizes are similar, especially the weight (grams, milligrams, or ounces) of each product.

Control Portion Sizes

Understanding the serving size on the nutrition facts label is important for controlling portions. Do not assume one bottle of soda is a serving. If you look at the label you may find the bottle actually has two or more servings and that you are doubling the amount of calories, fat, sugar, and salt you are eating.

Try dishing out a smaller amount on your plate or using smaller plates to avoid overeating. An average serving size of meat looks like a deck of cards. An average serving size of pasta or rice is about the size of a tennis ball. Here are some other ways to limit portions: split a meal or dessert with a friend at a restaurant, get a doggie bag for half of your meal, get in the habit of having one helping, and ask for salad dressing, butter, and sauces on the side so you can control how much you use.

Control Calories And Get The Most Nutrients

You want to stay within your daily calorie needs, especially if you are trying to lose weight, but you also want to get the most nutrients out of the calories, which means picking nutritionally rich foods. Children and adults should pay particular attention to getting adequate calcium, potassium, fiber, magnesium, and vitamins A, C, and E.

According to the Dietary Guidelines, there is room for what is known as a discretionary calorie allowance. This is for when people meet their recommended nutrient intake without using all their calories. The discretionary calorie allowance gives you some flexibility to have foods and beverages with added fats and sugars, but you still want to make sure you are getting the nutrients you need. For example, a 2,000-calorie diet has about 250 discretionary calories.

Know Your Fats

Fat provides flavor and makes you feel full. It also provides energy, and essential fatty acids for healthy skin, and helps the body absorb the fat-soluble vitamins A, D, E, and K. But fat also has nine calories per gram, compared to four calories per gram in carbohydrates and protein. If you eat too much fat every day, you may get more calories than your body needs, and too many calories can contribute to weight gain.

Too much saturated fat, trans fat, and cholesterol in the diet increases the risk of unhealthy blood cholesterol levels, which may increase the risk of heart disease. Saturated fat is found mainly in foods from animals. Major sources of saturated fats are cheese, beef, and milk. Trans fat results when manufacturers add hydrogen to vegetable oil to increase the food's shelf life and flavor. Trans fat can be found in vegetable shortenings, some margarine, crackers, cookies, and other snack foods. Cholesterol is a fat-like substance in foods from animal sources such as meat, poultry, egg yolks, milk, and milk products.

Most of your fats should come from polyunsaturated and monounsaturated fatty acids, such as those that occur in fish, nuts, soybean, corn, canola, olive, and other vegetable oils. This type of fat does not raise the risk of heart disease and may be beneficial when consumed in moderation.

Make Choices That Are Lean, Low Fat, Or Fat-Free

When buying meat, poultry, milk, or milk products, choose versions that are lean, low fat, or fat-free. Choose lean meats like chicken without the skin and lean beef or pork with the fat trimmed off.

If you frequently drink whole milk, switch to 1 percent milk or skim milk. Many people do not taste a difference. Some mix whole milk with lower-fat milk for a while so the taste buds can adjust. This does not mean you can never eat or drink the full-fat versions; they should be factored into your discretionary calories.

Other tips to reduce saturated fat include cooking with non-stick

> ### ✔ Quick Tip
> ### Smart Snacks
>
> - Unsalted pretzels
> - Applesauce
> - Low-fat yogurt with fruit
> - Grapes
> - Raisins
> - Nuts
> - Graham crackers
> - Gingersnap cookies
> - Unbuttered and unsalted popcorn
> - Apple slices with peanut butter
> - Low- or reduced-fat string cheese
> - Baked whole-grain tortilla chips with salsa
> - Whole-grain cereal with low-fat milk
> - Broccoli, carrots, or cherry tomatoes with dip or low-fat yogurt
>
> Source: "A Guide to Healthier Eating," U.S. Food and Drug Administration.

sprays and using olive, safflower, or canola oils instead of lard or butter. Eat more fish, which is usually lower in saturated fat than meat. Bake, grill, and broil food instead of frying it because more fat is absorbed into the food when frying. You could also try more meatless entrees like veggie burgers and add flavor to food with low-fat beans instead of butter.

Focus On Fruit

The Dietary Guidelines recommend two cups of fruit per day at the 2,000-calorie reference diet. Fruit intake and recommended amounts of other food groups vary at different calorie levels. An example of two cups of fruit includes: one small banana, one large orange, and one-fourth cup of dried apricots or peaches.

Eat a variety of fruits, whether fresh, frozen, canned, or dried, rather than fruit juice for most of your fruit choices. Whole fruit has more fiber, is more filling, and is naturally sweet. Can't live without juice? Some juices, such as orange and prune, are a good source of potassium.

Ways to incorporate fruit in your diet include adding it to your cereal, eating it as a snack with low-fat yogurt or a low-fat dip, or making a fruit smoothie for dessert by mixing low-fat milk with fresh or frozen fruit such as strawberries or peaches.

Eat Your Veggies

The Dietary Guidelines recommend two and one-half cups of vegetables per day if you eat 2,000 calories each day.

Try putting vegetables into foods such as meatloaf, lasagna, omelets, stir-fry dishes, and casseroles. Frozen chopped greens such as spinach, peas, carrots, and corn are easy to add. Also, add dark leafy green lettuce to sandwiches. Choose a variety of dark green vegetables such as broccoli, spinach, and greens; orange and deep yellow vegetables such as carrots, winter squash, and sweet potatoes; starchy vegetables like corn; legumes, such as dry beans, peas, chickpeas, pinto beans, kidney beans, and tofu; and other vegetables, such as tomatoes and onions.

Make Half Your Grains Whole

Like fruits and vegetables, whole grains are a good source of vitamins, minerals, and fiber. The Dietary Guidelines recommend at least three ounces of whole grains per day. One slice of bread, one cup of breakfast cereal, or one-half cup of cooked rice or pasta are each equivalent to about one ounce.

In general, at least half the grains you consume should come from whole grains. For many, but not all, whole grain products, the words "whole" or "whole grain" will appear before the grain ingredient's name. The whole grain must be the first ingredient listed in the ingredients list on the food package. The following are some whole grains: whole wheat, whole oats or oatmeal, whole-grain corn, popcorn, wild rice, brown rice, buckwheat, whole rye, bulgur or cracked wheat, whole-grain barley, and millet. Whole-grain foods cannot necessarily be identified by their color or by names such as brown bread, nine-grain bread, hearty grains bread, or mixed grain bread.

Lower Sodium And Increase Potassium

Higher salt intake is linked to higher blood pressure, which can raise the risk of stroke, heart disease, and kidney disease. The Dietary Guidelines recommend that people consume less than 2,300 milligrams of sodium per day (approximately one teaspoon of salt). There are other recommendations for certain populations that tend to be more sensitive to salt. For example, people with high blood pressure, African Americans, and middle-aged and older adults should consume no more than 1,500 milligrams of sodium each day.

Most of the sodium people eat comes from processed foods. Use the nutrition facts label on food products: 5%DV or less for sodium means the food is low in sodium and 20%DV or more means it's high. Compare similar products and choose the option with a lower amount of sodium. Most people won't notice a taste difference. Consistently consuming lower-salt products will help taste buds adapt, and you will enjoy these foods as much or more than higher-salt options.

Prepare foods with little salt. The DASH (Dietary Approaches to Stop Hypertension) eating plan from the National Heart, Lung, and Blood Institute recommends giving flavor to food with herbs, spices, lemon, lime, vinegar, and salt-free seasoning blends. Consult with your physician before using salt substitutes because their main ingredient, potassium chloride, can be harmful to some people with certain medical conditions.

Increase potassium-rich foods such as sweet potatoes, orange juice, bananas, spinach, winter squash, cantaloupe, and tomato puree. Potassium counteracts some of sodium's effect on blood pressure.

Limit Added Sugars

The Dietary Guidelines recommend choosing and preparing food and beverages with little added sugars. Added sugars are sugars and syrups added to foods and beverages in processing or preparation, not the naturally occurring

♣ It's A Fact!!
Teens And Fast Food

Teens who frequently eat fast food gain more weight and have a greater increase in insulin resistance in early middle age, according to a large study funded by the National Heart, Lung, and Blood Institute (NHLBI).

After 15 years, those who ate fast food more than twice each week, compared to less than once a week, had gained an extra ten pounds and had a greater increase in insulin resistance, a risk factor for type 2 diabetes. Diabetes is a major risk factor for heart disease.

One reason for the weight gain may be that a single meal of fast food often contains enough calories to satisfy a person's caloric requirement for an entire day. It is important to watch carefully what you eat, especially at a fast food restaurant. Knowing the nutritional content is important. Keep portion sizes small, and ask that high-fat sauces and condiments, such as salad dressing and mayonnaise, be "on the side," and use them sparingly to reduce calories.

Source: Excerpted from "Science in the News: New Study on Teens and Fast-Food," *FDA & You*," Issue #5, Winter 2005, U.S. Food and Drug Administration.

sugars in fruits or milk. Major sources of added sugars in the American diet include regular sodas, candy, cake, cookies, pies, and fruit drinks. In the ingredients list on food products, sugar may be listed as brown sugar, corn syrup, glucose, sucrose, honey, or molasses. Be sure to check the sugar in low-fat and fat-free products, which sometimes contain a lot of sugar.

Instead of drinking regular soda and sugary fruit drinks, try diet soda, low-fat or fat-free milk, water, flavored water, or 100 percent fruit juice.

For snacks and desserts, try fruit. You may be surprised how great fruit is for satisfying a sweet tooth. And if ice cream is calling your name, do not have it in the freezer. Make it harder to get by having to go out for it. Then it can be an occasional treat.

Chapter 25

Exercise Program Guidelines

Making A Commitment

The decision to carry out a physical fitness program requires a lifelong commitment of time and effort. This chapter provides guidelines intended for the average healthy teen. It tells you what your goals should be and how often, how long, and how hard you must exercise to achieve them. It also includes information that will make your workouts easier, safer, and more satisfying. The rest is up to you.

Checking Your Health

If you're under 35 and in good health, you do not need to see a doctor before beginning an exercise program. Some conditions that indicate a need for medical clearance include high blood pressure, heart trouble, family history of early stroke or heart attack deaths, frequent dizzy spells, extreme breathlessness after mild exertion, arthritis or other bone problems, severe muscular, ligament, or tendon problems, or other known or suspected disease.

Vigorous exercise involves minimal health risks for persons in good health or those following a doctor's advice. Far greater risks are presented by habitual inactivity and obesity.

About This Chapter: Information in this chapter is excerpted from "Fitness Fundamentals: Guidelines for Personal Exercise Programs," The President's Council on Physical Fitness and Sports, U.S. Department of Health and Human Services, October 2004.

Knowing The Basics

Cardiorespiratory Endurance: The ability to deliver oxygen and nutrients to tissues, and to remove wastes, over sustained periods of time. Long runs and swims are among the methods employed in measuring this component.

Muscular Strength: The ability of a muscle to exert force for a brief period of time. Upper-body strength, for example, can be measured by various weight-lifting exercises.

Muscular Endurance: The ability of a muscle, or a group of muscles, to sustain repeated contractions or to continue applying force against a fixed object. Pushups are often used to test endurance of arm and shoulder muscles.

Flexibility: The ability to move joints and use muscles through their full range of motion. The sit-and-reach test is a good measure of flexibility of the lower back and backs of the upper legs.

Body Composition: Often considered a component of fitness. It refers to the makeup of the body in terms of lean mass (muscle, bone, vital tissue, and organs) and fat mass. An optimal ratio of fat to lean mass is an indication of fitness, and the right types of exercises will help you decrease body fat and increase or maintain muscle mass.

A Workout Schedule

How often, how long, and how hard you exercise, and what kinds of exercises you do should be determined by what you are trying to accomplish. Your goals, your present fitness level, age, health, skills, interest, and convenience are among the factors you should consider. For example, an athlete training for high-level competition would follow a different program than a person whose goals are good health and the ability to meet work and recreational needs.

Your exercise program should include something from each of the four basic fitness components described previously. Each workout should begin with a warm-up and end with a cool down.

Here are the amounts of activity necessary for the average healthy person to maintain a minimum level of overall fitness. Included are some of the popular exercises for each category.

Quick Tip
Space your workouts throughout the week and avoid consecutive days of hard exercise.

Warm-Up: 5–10 minutes of exercise such as walking, slow jogging, knee lifts, arm circles, or trunk rotations. Low intensity movements that simulate movements to be used in the activity can also be included in the warm-up.

Muscular Strength: A minimum of two 20-minute sessions per week that include exercises for all the major muscle groups. Lifting weights is the most effective way to increase strength.

Muscular Endurance: At least three 30-minute sessions each week that include exercises such as calisthenics, pushups, sit-ups, pull-ups, and weight training for all the major muscle groups.

Cardiorespiratory Endurance: At least three 20-minute bouts of continuous aerobic (activity requiring oxygen) rhythmic exercise each week. Popular aerobic conditioning activities include brisk walking, jogging, swimming, cycling, rope jumping, rowing, cross-country skiing, and some continuous action games like racquetball and handball.

Flexibility: 10–12 minutes of daily stretching exercises performed slowly, without a bouncing motion. This can be included after a warm-up or during a cool down.

Cool Down: A minimum of 5–10 minutes of slow walking, low-level exercise, combined with stretching.

A Matter Of Principle

Specificity: Pick the right kind of activities to affect each component. Strength training results in specific strength changes. Also, train for the specific activity you are interested in.

Overload: Work hard enough, at levels that are vigorous, and long enough to overload your body above it's resting level to bring about improvement.

Regularity: You cannot hoard physical fitness. At least three balanced workouts a week are necessary to maintain a desirable level of fitness.

Progression: Increase the intensity, frequency, and/or duration of activity over periods of time in order to improve.

Some activities can be used to fulfill more than one of your basic exercise requirements. For example, in addition to increasing cardiorespiratory endurance, running builds muscular endurance in the legs, and swimming develops the arm, shoulder and chest muscles.

Measuring Your Heart Rate

Exercise that does not raise your heart rate to a certain level, and keep it there for 20 minutes, will not contribute significantly to cardiovascular fitness.

The heart rate you should maintain is called your target heart rate. There are several ways of arriving at this figure. One of the simplest is this: maximum heart rate (220) minus age, times x 70%. Thus, the target heart rate for a 15 year-old would be 144 (220 - 15 x .70 = 144).

Some methods for figuring the target rate take individual differences into consideration. Here is one of them:

- Subtract age from 220 to find maximum heart rate.
- Subtract resting heart rate (see below) from maximum heart rate to determine heart rate reserve.
- Take 70% of heart rate reserve to determine heart rate raise.
- Add heart rate raise to resting heart rate to find target rate.

When checking heart rate during a workout, take your pulse within five seconds after interrupting exercise because it starts to go down once you stop moving. Resting heart rate should be determined by taking your pulse after sitting quietly for five minutes.

Controlling Your Weight

The key to weight control is keeping energy intake (food) and energy output (physical activity) in balance. When you consume only as many calories as your body needs, your weight will usually remain constant. If you take in more calories than your body needs, you will put on excess fat. If you expend more energy than you take in you will burn excess fat.

Exercise plays an important role in weight control by increasing energy output, calling on stored calories for extra fuel. Recent studies show that not only does exercise increase metabolism during a workout, but it causes your metabolism to stay increased for a period of time after exercising, allowing you to burn more calories.

> ♣ **It's A Fact!!**
>
> The combination of exercise and diet offers the most flexible and effective approach to weight control.

How much exercise is needed to make a difference in your weight depends on the amount and type of activity and on how much you eat. Aerobic exercise burns body fat. A medium-sized young adult would have to walk more than 30 miles to burn up 3,500 calories, the equivalent of one pound of fat. Although that may seem like a lot, you do not have to walk the 30 miles all at once. Walking a mile a day for 30 days will achieve the same result, providing you do not increase your food intake to negate the effects of walking.

If you consume 100 calories a day more than your body needs, you will gain approximately 10 pounds in a year. You could take that weight off, or keep it off, by doing 30 minutes of moderate exercise daily.

Since muscle tissue weighs more than fat tissue, and exercise develops muscle to a certain degree, your bathroom scale will not necessarily tell you whether or not you are "fat." Well-muscled individuals, with relatively little body fat, invariably are "overweight" according to standard weight charts. If you are doing a regular program of strength training, your muscles will increase in weight, and possibly your overall weight will increase. Body composition is a better indicator of your condition than body weight.

Lack of physical activity causes muscles to get soft, and if food intake is not decreased, added body weight is almost always fat. Once-active people, who continue to eat as they always have after settling into sedentary lifestyles, tend to suffer from "creeping obesity."

Clothing

All exercise clothing should be loose-fitting to permit freedom of movement and should make the wearer feel comfortable and self-assured.

As a general rule, you should wear lighter clothes than temperatures might indicate. Exercise generates great amounts of body heat. Light-colored clothing that reflects the sun's rays is cooler in the summer, and dark clothes are warmer in winter. When the weather is very cold, it is better to wear several layers of light clothing than one or two heavy layers. The extra layers help trap heat, and it is easy to shed one of them if you become too warm.

In cold weather, and in hot, sunny weather, it is a good idea to wear something on your head. Wool watch or ski caps are recommended for winter wear, and some form of tennis or sailor's hat that provides shade and can be soaked in water is good for summer.

Never wear rubberized or plastic clothing; such garments interfere with the evaporation of perspiration and can cause body temperature to rise to dangerous levels.

The most important item of equipment for the runner is a pair of sturdy, properly fitting running shoes. Training shoes with heavy, cushioned soles and arch supports are preferable to flimsy sneakers and light racing flats.

> ✔ **Quick Tip**
> You should not exercise strenuously during extremely hot, humid weather or within two hours after eating. Heat and/or digestion both make heavy demands on the circulatory system, and in combination with exercise, can be an overtaxing double load.

When To Exercise

The hour just before the evening meal is a popular time for exercise. The late afternoon workout provides a welcome change of pace at the end of the school day and helps dissolve the day's worries and tensions.

Another popular time to work out is early morning, before the school day begins. Advocates of the early start say it makes them more alert and energetic at school or at work.

Among the factors you should consider in developing your workout schedule are personal preference, school and job responsibilities, availability of exercise facilities, and weather. It is important to schedule your workouts for a time when there is little chance that you will have to cancel or interrupt them because of other demands on your time.

Chapter 26

Getting Enough Sleep

Sleep is food for the brain. During sleep, important body functions and brain activity occur. Skipping sleep can be harmful, even deadly, particularly if you are behind the wheel. You can look bad, you may feel moody, and you perform poorly. Sleepiness can make it hard to get along with your family and friends and hurt your scores on school exams, on the court, or on the field. Remember: A brain that is hungry for sleep will get it, even when you do not expect it. For example, drowsiness and falling asleep at the wheel cause more than 100,000 car crashes every year. When you do not get enough sleep, you are more likely to have an accident, injury and/or illness.

What Are The Facts About Sleep And Teens?

- Sleep is vital to your well being, as important as the air you breathe, the water you drink, and the food you eat. It can even help you to eat better and manage the stress of being a teen.

- Biological sleep patterns shift toward later times for both sleeping and waking during adolescence—meaning it is natural to not be able to fall asleep before 11:00 p.m.

About This Chapter: Information in this chapter is from "Sleep and Teens." © 2006 National Sleep Foundation. All rights reserved. Reprinted with permission.

- Teens need about 9¼ hours of sleep each night to function best (for some, 8½ hours is enough). Most teens do not get enough sleep; one study found that only 15% reported sleeping 8½ hours on school nights.

- Teens tend to have irregular sleep patterns across the week. They typically stay up late and sleep in late on the weekends, which can affect their biological clocks and hurt the quality of their sleep.

- Many teens suffer from treatable sleep disorders such as narcolepsy, insomnia, restless legs syndrome, or sleep apnea.

✔ Quick Tip

- **Organize your life for sleep.** Make sleep a priority. Decide what you need to change to get enough sleep to stay healthy, happy, and smart.

- **A quick pick-me-up.** Naps can help pick you up and make you work more efficiently, if you plan them right. Naps that are too long or too close to bedtime can interfere with your regular sleep.

- **Create the right space.** Make your room a sleep haven. Keep it cool, quiet, and dark. If you need to, get eyeshades or blackout curtains. Let in bright light in the morning to signal your body to wake up.

- **You can't fake wake.** No pills, vitamins, or drinks can replace good sleep. Consuming caffeine close to bedtime can hurt your sleep, so avoid coffee, tea, soda/pop and chocolate late in the day so you can get to sleep at night. Nicotine and alcohol will also interfere with your sleep.

- **Drowsy driving is as dangerous as drunk driving.** When you are sleep deprived, you are as impaired as driving with a blood alcohol content of .08%, which is illegal for drivers in many states. Drowsy driving causes over 100,000 crashes each year. Recognize sleep deprivation and call someone else for a ride. Only sleep can save you!

- **Keep it constant.** Establish a bedtime and wake time and stick to it, coming as close as you can on the weekends. A consistent sleep schedule will help you feel less tired since it allows your body to get in sync with its natural patterns. You will find that it is easier to fall asleep at bedtime with this type of routine.

Sleep Deprivation Has Serious Consequences

Not getting enough sleep or having sleep difficulties can result in the following:

- Limit your ability to learn, listen, concentrate, and solve problems. You may even forget important information like names, numbers, your homework, or a date with a special person in your life.

- Make you more prone to pimples. Lack of sleep can contribute to acne and other skin problems.

- **Prepare your body.** Do not eat, drink, or exercise within a few hours of your bedtime. Do not leave your homework for the last minute. Try to avoid the TV, computer, and telephone in the hour before you go to bed. Stick to quiet, calm activities, and you will fall asleep much more easily.

- **Create a bedtime ritual.** If you do the same things every night before you go to sleep, you teach your body the signals that it is time for bed. Try taking a bath or shower (this will leave you extra time in the morning) or read a book.

- **Leave stress out of it.** Try keeping a diary or to-do lists. If you jot notes down before you go to sleep, you will be less likely to stay awake worrying or stressing.

- **Talk to your friends about your sleep.** When you hear your friends talking about their all-nighters, tell them how good you feel after getting enough sleep.

- **Understand your body.** Most teens experience changes in their sleep schedules. Their internal body clocks can cause them to fall asleep and wake up later. You cannot change this, but you can participate in interactive activities and classes to help counteract your sleepiness. Make sure your activities at night are calming to counteract your already heightened alertness.

- Lead to aggressive or inappropriate behavior such as yelling at your friends or being impatient with your teachers or family members.

- Cause you to eat too much or eat unhealthy foods like sweets and fried foods that lead to weight gain.

- Heighten the effects of alcohol and possibly increase use of caffeine and nicotine.

- Contribute to illness, not using equipment safely, or driving drowsy.

What Does Teen Sleep Have To Do With School Start Times?

Is your brain still on the pillow when school starts?

If teens need about 9¼ hours of sleep to do their best and naturally go to sleep around 11:00 p.m., one way to get more sleep is to start school later.

Teens' natural sleep cycle puts them in conflict with school start times. Most high school students need an alarm clock or a parent to wake them on school days. They are like zombies getting ready for school and find it hard to be alert and pay attention in class. Because they are sleep deprived, they are sleepy all day and cannot do their best.

Schools that have set later bell times find that students do not go to bed later, but get one hour more of sleep per school night, which means five hours more per week.

Enrollment and attendance improves, and students are more likely to be on time when school starts. Parents and teachers report that teens are more alert in the morning and in better moods; they are less likely to feel depressed or need to visit the nurse or school counselor.

Chapter 27

Stopping Germs At Home, School, And Work

What Are Microbes?

Microbes are tiny organisms—too tiny to see without a microscope, yet they are abundant on Earth. They live everywhere—in air, soil, rock, and water. Some of them live happily in searing heat, and others in freezing cold. Like humans, some microbes need oxygen to live, but others cannot exist with it. These microscopic organisms are in plants, animals, and in the human body.

Some microbes cause disease in humans, plants, and animals. Others are essential for a healthy life, and we could not exist without them. Indeed, the relationship between microbes and humans is very delicate and complex. In this chapter, we will learn that some microbes keep us healthy while others can make us sick.

Most microbes belong to one of four major groups: bacteria, viruses, fungi, or protozoa. A familiar, often-used word for microbes that cause disease is "germs." Some people refer to disease-causing microbes as "bugs." "I've got the flu bug," for example, is a phrase you may hear during the wintertime to describe an influenza virus infection.

About This Chapter: Information in this chapter is excerpted from "MICROBES in Sickness and in Health," National Institute of Allergy and Infectious Diseases, National Institutes of Health, July 2002.

Bacteria

Microbes belonging to the bacteria group are made up of only one cell. Under a microscope, bacteria look like balls, rods, or spirals. Bacteria are so small that a line of 1,000 could fit across the eraser of a pencil. Life in any form on Earth could not exist without these tiny cells.

Like humans, some bacteria (aerobic bacteria) need oxygen to survive, but others (anaerobic bacteria) do not. Amazingly, some can adapt to new environments by learning to survive with or without oxygen.

Like all living cells, each bacterium requires food for energy and building materials. There are countless numbers of bacteria on Earth. Most are harmless and many are even beneficial to humans. In fact, less than 1 percent of them cause diseases in humans. For example, harmless anaerobic bacteria, such as *Lactobacilli acidophilus*, live in human intestines, where they help to digest food, destroy disease-causing microbes, fight cancer cells, and give the body needed vitamins. Healthy food products, such as yogurt, sauerkraut, and cheese, are made using bacteria.

Some bacteria produce poisons called toxins, which also can make us sick.

Are Toxins Always Harmful?

Certain bacteria give off toxins that can seriously affect your health. Botulism, a severe form of food poisoning, affects the nerves and is caused by toxins from *Clostridium botulinum* bacteria. Under certain circumstances, however, bacterial toxins can be helpful. Several vaccines that protect us from getting sick are made from bacterial toxins. One type of pertussis vaccine, which protects infants and children from whooping cough, contains toxins from *Bordetella pertussis* bacteria. This vaccine is safe and effective and causes fewer reactions than other types of pertussis vaccine.

Viruses

Viruses are among the smallest microbes, much smaller even than bacteria. Viruses are not cells. They consist of one or more molecules of DNA or RNA, which contain the virus's genes surrounded by a protein coat. Viruses can be rod-shaped, sphere-shaped, or multisided. Some look like tadpoles.

Unlike most bacteria, most viruses do cause disease because they invade living, normal cells, such as those in the human body. They then multiply and produce other viruses like themselves. Each virus is very particular about which cell it attacks. Various human viruses specifically attack particular cells in the body's organs, systems, or tissues, such as the liver, respiratory system, or blood cells.

Fungi

A fungus is actually a primitive vegetable. Fungi can be found in air, in soil, on plants, and in water. Thousands, perhaps millions, of different types of fungi exist on Earth. The most familiar ones to us are mushrooms, yeast, mold, and mildew. Some live in the human body, usually without causing illness. In fact, only about half of all types of fungi cause disease in humans. Those conditions are called mycoses.

Some fungi have made our lives easier. Penicillin and other antibiotics, which kill harmful bacteria in our bodies, are made from fungi. Other fungi, like certain yeasts, also can be beneficial. For example, when a warm liquid, like water, and a food source are added to certain yeasts, the fungus ferments. The process of fermentation is essential for making healthy foods like some breads and cheeses.

Protozoa

Protozoa are a group of microscopic one-celled animals. Protozoa can be parasites or predators. In humans, protozoa usually cause disease. Some protozoa, like plankton, live in water environments and serve as food for marine animals, such as some species of whales. Protozoa also can be found on land in decaying matter and in soil, but they must have a moist environment to survive. Termites would not be able to do such a good job of digesting wood without these microorganisms in their guts.

Malaria is caused by a protozoan parasite. Another protozoan parasite, *Toxoplasma gondii*, causes toxoplasmosis in humans. This is an especially troublesome infection in pregnant women because of its effects on the fetus and in people with HIV infection or other immune deficiency.

Microbes Can Make Us Sick

According to health care experts, infectious diseases caused by microbes are responsible for more deaths worldwide than any other single cause. They estimate the annual cost of medical care for treating infectious diseases in the United States alone is about $120 billion.

Unfortunately, microbes are much better at adapting to new environments than people are. On Earth for billions of years, microbes are constantly challenging human newcomers with ingenious new survival tactics.

- Many microbes are developing new properties to resist drug treatments that once effectively combated them. Drug resistance has become a serious problem worldwide.

- Changes in the environment have put certain human populations in contact with newly identified microbes that cause diseases never seen before or that previously occurred only in isolated populations.

♣ **It's A Fact!!**

Common Diseases And Infections With Their Microbial Causes

- Athlete's foot—fungus
- Chickenpox—virus
- Common cold—virus
- Diarrheal disease—bacteria, protozoa, virus
- Flu—virus
- Genital herpes—virus
- Malaria—protozoa
- Meningitis—bacteria, virus
- Pneumonia—bacteria, fungus, virus
- Sinusitis—bacteria, fungus
- Skin diseases—bacteria, fungus, protozoa, virus
- Strep throat—bacteria
- Tuberculosis—bacteria
- Urinary tract infection—bacteria
- Vaginal infections—bacteria, fungus
- Viral hepatitis—virus

Source: "MICROBES in Sickness and in Health," National Institute of Allergy and Infectious Diseases.

- Newly emerging diseases are a growing global health concern. Since 1976, scientists have identified approximately 30 new pathogens.

Microbes Can Infect Us

You can get infected by germs in many different ways.

Some Microbes Can Travel Through The Air

Microbes can be transmitted from person to person through the air, as in coughing or sneezing. These are common ways to get viruses that cause colds or flu or the bacterium that causes tuberculosis (TB). Interestingly, international airplane travel can expose passengers to germs not common in their own countries.

Germs Can Be Passed Directly From Person To Person

Scientists have identified more than 500 types of bacteria that live in the human mouth. Some keep the oral environment healthy, while others cause gum disease, for example. One way to transmit oral bacteria from person to person is by kissing. Microbes such as HIV, herpes simplex virus 1, and gonorrhea bacteria are examples of germs that can be transmitted directly during sexual intercourse.

You Can Pick Up And Spread Germs By Touching Infectious Material

A common way for some microbes to enter the body, especially when caring for young children, is to unintentionally pass feces on your hand to your mouth or the mouths of young children. Infant diarrhea is often spread in this way. Day care workers, for example, can pass diarrhea-causing rotavirus or *Giardia lamblia* (protozoa) from one baby to the next between diaper changes and other childcare practices.

It also is possible to pick up cold viruses from shaking someone's hand or from touching surfaces such as a handrail or telephone.

A Healthy Person Can Be A Germ Carrier And Pass It On To Others

The story of "Typhoid Mary" is a famous example from medical history about how a person can pass germs on to others, yet not be affected by them.

The germs in this case were *Salmonella typhi* bacteria, which cause typhoid fever and are usually spread through food or water.

Mary Mallon, an Irish immigrant who lived at the turn of the 19th century, worked as a cook for several New York City families. More than half of the first family she worked for came down with typhoid fever. Through a clever deduction, a researcher determined that the family cook caused the disease. He concluded that although Mary had no symptoms of the disease, she probably had had a mild typhoid infection sometime in the past. Though not sick, she still carried the bacteria and was able to spread them to others through the food she prepared.

Germs From Your Household Pet Can Make You Sick

You can catch a variety of germs from animals, especially household pets. The rabies virus, which can infect cats and dogs, is one of the most serious and deadly of these microbes. Fortunately, the rabies vaccine prevents animals from getting rabies. Vaccines also protect people from accidentally getting the virus from an animal and prevent people who have been exposed to the virus, such as through an animal bite, from getting sick.

Dog and cat saliva can contain any of more than 100 different germs that can make you sick. *Pasteurella* bacteria, the most common, can be transmitted through bites that break the skin causing serious, and sometimes fatal, diseases such as blood infections and meningitis.

Warm-blooded animals are not the only ones that can cause you harm. Pet reptiles such as turtles, snakes, and iguanas can transmit *Salmonella* bacteria to their unsuspecting owners.

You Can Get Microbes From Tiny Critters

Mosquitoes may be the most common insect carriers (vectors) of pathogens. *Anopheles* mosquitoes can pick up *Plasmodium*, which causes malaria, from the blood of an infected person and transmit the protozoan to an uninfected person.

Fleas that pick up *Yersinia pestis* bacteria from rodents can then transmit plague to humans.

Ticks, which are more closely related to crabs than to insects, are another common vector. The tiny deer tick can infect humans with *Borrelia burgdorferi*, the bacterium that causes Lyme disease, which it picks up from deer.

Microbes In The Food You Eat Or Water You Drink Could Make You Sick

Every year, millions of people worldwide become ill from eating contaminated foods. Although many cases of food borne illness or "food poisoning" are not reported, the U.S. Centers for Disease Control and Prevention (CDC) estimates there are 76 million illnesses, 325,000 hospitalizations, and 5,200 deaths in the United States each year that are caused by food borne bacteria. Bacteria, viruses, and protozoa can cause these illnesses, some of which can be fatal if not treated properly.

Poor manufacturing processes or poor food preparation can allow microbes to grow in food and subsequently infect you. *Escherichia coli* (E. coli) bacteria sometimes persist in food products such as undercooked hamburger meat and unpasteurized fruit juice. These bacteria can have deadly consequences in vulnerable people, especially children and the elderly.

> ### ✔ Quick Tip
>
> When soap and water are not available, alcohol-based disposable hand wipes or gel sanitizers may be used. You can find them in most supermarkets and drug stores. If using gel, rub your hands until the gel is dry. The gel does not need water to work; the alcohol in it kills the germs on your hands.
>
> Source: Excerpted from "Stopping Germs at Home, Work and School," *FDA & You*, Issue #5, Winter 2005, U.S. Food and Drug Administration.

Cryptosporidia are bacteria found in fecal matter and can get into lake, river, and ocean water from sewage spills, animal waste, and water run-off. They can be released in the millions from infectious fecal matter. People who drink, swim, or play in infected water can get sick.

People, including babies, with diarrhea caused by *Cryptosporidia* or other diarrhea-causing microbes, such as *Giardia* and *Salmonella*, can infect others while using swimming pools, water parks, hot tubs, and spas.

You Can Prevent Catching Or Passing On Germs

Hand Washing

Hand washing is one of the simplest, easiest, and most effective ways to prevent getting or passing on many germs. Amazingly, it is also one of the most overlooked. Healthcare experts recommend scrubbing your hands vigorously for at least 15 seconds with soap and water, about as long as it takes to recite the English alphabet. This will wash away cold viruses and staph and strep bacteria as well as many other disease-causing microbes. This also will help prevent accidentally passing those germs on to others.

It is especially important to wash your hands in the following situations:

- Before preparing or eating food
- After coughing or sneezing
- After changing a diaper
- After using the bathroom

Healthcare providers should be especially conscientious about washing their hands before and after examining any patient. Day care workers, too, should be vigilant about hand washing around their young children.

♣ **It's A Fact!!**

The flu has caused high rates of absenteeism among students and staff in U.S. schools. Influenza is not the only respiratory infection of concern in schools—nearly 22 million school days are lost each year to the common cold alone.

Source: Excerpted from "Stopping Germs at Home, Work and School," *FDA & You*, Issue #5, Winter 2005, U.S. Food and Drug Administration.

Chapter 28

Hygiene Basics

Oily Hair, Body Odor, And Body Hair

Puberty causes all kinds of changes in your body. Your skin and scalp may suddenly get oily very easily. Every day it seems you have new hair growing in different places. At times, you seem to sweat for no reason, and you may notice there are odors where you never had them before. What should you do about it?

These bodily changes are a normal part of becoming an adult. Still, some of them can be a real source of anxiety. Who wants to worry about whether their underarms smell, anyway?

This chapter will provide information on some hygiene basics, and you will learn how to deal with greasy hair, perspiration, and body hair.

Oily Hair

The hormones that create acne are the same ones that make you feel like you have been styling your hair with a comb dipped in motor oil lately. Each

About This Chapter: This chapter begins with information under the heading "Oily Hair, Body Odor, and Body Hair," from "Hygiene Basics." It was provided by TeensHealth, one of the largest resources online for medically reviewed health information written for parents, kids, and teens. For more articles like this one, visit www.TeensHealth.org, or www.KidsHealth.org. © 2004 The Nemours Foundation. Additional information under the heading "Your Skin" is from GirlsHealth.gov, sponsored by The National Women's Health Information Center, U.S. Department of Health and Human Services, Office on Women's Health, August 2005.

strand of hair has its own sebaceous (oil) gland, which keeps the hair shiny and waterproof. But during puberty, when the sebaceous glands produce extra oil, it can make your hair look too shiny, oily, and greasy.

Washing your hair every day or every other day can help control oily hair. There are dozens of shampoos on drugstore and supermarket shelves for you to choose from. Most brands are pretty similar, although you might want to try one that is specially formulated for oily hair. Use warm water and a small amount of shampoo to work up lather. Do not scrub or rub too hard; this does not get rid of oil any better and can irritate your scalp or damage your hair. After you have rinsed, you can follow up with a conditioner if you like; again, one for oily hair might work best.

When you are styling your hair, pay close attention to the products you use. Some styling gels or lotions can add extra grease to your hair, which defeats the purpose of washing it in the first place. Look for formulas that are called "greaseless" or "oil free."

Sweat And Body Odor

Perspiration, or sweat, comes from sweat glands that you have always had in your body. But thanks to puberty, these glands not only become more active than before, they also begin to secrete different chemicals into the sweat that has a stronger smelling odor. You might notice this odor under your arms in your armpits. Your feet and genitals might also have new smells.

The best way to keep clean is to bathe or shower every day using a mild soap and warm water. This will help wash away any bacteria that contribute to the smells. Wearing clean clothes, socks, and underwear each day can also help you to feel clean. If you sweat a lot, you might find that shirts, T-shirts, socks, and underwear made from cotton or other natural materials will help absorb sweat more effectively.

If you are concerned about the way your underarms smell, you can try using a deodorant or deodorant with antiperspirant. Deodorants get rid of the odor of sweat by covering it up, and antiperspirants actually stop or dry up perspiration. They come in sticks, roll-ons, gels, sprays, and creams and are available at any drugstore or supermarket. All brands are similar (and ones that say they are made for a man or for a woman are similar, too, except for some perfumes that are added).

If you choose to use deodorant or antiperspirant, be sure to read the directions. Some work better if you use them at night, whereas others recommend that you put them on in the morning. But keep in mind that some teens do not need deodorants or antiperspirants, so why use them if you do not have to? Deodorant and antiperspirant commercials may try to convince you that you will have no friends or dates if you do not use their product, but if you do not think you smell, and you take daily baths or showers and wear clean clothes, you may be fine without them.

Body Hair

Body hair in new places is something you can count on; again, it is hormones in action. You may want to start shaving some places where body hair grows, but whether you do is up to you. Some guys who grow facial hair like to let it develop into a mustache and beard. Some girls may decide to leave the hair on their legs and under their arms as is. It is all up to you and what you feel comfortable with.

If you do decide to shave, whether you are a guy or girl, you have a few different choices. You can use a traditional razor with a shaving cream or gel, or you can use an electric razor. If you use a regular razor, make sure the blade is new and sharp to prevent cuts and nicks. Shaving cream and gel are often a better bet than soap because they make it easier to pull the razor against your skin. Some of the newer razors contain shaving gel right in the blade area, making even beginners feel comfortable shaving.

Whether you 're shaving your legs, armpits, or face, go slowly. These are tricky areas of your body with lots of curves and angles, and it is easy to cut yourself if you move too fast. An adult or older sibling can be a big help when you are learning to shave. Do not be afraid to ask for tips.

You might want to avoid shaving your pubic hair, because when it grows back in, the skin may be irritated and itchy. Also, guys may think twice about shaving their chests, and girls should not ever try shaving their faces because the hair will grow back stiffer and thicker and look pricklier, forcing you to shave over and over.

If you are a girl and you are worried about hairs on your upper lip, step back from the mirror, and you may see that the hair everyone really sees is probably not as bad as you think. If you do decide you want to get rid of unwanted facial hair, research the options and ask an adult or older sibling for advice. There are many products made for facial hair—everything from bleach to lessen its appearance to hair removers that are specially made for hair on the face. There are also some new oil-free facial moisturizers on the market that contain substances to make facial hair softer and less visible. You may want to try one before you opt for bleaching or hair removal. In the rare case where a girl's facial hair growth is enough to cause anxiety, a dermatologist or skin specialist can use permanent removal techniques such as electrolysis.

Your Skin

Your skin is just one more thing that changes when you go through puberty.

A few different skin problems are a part of acne: whiteheads, blackheads, and cystic acne. Whiteheads are made when a hair follicle (root) is plugged with oil and skin cells. If this plugged up stuff comes up to the surface of the skin and the air touches it, it turns black—a "blackhead." So, blackheads are not caused by dirt. If a plugged follicle breaks, the area swells and becomes a red bump. If this happens close to the surface of the skin, the bump most often becomes a pimple. If it breaks deep inside in the skin, nodules or cysts can form, which can look like larger pimples. This is cystic acne.

♣ **It's A Fact!!**

Acne often starts in your early teen years because your body is making more oil glands, which is normal.

Source: "Your Skin," GirlsHealth.gov, August 2005.

Acne is common among teens, but not everyone will have the same troubles. It may be worse in boys because they have more oils in their skin. Also, it can run in the family. If your mother or father had bad acne, the same may happen for you. Some people also just have more sensitive skin.

♣ It's A Fact!!
Do Girls Need To Douche?

No. The vagina actually cleans itself on the inside with natural fluids. The best way to clean the outside of your vagina is to wash with warm water and gentle, scent-free soap during a bath or shower. Products you might see on T.V. or at the drug store, such as feminine hygiene soaps, powders, and sprays, are not needed. And they may even be harmful to you.

Douching is rinsing or cleaning out the vagina by squirting water or other fluids (solutions made with vinegar or baking soda that you can buy at the drug store) into the vagina. Women douche to rinse away blood after their periods and to generally feel cleaner. Many women douche, but doctors do not recommend it. Douching changes the balance of natural chemicals in your vagina and can make it easier for you to get dangerous infections.

If you have any of the following problems, tell your doctor right away:

• Itching in, and near, your vagina

• Burning or pain in your vagina

• Pain when you go to the bathroom

• Discharge, or fluid from your vagina that is not normal, such as thick and white (like cottage cheese) or yellowish-green discharge that is foul smelling. Normal discharge changes throughout your menstrual cycle, but may normally look clear, cloudy white, and/or yellowish.

If you are not sure if the discharge or fluid is normal, have your doctor check you out.

Source: "Do You Need To Douche?" GirlsHealth.gov, March 2006.

How Is Acne Treated?

Wash your face regularly. If the acne does not go away, there are over-the-counter products (you can buy these without a doctor's order) available in different forms, such as gels, lotions, creams, and soaps. Common ingredients used in these products to fight acne are benzoyl peroxide, resorcinol, salicylic acid, and sulfur. If you have a bad skin reaction to any products you buy on your own, tell your doctor. Also, it can take time for these products to work. If they do not make your acne better after two months, ask your doctor for help. The doctor can give you stronger medicines, including antibiotics or other pills and creams that have either retinoids or adapalene in them. Retinoids can make you very sensitive to the sun, so avoid those rays or use a strong sunscreen to protect yourself. Another word of caution: the medicine isotretinoin (the product is called Accutane) can cause birth defects and miscarriages (losing a baby while pregnant) if taken when a woman is pregnant.

What Can Make Acne Worse?

- Oil-based makeup, suntan oil, hair gels, and sprays
- Stress
- Your period
- Picking at your pimples
- Scrubbing your skin too hard
- Getting too much sun

What Doesn't Cause Acne?

Dirt, fried foods or chocolate, and sexual activity do not cause acne. These are myths.

Chapter 29

Girls And Hair Removal

As you browse the aisles of your local drugstore, you may feel a little dizzy. There are hundreds of products devoted to making the hair on your head more lustrous, clean, fragrant, and full—and just steps away, dozens more promise to get rid of your unwanted hair just as easily. Which ones work best? How do they work? And do you need any of them?

Different Types Of Hair

Before removing hair, it helps to know about the different types of hair on our bodies. All hair is made of keratin, a hard protein that is also found in your fingernails and toenails. Hair growth begins beneath the surface of your skin at a hair root inside a hair follicle, a small tube in the skin.

You have two types of hair on your body. Vellus hair is soft, fine, and short. Most women have vellus hair on the chest, back, and face. It can be darker and more noticeable in some women than others, especially women with darker complexions. Vellus hair helps the body maintain a steady temperature by providing some insulation.

About This Chapter: Information in this chapter is from "Hair Removal." This information was provided by TeensHealth, one of the largest resources online for medically reviewed health information written for parents, kids, and teens. For more articles like this one, visit www.TeensHealth.org, or www.KidsHealth.org. © 2004 The Nemours Foundation.

Terminal hair is coarser, darker, and longer than vellus hair and is the type of hair that grows on your head. When a teen reaches puberty, terminal hair starts to grow in the armpits and pubic region. On guys, terminal hair begins to grow on the face and other parts of the body such as the chest, legs, and back. Terminal hair provides cushioning and protection.

In some cases, excess hair growth, called hirsutism (pronounced: hur-suh-tih-zum), may be the result of certain medical conditions. In girls, poly-cystic ovary syndrome and other hormonal disorders can cause dark, coarse hair to grow on the face, especially the upper lip, and on the arms, chest, and legs. Some medications, like anabolic steroids, can also cause hirsutism.

Getting Rid Of Hair

Shaving

How It Works: Using a razor, a person removes the tip of the hair shaft that has grown out through the skin. Some razors are completely disposable, some have a disposable blade, and some are electric. Guys often shave their faces, and women often shave their underarms, legs, and bikini areas.

How Long It Lasts: It lasts one to three days.

Pros: Shaving is fairly inexpensive. All you need is some warm water, a razor, and if you choose, shaving gel or cream. You do not need an appointment. Shaving is a do-it-yourself endeavor, resulting in smooth, hairless skin.

Cons: Razor burn, bumps, nicks, cuts, and ingrown hairs are side effects of shaving. Ingrown hairs occur when hairs are cut below the level of the skin. When the hair begins to grow, it grows within the surrounding tissue rather than growing out of the follicle. The hair curls around and starts growing into the skin, and irritation, redness, and swelling can occur at the hair follicle.

Tips: Look for blades that have safety guard wires; they minimize nicks and cuts. Also, you will get a closer shave if you shave in the shower after your skin has been softened by warm water. Go slowly, change your blades often to avoid nicks, and use a moisturizing cream to soften the hair. Although most people shave in the opposite direction from the hair growth, if you want to avoid ingrown hairs it can help to shave in the direction the hair grows. If you have an ingrown hair, try exfoliating (removing dead skin cells with a loofah), sterilizing a pointed pair of tweezers with rubbing alcohol, and attempting to pluck out the ingrown hair.

Plucking

How It Works: Using tweezers, a person stretches the skin tightly, grips the hair close to the root, and pulls it out.

How Long It Lasts: It lasts three to eight weeks.

Pros: Plucking is time-consuming because you can only remove one hair at a time. However, it is inexpensive because all you need are tweezers.

Cons: Plucking can be painful, so it is best to do it only on small areas, such as the eyebrows, upper lip, and chin. If the hair breaks off below the skin, a person may get an ingrown hair. After plucking, you may notice temporary red bumps because the hair follicle is swollen and irritated.

Tips: Make sure you sterilize your tweezers with rubbing alcohol before and after use to reduce the chance of infection.

Depilatories

How They Work: A depilatory is a cream or liquid that removes hair from the skin's surface. They work by reacting with the protein structure of the hair, so the hair dissolves and can be washed or wiped away.

How Long They Last: They last several days to two weeks.

Pros: Depilatories work quickly, are readily available at drugstores and grocery stores, and are inexpensive. They are best on the leg, underarm, and bikini areas. Special formulations may be used on the face and chin.

Cons: Applying depilatories can be messy, and many people dislike the odor. If you have sensitive skin, you might have an allergic reaction to the chemicals in the depilatory, which may cause a rash or inflammation. Depilatories may not be as effective on people with coarse hair.

Tips: Read product directions carefully and be sure to apply the product only for the recommended amount of time for best results.

✔ **Quick Tip**

The Food and Drug Administration (FDA) has received complaints about skin burns and scarring from some chemical hair removal products. If you use this type of product, always do a patch test in accordance with the directions, do not use it on broken or irritated skin, and keep the product away from eyes. Cosmetics do not go through FDA approval before they are marketed, though the FDA can take action to get unsafe products off the market.

Source: Excerpted from "Summer Safety Savvy," *FDA & You*, Issue #6, Spring 2005, Updated June 2005, U.S. Food and Drug Administration.

Waxing

How It Works: A sticky wax is spread on the area of skin where the unwanted hair is growing. A cloth strip is then applied over the wax and quickly pulled off, taking the hair root and dead skin cells with it. The wax can be warmed or may be applied cold. Waxing can be done at a salon or at home.

How Long It Lasts: It lasts three to six weeks.

Pros: Waxing leaves the area smooth and is long lasting. Waxing kits are readily available in drugstores and grocery stores. Hair re-growth looks lighter and less noticeable than it is after other methods of hair removal, such as shaving.

Cons: Many people mention that the biggest drawback to waxing is the pain when the hair is ripped out by the root. A person may notice temporary redness, inflammation, and bumps after waxing. Professional waxing is also expensive compared to other hair removal methods.

People with diabetes should avoid waxing because they are more susceptible to infection. Also, teens who use acne medications such as tretinoin and isotretinoin may want to skip the wax because those medicines make the skin more sensitive. Teens with moles or skin irritation from sunburn should also avoid waxing.

Tips: For waxing to work, hair should be at least ¼ inch (about 6 millimeters) long, so skip shaving for a few weeks before waxing. Waxing works best on legs, bikini areas, and eyebrows.

Electrolysis

How It Works: Over a series of several appointments, a professional electrologist inserts a needle into the follicle and sends an electric current through the hair root, killing it. A small area such as the upper lip may take a total of 4 to 10 hours and a larger area, such as the bikini line, may take 8 to 16 hours.

How Long It Lasts: It is permanent.

Pros: Electrolysis is the only type of hair removal that is permanent.

Cons: Electrolysis takes big bucks and lots of time, so it is usually only used on smaller areas such as the upper lip, eyebrows, and underarms. Many people describe the process as painful, and dry skin, scabs, scarring, and inflammation may result after treatment. Infection may be a risk if the needles and other instruments are not properly sterilized.

Tips: Talk to your doctor if you are interested in this method. He or she may be able to recommend an electrologist with the proper credentials.

Laser Hair Removal

How It Works: A laser is directed through the skin to the hair follicle, where it stops growth. It works best on light-skinned people with dark hair because the melanin (colored pigment) in the hair absorbs more of the light, making treatment more effective.

How Long It Lasts: It lasts six months.

☞ Remember!!

Deciding to remove body hair is a personal choice.
Getting rid of body hair does not make a person healthier,
and you should not feel pressured to do so if you do not want to.
Some cultures view body hair as beautiful and natural, so do what
feels right to you.

Source: © 2004 The Nemours Foundation.

Pros: This type of hair removal is long lasting, and large areas of skin can be treated at the same time.

Cons: A treatment session may cost $500 or more. Side effects of the treatment may include inflammation and redness.

Tips: Using cold packs may help diminish any inflammation after treatment. Avoiding the sun before a treatment may make results more effective.

Prescription Treatments

A cream called eflornithine is available by prescription to treat facial hair growth (generally in women). The cream is applied twice a day until the hair becomes softer and lighter—more like vellus hair. Side effects may include skin irritation and acne. Talk to your doctor or dermatologist if you are concerned about hair growth and removal.

Antiandrogen medications are another method that doctors prescribe to reduce the appearance of unwanted hair. Because the hormone androgen can be responsible for hair growth in unwanted areas, antiandrogens can block androgen production. Oral contraceptives are frequently used in conjunction with these medications to enhance their effect and to help regularize the menstrual cycle in girls who need it.

Chapter 30

Guys And Shaving

You looked different this morning. While brushing your teeth, you gazed into the mirror, and there it was—hair sprouting all over your face. It is definitely cool, but you are not quite sure whether you want to grow that big bushy beard and moustache just yet. It is time to start shaving (as if you did not have enough things to do first thing in the morning).

Actually, shaving is no big deal once you get the hang of it. It is quick, easy, and if you follow the tips outlined below, absolutely painless.

Razor Basics

Shaving is simply using a razor to remove the tip of the hair shaft that has grown up through the skin. Razors come in a bunch of different forms. There are standard razors that are either completely disposable or have a disposable blade that needs to be replaced regularly, and there are electric razors.

Using an electric razor can be quick and convenient, but many guys find that it may not give the close and accurate shave that a standard razor can.

About This Chapter: Information in this chapter is from "Shaving." This information was provided by TeensHealth, one of the largest resources online for medically reviewed health information written for parents, kids, and teens. For more articles like this one, visit www.TeensHealth.org, or www.KidsHealth.org. © 2004 The Nemours Foundation.

Although using an electric razor is pretty easy (just turn it on and move it around your face), shaving with a standard razor has a few rules to follow.

When you are using a standard razor, the most important item you need is a clean, sharp blade (the best razors have at least two blades and a movable head). Try to avoid shaving with a dull or blunt blade. At best, a dull blade will give you an uneven shave and leave you with redness, blotches, and patches of unshaven hair on your face and neck. At worst, a dull blade will remove a fair amount of your skin along with the hair. Do not be afraid of changing the blade (or the razor, if you are using the disposable kind) often. You will be glad you did.

Shaving scrapes natural oils off your face, so the next most important item is some sort of shaving gel to keep your skin from becoming too dry and reduce friction from the razor. Pick a gel you think sounds good and give it a try. If you choose a shaving gel that is mentholated (it will say that on the label), be aware that menthol can sometimes cause a slight reaction with some types of skin and may result in red blotches. If this happens to you, do not worry. Just switch to a non-mentholated shaving cream.

Ouch!

Cuts and nicks are a part of shaving. They will not happen to you every time, but they will happen. When you nick or cut yourself, be sure to grab a clean tissue or cloth and apply direct pressure to stop the bleeding.

> **✔ Quick Tip**
>
> If you have a zit or a cut right in the middle of the area you are going to shave, it is a good idea to drop the standard razor for a while and use an electric razor or give shaving a break altogether for a few days.

Also, some guys might get ingrown hairs after shaving, in that the hair grows back into the skin. It can pierce the hair follicle, which in turn causes razor bumps. Called folliculitis, this condition can sometimes be handled by using a special safety razor, but this does not always work for every guy. If you experience folliculitis, talk to a dermatologist about the best way to remove your beard and moustache.

How To Shave

Before you begin, be sure to remember to rinse your razor after every few strokes. That way, the razor is cleared of any shaving cream or hair that might clog it up. Also, because the hair on different parts of your face grows in different directions, always try to shave in the direction your hair is growing (shaving against the direction your hair is growing can cause razor burn, redness, and rashes).

Now let's shave. Here is how to do it:

- First, wet your face with hot or warm water. This makes the hair on your face softer and opens your skin's pores, getting you ready for a closer and easier shave. Even better, try to shave right after you get out of the shower.

- Squirt some shaving gel into your hand, then apply it to your face, making sure to cover the sides of your face, chin, mouth area (around your lips), neck, and throat.

- Press the razor to the area you want to shave (it is a good idea to start with the sides of your face as they are easy to handle). Use short, slow strokes and remember to move the razor in the direction your hair is growing. Do not press too hard but do not be too gentle. Find the right touch by making sure the razor is cutting the hair and not your skin. You will know if you are being too gentle if you only remove the shaving cream and the hair is still there.

- When the sides of your face are finished, move on to the more tricky spots. For areas like your upper lip/moustache area, bottom lip/chin area, and neck/throat area, you will have to work a little. Try to stretch your skin a bit to make a flat surface, and glide the razor over those tricky areas.

- When you are finished, rinse your clean, smooth face with cold water. If you want to, put on some aftershave. Depending on how fast you grow that beard and moustache, repeat the entire process in one to three days.

Chapter 31

Oral Hygiene: Keep Your Teeth Clean And Bright

What is oral health?

Oral refers to the mouth, which includes the teeth, gums, and supporting tissues. The health of your mouth can be a sign of your overall health.

How are problems with the tissues in your mouth linked to health problems in other places in your body?

Many serious diseases, such as diabetes, HIV, and some eating disorders, show their first signs as symptoms in the mouth. This is why it is important to have complete, regular oral exams.

Most of us think of problems with the mouth in terms of cavities, toothaches, and crooked or stained teeth. Lacking healthy teeth and gums has an effect on how we look, but it also affects the health of our bodies. The following are some examples:

- If you have gum disease, you may be more likely to get heart disease.

- Having missing teeth can affect your mental health since it can lead to feeling badly about yourself.

About This Chapter: Information in this chapter is excerpted from "Oral Health," The National Women's Health Information Center, U.S. Department of Health and Human Services, Office On Women's Health, August 2004.

- If you have diabetes, you may be more likely to get gum disease.

- If you have both diabetes and gum disease, you can have more problems controlling your blood sugar levels.

What are the most common oral health problems?

Dental Cavities: Everyone is at risk for getting cavities throughout life. By the time most people are adults, 85% of people will have had a cavity.

This is how it happens. You naturally have bacteria (germs) in your mouth. The bacteria mix with your saliva and bits of food in your mouth to form a coating (dental plaque) that sticks to your teeth. There are acids in the plaque that wear away the teeth. These acids can get inside the teeth and create holes in the teeth, which are called cavities.

Gum Diseases: Gum disease is caused by infection or plaque around your teeth and is a common cause of tooth loss after age 35. The first stage, and most common type of gum disease, is gingivitis (jin-ji-vie-tus). Gingivitis irritates the gums and causes them to bleed and swell. Gum diseases are more often seen as people age, with most people showing signs of them by their mid-30s.

Periodontitis (pear-ee-o-don-tie-tus) is a more serious type of gum disease that, if left untreated, gets worse as pockets of infection form between the teeth and gums. This causes your gums to grow away from teeth and lose supporting bone. If the teeth cannot be supported, they could fall out. This disease results from bacteria in your mouth. You may be more likely to be infected with these bacteria if the following is true: someone else in your family has periodontitis; you are a smoker; you have a disease like diabetes or HIV.

What are some other problems you might have with your mouth?

Cold sores (herpes simplex virus type 1 (HSV-1) infections): If you have ever had a cold sore, you are not alone. A half million people get one every year. Once exposed to this virus, it can hide in the body for years. Getting too much sun, having mild fevers that occur with a cold, or stress can trigger the virus and cause tiredness, muscle aches, sore throat, enlarged and tender lymph nodes, and cold sores. These sores are very contagious and usually form on the lips, and sometimes under the nose or under the chin. The sores heal in about seven to ten days without scarring. You can buy medicines at the drug store or grocery store to put on the cold sore to numb or relieve the pain. If cold sores are a problem for you, talk with your doctor or dentist about a prescription for an antiviral drug to help lower your chances of getting these kinds of viral infections.

Canker sores: These common, but mostly harmless, sores appear as ulcers with a white or gray base and a red border inside the mouth. They occur in women more often than men, often during their periods. The reason why they appear is unknown, but some experts believe that problems with the immune system, the system in our bodies that fights disease, bacteria, or viruses may be involved. Fatigue, stress, or allergies can increase your chances of getting a canker sore. You also might get one if you have a cut inside your cheek or on your tongue. Canker sores tend to be tiny and heal by themselves in one to three weeks. If you get a large sore (larger than 1 centimeter) though, it may need to be treated with medicine.

Oral fungal or yeast infections (candidiasis [can-di-die-uh-sis]): These infections appear as red or white lesions, flat or slightly raised, in the mouth. They are common among denture wearers and occur most often in people who are very young, elderly, or who have a problem with their immune system.

Dry mouth syndrome: This is common in many adults, especially as they age. It may make it hard to eat, swallow, taste, and speak. It happens when salivary glands fail to work right.

Oral cancer: This cancer most often occurs in people over the age of 40. It is often found at late stages when it is harder to treat. This is because oral cancer is not usually painful, so you may not know you have it. And many people do not visit their dentists often enough to find the cancer early. The most common sites of oral cancer are on the tongue, lips, and floor of the mouth. Use of tobacco, especially with alcohol, is the main cause for these cancers.

Oral problems from cancer therapies: Treatments like chemotherapy or radiation to the head and neck can cause dry mouth, tooth decay, painful mouth sores, and cracked, peeling lips.

✔ **Quick Tip**

What type of toothpaste or mouthwash should you use?

There are so many types of toothpastes to choose from. Some say they are made for whitening, others for reducing gingivitis and plaque, and others for sensitive teeth. You should feel good choosing whatever brand and flavor you like if you know these basics:

- As long as the toothpaste contains fluoride and its box has the American Dental Association's (ADA) seal of acceptance, it is good for your oral health. Beyond that, choosing toothpastes based on what they claim to do is a personal choice.

- Mouthwashes claim to freshen your breath, but they really only mask breath odor for a few hours. If you must constantly use a breath freshener to hide bad mouth odor, see your dentist.

- If you need extra help controlling plaque, your dentist might suggest using an antiseptic mouth rinse. Many of these products are accepted by the ADA because they reduce plaque and gum disease, and help kill the germs that cause bad breath.

- You also may want to use a fluoride mouth rinse, along with brushing and flossing, to help prevent tooth decay.

How can you safely whiten your teeth?

You might want to whiten teeth more than is possible through regular brushing, flossing, and check ups. There are several options that vary in price and in how well they work:

- **Chair side bleaching or "power bleaching:"** In your dentist's office, he or she applies a gel or rubber shield to protect your gums and oral tissues, and then puts a bleach on your teeth. With this method you may have to go for more than one visit. You will see results right away (about 5 shades brighter). It works well on a range of stains.

- **Professional dispensed bleaching solutions:** These products are for use at home, and you get them from your dentist. They contain peroxide(s), to bleach the tooth enamel. Most come in a gel and are placed in a mouth guard or tray that fits inside your mouth around your teeth. Some products are used for about twice a day for two weeks, and others are used overnight for one to two weeks.

- **Over-the-counter, TV, and internet products:** These products are for use at home and include whitening strips, paint-on products, and gels and trays. They have a low amount of peroxide. They have limited results without first having professional removal of the stains, but they can help prolong the results you get from professional removal.

- **Whitening toothpastes:** All toothpastes help remove surface stain. "Whitening" toothpastes that have the American Dental Association seal have special polishing agents that remove more stains. These products do not change the actual color of teeth. They help slight surface stains only.

Options offered by your dentist can be expensive, so be certain to ask your dentist to fully explain what results you can really expect. Keep in mind that whitening your teeth alone does not make your mouth any healthier.

What small, easy steps can you take to have a healthy smile?

1. Brush your teeth at least twice each day.

Aim for first thing in the morning and before going to bed. Once a day, use floss or an interdental cleaner to clean between teeth to remove food that your toothbrush missed. Make sure you do the following:

- Drink fluoridated water if you can.

- Gently brush all sides of your teeth with a soft bristled brush and fluoride toothpaste. Circular and short back-and-forth strokes work best.

- Take time to brush along the gum line, and lightly brush your tongue to help remove plaque and food debris.

- Ask your dentist or dental hygienist to show you the best way to floss your teeth.

- Change your toothbrush at least every three months or earlier if the toothbrush looks worn. A new toothbrush can remove more plaque than one that is more than three months old.

2. Have a healthy lifestyle.

- Eat healthy meals. Cut down on tooth decay by brushing after meals and not snacking on sugary or starchy foods between meals.

- Do not smoke. Smoking raises your risk for getting gum disease, oral and throat cancers, and oral fungal infections.

3. Get regular check ups.

- During regular check ups, dentists and other types of dental providers can find signs of nutritional deficiencies, diseases, infections, immune disorders, injuries, and some cancers.

- Make an appointment right away if your gums bleed often, if you see any red or white patches on the gums or tongue, have mouth/jaw pain that will not go away, have sores that do not heal within two weeks, or if you have problems swallowing or chewing.

- Besides your dentist, here are some other types of dental providers:

    - *Dental hygienists:* They clean gums and teeth, and instruct patients on ways to prevent oral disease and to maintain oral health.

    - *Periodontists:* Dentists who treat gum disease and place dental implants, or artificial teeth, to replace lost teeth.

    - *Oral surgeons:* Dentists who can perform biopsies or surgery on your mouth and supporting tissues if you have a serious problem.

4. Follow your dentist's advice.

Your dentist may suggest that you do different things to keep your mouth healthy. He or she can teach you how to properly floss or brush, and how often. He or she might suggest preventive steps or treatments to keep your mouth healthy.

5. If you have another health problem, think how it may affect your oral health.

For instance, if you take medicines that give you a dry mouth, ask your doctor or nurse if there is another drug you can use instead. Have an oral exam before beginning cancer treatment. And know that if you have diabetes, good oral hygiene to prevent gum disease is very important.

Chapter 32

Straight Talk About Braces

Today's braces are a lot different from the metal-mouth look of a genera-tion ago. "They are more aesthetic and more efficient," says Donald Joondeph, D.D.S., an associate professor of orthodontics at the University of Washing-ton in Seattle. And they are more comfortable to wear and better at reposi-tioning teeth, he adds.

Braces used to be put on only after all the permanent teeth came in. Today, a multitude of dental devices, or orthodontic appliances, are being used at an early age to simplify later treatment, provide a better outcome, and, in some cases, avoid braces altogether.

Not Just For Looks

Braces are more than the means to a stunning smile; they can improve dental health and function, says Susan Runner, D.D.S., chief of the Dental Devices Branch in the U.S. Food and Drug Administration (FDA)'s Center for Devices and Radiological Health. "They can be used to move teeth that are overcrowding," Runner says. Crowded or crooked teeth are harder to brush and floss, and improper cleaning can lead to tooth decay and other dental problems.

About This Chapter: Information in this chapter is excerpted from "Straight Talk On Braces," *FDA Consumer Magazine*, by Linda Bren, January-February 2005, U.S. Food and Drug Administration.

"Braces can correct severe bite problems that would hamper eating and give a greater risk of gum disease and tooth and bone loss," says Runner. Bite problems may occur when the upper and lower jaw do not come together properly. Uncorrected bite problems can cause teeth to wear down, make for difficult chewing, and put stress on the jawbone, producing pain.

Causes Of Crooked Teeth

Heredity and environmental factors are the two causes of crooked teeth and bite problems, says Terry Pracht, D.D.S., president of the American Association of Orthodontists (AAO) and an orthodontist in Westerville, Ohio. Crowding of teeth, too much space between teeth, and upper teeth that do not match lower teeth when biting down are usually inherited. Also, jaw-jolting accidents, as well as habits such as tongue thrusting and thumb sucking, can cause crooked teeth.

Tongue thrusting is the abnormal tendency to push the tongue onto the back of the front teeth during swallowing, causing the teeth to protrude over time.

♣ **It's A Fact!!**
Most people do not have naturally straight teeth. The American Association of Orthodontists (AAO) estimates that up to 75 percent of people could benefit from orthodontic care.

Thumb sucking is normal in young children and is not an orthodontic problem unless it persists when the permanent teeth come in, says Pracht. "If a child is still thumb sucking at about age 7 when the upper front teeth start to erupt, it can not only affect the teeth, but the shape of the jawbone," he says.

Then And Now

Braces work by putting pressure against the teeth, moving them gradually over time. A metal wire, called an arch wire that runs on the outside of the teeth, applies most of the pressure. "Rubber" bands, actually made from surgical latex, put additional pressure on the teeth that the arch wire alone cannot do.

Earlier types of braces had an arch wire connected to large metal bands that were individually wrapped and cemented around each tooth. "The metal bands were uncomfortable," says Pracht, adding that it used to hurt to have braces put on and adjusted. "There was a lot of pushing and shoving."

Today, the arch wire is attached to tiny brackets made of metal or ceramic. The brackets are bonded with a glue-type agent to the front of the teeth. Some of the bonding agents continuously release fluoride to help protect the enamel of the teeth underneath the brackets. Metal bands may still be used on the back teeth, but they are smaller and lighter than bands used previously.

The arch wire requires periodic adjustment or replacement by the orthodontist to apply continuous pressure. Today's arch wires are active over longer periods of time, meaning patients do not have to visit the orthodontist as often to get their braces adjusted. "It used to be every three to four weeks; now it is every six to eight weeks," says Pracht. Arch wires are much gentler. "There is some sensitivity when eating for only a day or two after an adjustment."

Arch wires now are made from a heat-activated, nickel-titanium mixture originally developed by NASA to activate solar panels of spacecraft in orbit. At room temperature, the wires are very flexible, allowing them to be attached to the teeth more easily. When they warm to mouth temperature, they apply gradual and constant pressure on the teeth.

Today's braces come with more options to make them less obvious; or, if a person chooses, more obvious, with an element of fun and fashion. With colored braces, the colors are mainly on the elastic ties that attach the arch wire to the brackets, and they can be changed when the arch wire is adjusted. Arch wires and rubber bands also come in a variety of hues.

Colored braces are a popular with children and teens, who will often choose the colors of their school, a favorite sports team, or holiday colors, such as pink and red for Valentine's Day and orange and black for Halloween.

For complete invisibility, braces can be fitted onto the inside of the teeth. These "lingual braces" have limitations, says Joondeph. "They can be tougher on a patient. They affect speech more and may irritate the tongue." Treatment times may also be longer than with standard braces, he says, adding that patients should talk with their orthodontists to find out if lingual braces or other options are appropriate for them.

Innovations in materials and designs have brought braces a long way since the "tin-grin" look of the past, but one thing that has not changed significantly is the length of time they are worn. "It is important to move the teeth gradually," says Runner. "If you move the teeth too fast, it can result in severe loosening of the teeth or tooth loss."

Braces, on average, are left on between 20 and 24 months, says Joondeph.

To keep teeth straight after braces are removed, people must wear retainers. These appliances hold the teeth in their corrected position until the bones grow around the teeth to stabilize them. Since teeth tend to shift as a person ages, wearing retainers periodically may be a life-long requirement.

Retainers can be all plastic, or plastic with some metal wire. They are either fixed permanently in the mouth or are removable. Like braces, retainers come in different colors and designs. They can be roof-of-the-mouth pink or personalized with such items as sports team logos, pictures of pets, or a person's or orthodontist's phone number in case of loss.

A Commitment

Having braces or any other orthodontic appliance requires more frequent brushing, flossing, and general care. "Orthodontics is a serious treatment commitment," says Janie Fuller, D.D.S., M.P.H., a regulatory review officer in the FDA's Office of Surveillance and Biometrics.

"If you have poor oral hygiene, you are trading one problem for another," adds Joondeph. "Your bite may be better and your teeth straighter, but there will be significant decay."

People with braces must avoid "hard, sticky, or gooey foods," says Joondeph, such as jawbreakers, peanuts, ice cubes, caramel, and taffy. These foods can break brackets, bend wires, or get caught in the braces, causing cavities.

♣ It's A Fact!!
About 4.5 million people in the United States are wearing braces or other appliances to achieve a beautiful smile and healthy teeth, according to the American Association of Orthodontists (AAO).

Another Straightening Option

An alternative to braces, Invisalign, was cleared by the FDA to straighten crooked teeth in people who have all of their second molars, permanent teeth that usually come in by the late teens. Invisalign uses a series of clear removable aligners instead of wires and brackets. An orthodontist takes impressions of the teeth and sends these models to the maker of Invisalign, Align Technology Inc., of Santa Clara, California. The company uses a computer-generated simulation of the desired movement of the teeth to custom make the aligners for each patient. Each aligner is worn for about two weeks.

The aligners are removable for eating, brushing, and flossing, so unlike people who wear braces, Invisalign-wearers are not restricted from eating hard or chewy foods. They still must visit their orthodontist every six weeks during treatment to ensure proper progress.

The total treatment time with Invisalign averages between nine and 15 months and the average number of aligners worn during treatment is between 18 and 30, according to Align Technology. For some people, a combination of braces and Invisalign is successful, requiring less time in traditional braces.

"They have a place in the spectrum of orthodontic treatments for mild to moderate cases," Joondeph says. "But they cannot give us the sophisticated tooth movement and control of braces."

Appliances For Children

Other orthodontic appliances besides braces are available to help correct a broad range of tooth and jaw problems in growing children, from closing up a gap to widening the jaw to make room for new teeth to grow in properly. Some of these "functional orthodontics" are fixed in place; others are removable for brushing, eating, and sleeping.

Some children require headgear to guide the development of an improperly growing upper jaw. To move the jaw, wires must connect the upper teeth to another fixed point. Since no other teeth are strong enough to serve as a fixed point, headgear is used to anchor the upper teeth to a point outside the mouth: the head or neck. Elastic is wrapped around the top of the head or the back of the neck and connects an arch wire to the upper teeth.

"Make sure the orthodontist demonstrates how to place the device and how to remove it," cautions Fuller. In one case reported to the FDA, a child was blinded in one eye and injured in the other when removing headgear improperly, causing the metal prongs from the mouthpiece to snap back into the child's face in a slingshot-like fashion.

"Never leave the office with headgear, or any other removable appliance, until you have demonstrated to the staff that you know how to remove the device safely and put it back in safely to avoid injury and to optimize treatment," says Fuller.

> ✔ **Quick Tip**
> ## What You Should Take Home From An Orthodontic Consultation
>
> - The reason that treatment is needed
> - The best time for starting treatment
> - The treatment approach that will be used
> - The length of treatment
> - The expected appearance when treatment is completed
> - The success rate with other patients
> - The pros and cons of treatment
> - The treatment cost and payment plan
>
> Source: William J. Trepp, D.D.S. *FDA Consumer Magazine*, January-February 2005, U.S. Food and Drug Administration.

In some cases, a dental implant can replace the need for headgear. The implant contains a screw or pin that is inserted into the jawbone, allowing a post to protrude. The post serves as a point of stabilization to which a tooth-moving appliance is attached.

Functional orthodontics are ineffective after about age 16 for women and after age 18 for men. At these ages, the permanent teeth are in place and the jaw is set, so only braces or jaw surgery can produce straight teeth or a normal bite.

Chapter 33

Preventive Health Care Checkups

You may think that going to the doctor is only for when you are not feeling well, but did you know that it is important to visit the doctor every year? This "while-you're-healthy" visit is called a physical, or a well-child exam, and it is to make sure that your body is on the right track. Some people get nervous when they go to the doctor, but you do not have to be one of them. Here is what to expect.

A nurse will call your name in the waiting room and take you back to the offices. You may bring your parent or caregiver in with you or not. It is your decision. The nurse will weigh and measure your height and write that information in your folder. In this way, your doctor keeps track of how fast you are growing. Then the nurse will take you to a small room where you will wait for the doctor.

When the doctor comes in, she will ask you some general questions about your health and your lifestyle. These could include questions about how much sleep you usually get, how often you exercise, what you are eating, and if you have had any problems. Answer with the truth; your doctor is just trying to find out if you are healthy and happy.

About This Chapter: Information in this chapter is from "What To Expect When You Visit the Doctor," Girl Power, sponsored by the U.S. Department of Health and Human Services, December 2005.

The doctor may also ask if your parents have talked to you about things like puberty, smoking, drugs, and drinking. Now is also a good time to ask any questions you may have.

You can talk about problems seeing the blackboard at school, trouble at home, or anything that may be worrying you, even if you do not think it is health related. Your doctor will most likely be able to help or tell you about someone who can.

✔ Quick Tip
Do not be afraid to ask your doctor questions. Doctors have been asked everything, and there are no stupid or silly questions.

When she is finished talking to you, your doctor will examine your body and take measurements. She will write them down in her chart so she can keep track of your progress over the years. Here are some of the things she will measure:

- **Body temperature:** Your doctor will use a thermometer, usually in your mouth, ear, or under your arm to check your temperature. You may have heard that the normal temperature is 98.6 degrees. Actually, your temperature is normal if it is below 100 degrees Fahrenheit. Anything above 100 degrees means that you have a fever, which is your body's way of fighting infection.

- **Heart and lungs:** A stethoscope is a tool that lets doctors listen. It has a round part that is pressed to your body and tubes going up to ear pieces that the doctor puts in her ear. The doctor will press the stethoscope against your chest in different places to listen to your heart and make sure it is beating correctly. She also may take your pulse (how often your heart beats) by feeling the inside of your wrist or your neck under your jawbone. Then she will press it against your back and ask you to take some deep breaths so she can listen to your lungs.

- **Blood pressure:** To measure how hard your heart pumps blood through your body, your doctor will use a sphygmomanometer (pronounced sfig'-mo-ma-nom-e-ter), which has a cuff that goes around your arm, a dial, a pump, and a valve. The doctor will pump up the cuff, which will feel tight, and place the stethoscope under the cuff to listen. She will then let the air out and look at the dial while listening to your arm. The measurement will be two numbers, like "130 over 80."

- **Reflexes:** You may remember something like this from your toy doctor sets. To test reflexes, your doctor will use a little rubber hammer to tap your joints at the knees and elbows. Your arms and legs will jerk out; this is a good thing. It means that your brain is sending signals to your arms and legs, and the arms and legs are getting them.

- **Eyes, ears, nose, and throat:** To make sure that everything is okay and there is no irritation, your doctor will shine a light into your eyes, ears, nose, and throat. It may seem strange that someone wants to look up your nose, but it is important.

- **Genital exam:** Your doctor will look between your legs to make sure that you are developing okay. You may feel strange about this, but it is normal, so you do not need to be embarrassed.

- **Spine:** By feeling along your back while you bend over, your doctor can check to make sure your spine is straight. If your spine is curved, it may mean that you have scoliosis, which is a side-to-side curve in the spine that cannot be corrected just by standing up straight.

- **Hearing tests:** You will be asked to wear headphones and listen to some noises, some high pitched and some low pitched. Your doctor will ask you to raise your hand when you can hear a sound. It is okay to not hear every sound, but your doctor needs to know what you can hear so next time, she can check to make sure you can still hear as well.

- **Immunizations:** You probably got most of your shots when you were too young to remember. You may need boosters to keep the protection strong, but you will not need them every year.

- **Vision screening:** There will be a chart on the wall with different-sized letters. Your doctor will ask you to cover one eye and read the chart, and then do the same with the other eye. If you have trouble, you may be sent to a special eye doctor to be tested for glasses.

- **Blood tests:** The doctor may want to check your blood every once in a while, though not every time, to make sure nothing is wrong. She will use a needle to take blood out of your arm or finger. Do not worry about losing the blood; it is only a little bit compared to how much is in your body, and the initial prick may sting a little. Your body will make more blood to fill you back up.

Going to the doctor is not only necessary to stay healthy; it is also a good way to learn about your body. You can ask your doctor questions about how your body works, or how she measures things about your body. It is important for you to know about your body and what is normal for it, so you can tell if something is wrong.

Chapter 34

Your First Gynecological Visit

Going to the doctor's office for an annual gynecological examination is not exactly something that women eagerly anticipate; and if you add in the fact that it is a young woman's first gynecological exam, that heightens anxiety even more.

What To Do Before The Exam

Many times, young women wonder what the exam itself is like. "The most important piece of information you can give to young women to put them more at ease about this exam is that it does not hurt," says Karen Nichols, D.O., an osteopathic internist in Arizona. "They also should know that they have the right to ask for explanations of procedures at any point during the exam." Because the exam can be a bit intimidating, women may forget some of the questions they had intended to ask their physicians. Dr. Nichols suggests that women write down their questions and bring that list to the appointment.

She encourages patients to ask about anything, even embarrassing or uncomfortable issues, because such matters are probably the most important ones to address. "When dealing with your health, no question can be considered stupid," Dr. Nichols stresses.

About This Chapter: Information in this chapter is from "My First Gynecological Visit." Reprinted with the consent of the American Osteopathic Association. © American Osteopathic Association. Available online at http://www.osteopathic.org. Accessed March 22, 2006.

During the appointment, it is important that women be ready with information about their family medical history, especially patterns of breast disease or cancers of the reproductive organs. In addition to inquiring about the family, the physician will ask questions about personal health. Among the most common questions are the following:

- At what age did you start menstruating?

- When did your last period start?

- On what date did your last period begin?

- How long does your period usually last?

- Do you tend to have a light, medium, or heavy flow?

- How many pads or tampons do you use the first day of your period?

When To Schedule A Visit

Dr. Nichols emphasizes a few points to keep in mind when scheduling a gynecological exam. First of all, young women should get this exam when they become sexually active or reach age 18, whichever comes first. Also, women need to remember to make an appointment when they will be in between their menstrual cycles. A Pap smear cannot be done during the menstrual period because the blood covers up the cells the physician needs to examine. The Pap smear is important because it can detect pre-cancerous and cancerous cells in the cervix.

Women should immediately make an appointment if they experience any of the following problems:

- Severe pain in the abdomen or pelvis

- Unusual pain in the vagina

- Unusual discharge, itching, or bumps in or around the vagina

- Exposure to a sexually transmitted disease (STD)

- Severe pain during periods or irregular periods

- Breast discharge, changes in breast size, or changes in the skin of the breast

- Pain during intercourse

It's Exam Day—What Can You Expect?

The exam consists of a variety of steps. First, you sit down with the physician and talk about your medical history, both personal and family. During this time, you can also bring up any questions you may have about birth control, sexually transmitted diseases (STDs), menstruation, or other issues.

Carol Henwood, D.O., an osteopathic family physician in Pennsylvania, encourages open dialogue with her patients. In fact, when she sees patients for their first gynecological visit, she sits down with them to remind them that she was once in the very same position, and she understands that they are scared. "While they view it as a scary situation, I tell my patients the gynecological exam is a necessity to ensure their health," says Dr. Henwood. "Also, I make sure they have all the sexual health information they need, especially if they are sexually active."

The next step is that you change into an examination gown. Usually, you will be given a sheet to drape over yourself as well. When the physician returns to the room, he or she will perform a breast exam to look for lumps that may be a sign of cancer. If you have never done a self-exam, the physician can show you how to do it and tell you what to look for.

Dr. Henwood strongly recommends performing self-examinations on a monthly basis. She adds that the best time for a self-exam is about 10 days after your period.

According to the American Cancer Society, breast cancer is the second leading cause of cancer deaths among women. In the next year, an estimated 203,000 new cases of invasive breast cancer will be diagnosed. Women over the age of 20 should get a clinical breast exam performed by a physician or a nurse every year and should perform a self-exam every month.

The Dreaded Pelvic Exam

Next comes that part that you probably have been dreading the most—the pelvic exam. Dr. Henwood makes it a point to explain this procedure beforehand, as well as during the exam. However, if your physician does not provide explanations, and you want some answers, just ask. At this point, you will be instructed to slide to the end of the table and place your feet into stirrups. Staying relaxed is very important because you will be more comfortable, and the exam can be more complete.

The first step in the pelvic exam is for the physician to examine the external genital area for any signs of irritation, discharge, cysts, genital warts, or other problems. Next, the physician inserts a speculum. This instrument, which is made of metal or plastic, is used to separate the walls of the vagina. Once placed inside, it is opened up so that the doctor can examine the cervix and the vaginal walls.

☞ **Remember!!**
If you are at risk for any STDs, you need to tell your physician up front.

If you need to be tested for any STDs, the physician will collect cervical mucus on a cotton swab.

"It is so important for patients to be honest about their sex lives and their risk for contracting STDs," stresses Dr. Henwood. "For instance, human papilloma virus (HPV), more commonly known as genital warts, causes 95 percent of cervical cancers."

The American Cancer Society estimated that, in the year 2002, 13,000 new cases of invasive cervical cancer would be diagnosed and approximately 4,000 women would succumb to this disease.

If tests do not need to be conducted for STDs, a Pap smear will be done. This involves using a small brush or spatula to collect cells from the cervix. This test can detect the presence of pre-cancerous or cancerous cells, infections of the cervix, and thinning of the vaginal walls due to lack of estrogen.

With the speculum now removed, you have reached the halfway point of the exam. Next, the doctor inserts gloved fingers into the vagina while pressing on your abdomen to examine your internal organs—the uterus, the fallopian tubes, and the ovaries.

Lastly, the physician will insert a gloved finger into the rectum to check the condition of the muscles in between the vagina and the rectum. Sometimes the doctor will have one finger in the rectum and one in the vagina for a more thorough exam.

When that test is completed, you will have successfully completed your first gynecological examination. Results from the Pap smear are usually ready in 7–10 working days. If the results come back normal, you will not need another exam until the next year. If the results are abnormal, your physician will schedule you for follow-up exams and possibly advise you about other treatments.

Knowing what to expect during the first gynecological exam can alleviate many anxieties young women have. Not only does this exam provide an opportunity to catch health problems in their early stages, it is also an opportunity to learn about ways to maintain good gynecological health.

♣ It's A Fact!!
Did You Know...?

- The best time for a gynecological exam is one week after your menstrual cycle.

- Women should not douche or use vaginal creams for at least 72 hours before the exam.

- For 24 percent of women, the gynecological exam is the only regular exam they undergo.

- Every three minutes, a woman in the United States is diagnosed with breast cancer.

- After the age of 20, women should perform a self-breast exam every month.

- Ovarian cancer accounts for nearly four percent of all cancers among women with an estimated 23,000 new cases diagnosed in the United States in 2002.

Chapter 35

Testicular Exams

Medical exams, whether they are for school, a sport, or camp, are usually pretty straightforward. Many parts of the exam make sense to most guys. The scale is used to weigh you, and the stethoscope is used to listen to your heartbeat.

But why does the doctor need to touch and feel your testicles? What could be going on down there, and isn't there a better, less embarrassing way for him or her to check things out?

When you are healthy and going for a physical exam, the doctor is interested in finding out specific things about your body and your health. He or she will check your height and weight and take your blood pressure. You will have your heart listened to, and you may be asked to breathe deeply or cough, so the doctor can hear sounds or problems with your lungs. He or she will examine your eyes, ears, nose, and throat; test your reflexes by tapping your knees and ankles; and take your temperature. For all these parts of the exam, the doctor relies on tools and equipment to get the information that is needed.

About This Chapter: Information in this chapter is from "Why Do I Need Testicular Exams?" This information was provided by TeensHealth, one of the largest resources online for medically reviewed health information written for parents, kids, and teens. For more articles like this one, visit www.TeensHealth.org, or www.KidsHealth.org. © 2004 The Nemours Foundation.

However, for other parts of your body, the doctor must rely on his or her sense of touch and training in knowing how things should feel. During the physical, the doctor will touch your belly to feel for any problems with your liver or spleen. He or she will feel the lymph nodes in your neck, armpits, and groin to detect if there is any swelling, which can indicate an infection or other problem. And he or she will also need to feel the testicles and the area around them to detect two important things: a hernia or a tumor.

Hernias

A hernia can occur when a part of the intestine pushes out from the abdomen and into the groin or scrotum (the sac of skin that the testicles hang in). Some people believe that this can only happen when a person lifts something heavy, but usually this is not the case. Most hernias occur because of a weakness in the abdominal wall that the person was born with. If a piece of intestine becomes trapped in the scrotum, it can cut off the blood supply to the intestine and cause serious problems if the situation is not quickly corrected.

A doctor is able to feel for a hernia by using his or her fingers to examine the area around the groin and testicles. The doctor may ask you to cough while he or she is pressing on, or feeling the area. Sometimes, the hernia causes a bulge that the doctor can detect; if this happens, surgery almost always repairs the hernia completely.

Testicular Cancer

Although testicular cancer is unusual in teen guys (it occurs in 3 out of 100,000 guys between the ages of 15 and 19 in the United States), it is the second most common cancer seen during the teen years. It is the most common cancer in guys 20 to 34 years of age. Comedian Tom Green and Tour de France champion bicyclist Lance Armstrong have both successfully won recent battles with testicular cancer.

It is very important that your doctor examines your testicles at least once a year. When examining your testicles, your doctor will grasp one testicle at a time, rolling it gently between his or her thumb and first finger. He or she will feel for lumps and also pay attention to whether the testicle is hardened or enlarged. The doctor will explain how to do testicular self-exams.

If you are a teen guy, learning how to examine yourself at least once a month for any lumps or bumps on your testicles is very important. A tumor (growth or bump) on the testicles could be cancer. Knowing how your testicles feel when they are healthy will help you know when something feels different and possibly abnormal down there.

Finally, keep in mind that even though it might feel weird to have a doctor checking out your testicles, it is no big deal to him or her. Sometimes when a doctor is examining that area, you might get an erection, something you cannot control. This is a normal reaction that happens frequently during genital exams on guys. If it happens, it will not upset or bother the doctor, so there is no need to feel embarrassed.

> ## ♣ It's A Fact!!
>
> Noticing any new testicular lumps or bumps as soon as possible gives the best chances for survival and total cure if it turns out to be cancer.

Chapter 36

All About Vaccines

Why do we need vaccines?

Vaccines save lives by protecting us against infectious diseases like measles, mumps, and whooping cough.

How do vaccines work?

When you receive a vaccine it helps your body create antibodies. Antibodies are your body's defensive cells that fight off germs. Sometimes your body can create antibodies on its own, but the diseases you get vaccines for are very dangerous. Most people get very sick and some die before enough antibodies are produced.

What are some of the infectious diseases vaccines offer protection from?

Hib: This vaccine protects us from the *Haemophilus influenzae* type b bacteria that cause meningitis.

Meningitis is an inflammation of the cover that surrounds the brain and can cause brain damage. Also, these bacteria can infect the blood, joints, bones, muscles, throat, and the cover surrounding the heart. This is especially dangerous for babies.

About This Chapter: Information in this chapter is excerpted from "All About Vaccines," *FDA & You*, Issue #4, Fall 2004, U.S. Food and Drug Administration.

Diphtheria Tetanus Pertussis (DTP): Diphtheria is an infection that attacks the throat, mouth, and nose. This is a very contagious disease, but rare ever since the vaccine was created. Diphtheria can form a gray web that may completely cover the windpipe and can prevent breathing.

If this disease is not treated right away it could cause pneumonia, heart failure, or paralysis.

Tetanus is an infection caused by a bacteria found in dirt, gravel, and rusty metal. It usually enters the body through a cut. Tetanus bacteria cause the muscles to move suddenly and sometimes uncontrollably. If tetanus attacks the jaw muscles, it causes lockjaw, the inability to open and close your mouth. Tetanus can also cause the breathing muscles to spasm and can be deadly.

You may know pertussis by its more common name, whooping cough. Pertussis is a bacteria that clogs the lungs with a thick, slimy mucous. This can cause a severe cough that sounds like a "whoop." The cough can last for two months and allows for other bacteria such as pneumonia and bronchitis to attack the body.

♣ It's A Fact!!

Edward Jenner laid the foundation for modern vaccines by discovering one of the basic principles of immunization. He had used a relatively harmless microbe, cowpox virus, to bring about an immune response that would help protect people from getting infected by the related but deadly smallpox virus.

Dr. Jenner's discovery helped researchers find ways to ease human disease suffering worldwide. By the beginning of the 20th century, doctors were immunizing patients with vaccines for diphtheria, typhoid fever, and smallpox.

Source: Excerpted from "MICROBES in Sickness and in Health," National Institute of Allergy and Infectious Diseases, National Institutes of Health, July 2002.

Polio: Polio can paralyze the legs and chest making walking and breathing difficult or impossible. The first symptoms of polio are fever, sore throat, headache, and a stiff neck. Polio is very rare since the vaccine became available.

MMR: The first M in MMR stands for measles. Measles is a highly contagious disease that causes a high fever, cough, and a spotty rash all over. It may also cause ear infections and pneumonia.

The second M in MMR stands for mumps. Mumps causes painful swollen salivary glands, which are under the jaw, as well as a fever and a headache. Mumps also may cause meningitis or hearing loss.

The R in MMR stands for rubella. Rubella is also called German measles. It is most dangerous for women who are pregnant. Rubella can cause a mother to have a miscarriage or deliver a baby with heart disease, blindness, hearing loss, or learning problems.

Rubella is a mild disease in kids.

Hepatitis B: Hepatitis B causes extreme tiredness and jaundice. Jaundice is when all the white parts on your body, like your eyes, teeth, and nails, turn yellow. Hepatitis B may also cause the liver to stop working.

Chicken Pox: Chicken pox is a virus. It causes an itchy rash and a fever. You can catch it from someone who already has it if you touch an open blister on that person's skin or if that person sneezes or coughs around you. Not everyone gets the vaccine, so lots of kids still get chicken pox.

Hepatitis A: A serious liver disease caused by the hepatitis A virus (HAV).

Meningococcal: Meningococcal disease is an illness caused by bacteria. Meningitis is an infection of the brain and spinal cord coverings that can also cause blood infections.

Rabies: Rabies infection is serious, and often fatal, if it is not prevented. Vaccination induces active immunity against rabies virus either before (pre-exposure immunization) an exposure occurs or after (post-exposure prophylaxis) an exposure. Rabies shots need to be given as soon as possible after a bite has occurred, before symptoms appear.

Pneumococcal: Streptococcus pneumonia bacteria can cause serious illness and death—approximately 200 deaths each year among children under 5 years old. The pneumococcal vaccine helps prevent pneumococcal disease.

Influenza: Influenza is a virus that infects the respiratory tract that can cause severe illness and life-threatening complications in many people. The flu kills an estimated 36,000 people and causes more than 200,000 hospitalizations per year in the United States. Annual flu vaccination is the best way to reduce the chances that you will get the flu.

> **✔ Quick Tip**
>
> More people travel all over the world today. So, finding out which immunizations are recommended for travel to your destination(s) is even more important than ever. Vaccines can prevent yellow fever, polio, typhoid fever, hepatitis A, cholera, rabies, and other bacterial and viral diseases that are more prevalent abroad than in the United States.
>
> Source: Excerpted from "MICROBES in Sickness and in Health," National Institute of Allergy and Infectious Diseases, National Institutes of Health, July 2002.

Abbreviated Notes for Figure 36.1

The following comments, which focus on items of concern to teens, are excerpted from the complete notes to the Recommended Childhood and Adolescent Immunization Schedule. (The full text can be found online at http://www.cdc.gov/NIP/recs/child-schedule.htm.)

2. **Diphtheria and tetanus toxoids and acellular pertussis vaccine (DTaP).** Adolescents 13–18 years who missed the 11–12-year Td/Tdap booster dose should receive a single dose of Tdap if they have completed the recommended childhood DTP/DTaP vaccination series. Subsequent **tetanus and diphtheria toxoids (Td)** are recommended every 10 years.

4. **Measles, mumps, and rubella vaccine (MMR).** Those who have not previously received the second dose should complete the schedule by age 11–12 years.

5. **Varicella vaccine.** Susceptible persons (those who lack a reliable history of chickenpox or previously completed vaccination) aged 13 years and older should receive 2 doses administered at least 4 weeks apart.

Vaccine ▼ Age ▶	Birth	1 month	2 months	4 months	6 months	12 months	15 months	18 months	24 months	4-6 years	11-12 years	13-14 years	15 years	16-18 years
Hepatitis B[1]	HepB	HepB	HepB	HepB[1]	HepB						HepB Series			
Diphtheria, Tetanus, Pertussis[2]			DTaP	DTaP	DTaP		DTaP	DTaP		DTaP	Tdap		Tdap	
Haemophilus influenzae type b[3]			Hib	Hib	Hib[3]	Hib	Hib							
Inactivated Poliovirus			IPV	IPV	IPV	IPV	IPV			IPV				
Measles, Mumps, Rubella[4]						MMR	MMR			MMR	MMR			
Varicella[5]						Varicella	Varicella				Varicella			
Meningococcal[6]									MPSV4		MCV4		MCV4	MCV4
Pneumococcal[7]			PCV	PCV	PCV	PCV	PCV		PCV		PPV			
Influenza[8]					Influenza (Yearly)	Influenza (Yearly)					Influenza (Yearly)			
Hepatitis A[9]									HepA Series					

Vaccines within broken line are for selected populations

This schedule indicates the recommended ages for routine administration of currently licensed childhood vaccines, as of December 1, 2005, for children through age 18 years. Any dose not administered at the recommended age should be administered at any subsequent visit when indicated and feasible. ▆ Indicates age groups that warrant special effort to administer those vaccines not previously administered. Additional vaccines may be licensed and recommended during the year. Licensed combination vaccines may be used whenever any components of the combination are indicated and other components of the vaccine are not contraindicated and if approved by the Food and Drug Administration for that dose of the series. Providers should consult the respective ACIP statement for detailed recommendations. Clinically significant adverse events that follow immunization should be reported to the Vaccine Adverse Event Reporting System (VAERS). Guidance about how to obtain and complete a VAERS form is available at www.vaers.hhs.gov or by telephone, **800-822-7967.**

▨ Range of recommended ages   ▆ Catch-up immunization   ▨ 11-12 year old assessment

Figure 36.1. Recommended Childhood and Adolescent Immunization Schedule, United States, 2006 (Centers for Disease Control and Prevention).

CATCH-UP SCHEDULE FOR CHILDREN AGED 7 YEARS THROUGH 18 YEARS			
	Minimum Interval Between Doses		
Vaccine	Dose 1 to Dose 2	Dose 2 to Dose 3	Dose 3 to Booster Dose
Tetanus, Diphtheria[8]	4 weeks	6 months	**6 months** if first dose given at age <12 months and current age <11 years; otherwise **5 years**
Inactivated Poliovirus[9]	4 weeks	4 weeks	IPV[2,9]
Hepatitis B	4 weeks	8 weeks (and 16 weeks after first dose)	
Measles, Mumps, Rubella	4 weeks		
Varicella[10]	4 weeks		

Figure 36.2. Recommended Immunization Schedule for Children and Adolescents Who Start Late or Who Are More Than 1 Month Behind. This table gives a catch-up schedule and minimum intervals between doses for children who have delayed immunizations. There is no need to restart a vaccine series regardless of the time that has elapsed between doses.

6. **Meningococcal vaccine (MCV4).** Meningococcal conjugate vaccine (MCV4) should be given to all children at the 11–12 year-old visit as well as to unvaccinated adolescents at high school entry (15 years of age). Other adolescents who wish to decrease their risk for meningococcal disease may also be vaccinated. All college freshmen living in dormitories should also be vaccinated, preferably with MCV4, although **meningococcal polysaccharide vaccine (MPSV4)** is an acceptable alternative.

8. **Influenza vaccine.** Influenza vaccine is recommended annually for children aged 6 or older months with certain risk factors (including, but not limited to, asthma, cardiac disease, sickle cell disease, human immunodeficiency virus [HIV], diabetes, and conditions that can compromise respiratory function or handling of respiratory secretions or that can increase the risk for aspiration) or in close contact with persons in groups at high risk. For healthy persons aged 5–49 years, the intranasally administered, live, attenuated influenza vaccine (LAIV) is an acceptable alternative to the intramuscular trivalent inactivated influenza vaccine (TIV). Children aged 8 years or younger who are receiving influenza vaccine for the first time should receive 2 doses (separated by at least 4 weeks for TIV and at least 6 weeks for LAIV).

9. **Hepatitis A vaccine (HepA).** HepA is recommended for all children at 1 year of age (i.e., 12–23 months). The 2 doses in the series should be administered at least 6 months apart. States, counties, and communities with existing HepA vaccination programs for children 2–18 years of age are encouraged to maintain these programs. In these areas, new efforts focused on routine vaccination of 1 year-old children should enhance, not replace, ongoing programs directed at a broader population of children.

Abbreviated Notes for Figure 36.2

8. **Td.** Adolescent tetanus, diphtheria, and pertussis vaccine (Tdap) may be substituted for any dose in a primary catch-up series or as a booster if age appropriate for Tdap. A five-year interval from the last Td dose is encouraged when Tdap is used as a booster dose. See Advisory Committee on Immunization Practices (ACIP) recommendations for further information (http://www.cdc.gov/nip/acip).

9. **IPV.** Vaccine is not generally recommended for persons aged 18 years or older.

10. **Varicella.** Administer the 2-dose series to all susceptible adolescents aged 13 years or older.

For additional information about vaccines, including precautions and contraindications for immunization and vaccine shortages, please visit the National Immunization Program Website at www.cdc.gov/nip or contact 800-CDC-INFO (800-232-4636). (In English, En Español—24/7).

> ✔ **Quick Tip**
> Report adverse reactions to vaccines through the federal Vaccine Adverse Event Reporting System. For information on reporting reactions following immunization, please visit www.vaers.hhs.gov or call the 24-hour national toll-free information line 800-822-7967.

Part Five

How To Maintain Mental And Emotional Wellness

Chapter 37

Handling Stress

What is stress?

Stress is what you feel when you react to pressure from others or from yourself. Pressure can come from anywhere, including school, work, activities, friends, and family members. You can also feel stress from the pressure of wanting to get good grades or wanting to feel like you belong. Stress comes in many forms and everyone feels stress.

How does my body handle stress?

Your body has a built-in response to handle stress. When something stressful happens, you may experience sweaty palms, dry mouth, or knots in your stomach. This is totally normal and means that your body is working exactly as it should. Other signs of stress include emotional signs such as feeling sad or worried, behavioral (your actions) signs such as not feeling up to doing things, and mental (your mind) signs such as not being able to concentrate or focus.

What causes stress?

Just being a teen can be stressful. There is so much going on and so many changes that are happening all at once.

About This Chapter: Information in this chapter is from "Handling Stress," GirlsHealth.gov, sponsored by The National Women's Health Information Center, U.S. Department of Health and Human Services, Office on Women's Health, March 2006.

The following are some things that might cause stress:

- Schoolwork

- Not feeling good about yourself

- Changes in your body or weight

- Body shape or size

- Problems with friends, boyfriends, or other kids at school

- Living in a dangerous neighborhood

- Peer pressure from friends to dress or act a certain way, or smoke, drink, or use drugs

- Not fitting in or being part of a group

- Moving or friends moving away

- Separation or divorce of parents

- A family member who is ill

- Death of a loved one

- Changing schools

- Taking on too many activities at once

- Not getting along with your parents or having problems at home

- Feeling lonely

There may be other things that cause stress for you that are not on this list. Also, it can be very tough when more than one stressful event happens at the same time or stress is ongoing.

Is stress always a bad thing?

No. A little bit of stress can work in a positive way. For instance, during a sports competition, stress might push you to perform better. Also, without the stress of deadlines, you might not be able to finish schoolwork or get to where you need to be on time.

What are signs that you have too much stress or are stressed out?

The following are signs that you are stressed out:

- Feeling down, edgy, guilty, or tired

- Having headaches or stomachaches

- Having trouble sleeping

- Laughing or crying for no reason

- Blaming others for bad things that happen to you

- Wanting to be alone all the time (withdrawal)

- Not being able to see the positive side of a situation

- Not enjoying activities that you used to enjoy

- Feeling resentful of people or things you have to do

- Feeling like you have too many things you need to do

Are you stressed about your body?

During adolescence, your body is going through many changes that are happening at a fast pace. These changes might make you feel unsure of yourself at times, or stressed. They might make you worry about your size and wanting to fit in with the rest of the crowd.

During puberty, not only will you get taller, you will also see other changes in your body such as wider hips, bottoms, and thighs. Because your body is starting to produce new hormones (like estrogen), your weight may change and your body, which has both muscle and fat, will also start to have more fat compared to muscle than it did before. Changes in estrogen levels can also cause mood swings, especially around your period.

Try not to worry. Each woman changes at her own pace, and all of these new changes are normal. While you are experiencing these changes keep your self- confidence up by taking good care of yourself, eating healthy foods, and getting regular exercise. Remember, you are unique and beautiful just as you are.

✔ Quick Tip
Tips For Dealing With Stress

Put your body in motion. Moving from the chair to the couch while watching TV is not being physically active. Physical activity is one of the most important ways to keep stress away by clearing your head and lifting your spirits. Physical activity also increases endorphin levels, the natural "feel-good" chemicals in the body that leave you with a naturally happy feeling.

Fuel up. If your body were a car, you would not go for a long drive without filling up the gas tank first. Likewise, begin each day by eating breakfast to give you the energy you need to tackle the day. Eat regular meals and take time to enjoy them. Make sure to fuel up with fruits, vegetables, proteins (peanut butter, a chicken sandwich, or a tuna salad) and grains (wheat bread, pasta, or some crackers). These will give you the power you need to make it through those hectic days. Do not be fooled by the jolt of energy you get from sodas and sugary snacks. This only lasts a short time, and once it wears off, you may feel sluggish and more tired than usual. For that extra boost of energy to sail through history notes, math class, and after school activities, grab a banana, some string cheese, or a granola bar for some power-packed energy.

LOL (Laugh out loud). Some say that laughter is the best medicine. In many cases, it is. Did you know that it takes 15 facial muscles to laugh? Lots of laughing can make you feel good; and that good feeling can stay with you even after the laughter stops. So, head off stress with regular doses of laughter by watching a funny movie or cartoons, reading a joke book (you may even learn some new jokes), or even make up your own riddles. Laughter can make you feel like a new person.

Have fun with friends. Being with people you like is always a good way to ditch your stress. Get a group together to go to the movies, shoot some hoops, listen to music, play a board game, or just hang out and talk. Friends can help you work through your problems and let you see the brighter side of things.

Spill to someone you trust. Instead of keeping your feelings bottled up inside, talk to someone you trust or respect about what is bothering you. It could be a friend, a parent, a friend's parent, someone in your family or from your religious community, or a teacher. Talking out your problems and seeing them from a different view might help you figure out ways to deal with them. Just remember, you do not have to go at it alone.

Take time to chill. Pick a comfy spot to sit and read, daydream, or even take a snooze. Listen to your favorite music. Work on a relaxing project like putting together a puzzle or making jewelry.

Get some sleep. Fatigue is a best friend to stress. When you do not get enough sleep, it is hard to deal with things. When you are overtired, a problem may seem much bigger than it actually is. You may have a hard time doing a school assignment that usually seems easy, you do not do your best in sports or any physical activity, or you may have an argument with your friends over something really stupid. Most teens need between 8.5 and just over 9 hours of sleep each night. Because your body (and mind) is changing and developing, it requires more sleep to re-charge for the next day. So do not resist, and get some sleep.

Keep a journal. If you are having one of those crazy days when nothing goes right, it is a good idea to write things down in a journal to get it off your chest—like how you feel, what is going on in your life, and things you would like to accomplish. You could even write down what you do when you are faced with a stressful situation, and then look back and think about how you handled it. So, find a quiet spot, grab a notebook and pen, and start writing.

Get it together. Too much to do but not enough time? Forgot your homework? Feeling overwhelmed or forgetful? Being unprepared for school, practice, or other activities can make for a very stressful day.

Getting everything done can be a challenge, but all you have to do is plan a little and get organized.

Lend a hand. Get involved in an activity that helps others. It is almost impossible to feel stressed out when you are helping someone else. It is also a great way to find out about yourself and the special talents you never knew you had.

Learn ways to better deal with anger. It is totally normal to be angry sometimes. Everyone gets mad at some point. And as a teen, the changing hormones in your body can cause you to feel mad for what seems like no good reason sometimes. The important thing is to deal with your anger in a healthy way. It will help to cool down first, and then focus on positive solutions to problems. This will help you to communicate better with the people in your life, and you can even earn more respect along the way.

Source: From "11 Tips for Dealing with Stress," GirlsHealth.gov, March 2006.

What are ways you can handle stress?

Different things stress different people. Here are some examples:

- You might get upset or stressed when you do not make good grades, but your friend might not.

- You might be able to handle doing homework and being involved in after-school activities, but your sister or friend might feel they cannot do both.

- Your friend might see moving to a new house as a stress, but you might view it as an adventure.

There are no right or wrong things to stress over. There are just differences in what we consider to be stressful. No matter what stresses you out, there are many things you can try to help you deal with it.

Can stress lead to more serious problems?

Yes. Struggling with major stress and low self-esteem issues can contribute to more serious problems such as eating disorders, hurting yourself, depression, alcohol and drug abuse, and even suicide. Continued depression and thoughts about hurting or killing yourself are signs that it is time to seek help. Talk to an adult you trust right away.

Chapter 38

Dealing With Depression

As a teenager, there are so many changes taking place in your body and with your emotions that it can be very overwhelming. You might feel like you are in a great mood one minute and a bad one the next. This roller coaster of emotions is normal. It is okay to have the blues sometimes, and there are things you can do to feel better. Try these tips to improve your mood:

- Know that what you are going through is very common.

- Find a way to relax, such as sitting down and taking a deep breath or taking a shower.

- Talk to your friends, parents/guardians, teachers, counselors, or doctors about what you are feeling. They can help you sort through your emotions.

- Get some exercise. When you exercise, your body makes more special chemicals called endorphins. Endorphins can help improve your mood.

- Make sure that you get enough rest. Being tired can make you feel more stressed.

There is a big difference between having the blues and having depression. Depression is a serious illness that affects many young people. The good news is that depression can be treated.

About This Chapter: Information in this chapter is from "Depression or Feeling Blue," GirlsHealth.gov, sponsored by The National Women's Health Information Center, U.S. Department of Health and Human Services, Office on Women's Health, March 2006.

♣ It's A Fact!!
Treatment Options

There are two common types of treatment for depression—medicine and talk therapy. Ask your doctor which type is best for you. Some people need both treatments to feel better.

Medicine: Medicines for depression are called antidepressants. Your regular doctor or a psychiatrist (a medical doctor trained in helping people with depression) can prescribe them for you.

Antidepressants may take a few weeks to work. Be sure to tell the doctor how you are feeling. If you are not feeling better, you may need to try different medicines to find out what works best for you.

Medicines sometimes cause unwanted side effects. You may feel tired, have blurred vision, or feel sick to your stomach. Tell the doctor if you have these or any other side effects.

Talk Therapy: Talk therapy involves talking to someone such as a psychologist, social worker, or counselor. It helps you learn to change how depression makes you think, feel, and act. Ask your doctor or psychiatrist whom you should go to for talk therapy.

Source: Excerpted from *Stories of Depression: Does this sound like you?* National Institute of Mental Health, National Institutes of Health, U.S. Department of Health and Human Services, November 2002.

How will I know if I have depression?

While some signs of depression can seem a lot like just having the blues, there is a way to know if you need to talk to your doctor about depression. See your doctor about depression if you have five or more of the following symptoms for at least two weeks, or any one of these symptoms gets in the way of school or family life:

- Sadness or crying that you cannot explain

- Major changes in the way you eat, such as not eating or overeating

- Being crabby, angry, worried, or nervous

- Feeling negative or not caring about anything

- Feeling guilty or worthless

- Thinking about death or committing suicide

- Sleep changes, such as sleeping more or having trouble sleeping

- Not being able to focus or make a decision

- Not being able to enjoy the things you usually enjoy

- Not wanting to spend time with your friends

- Feeling restless or tired most of the time

✔ Quick Tip

Make sure to talk to your doctor or school counselor about any worries you have about depression.

Source: GirlsHealth.gov.

If your doctor decides that you do have depression, there are many ways it can be treated. The important thing is to get help.

Chapter 39

Eating Disorders

What Are Eating Disorders?

Eating disorders are extreme expressions of food and weight issues experienced by many individuals, particularly girls and women. They include anorexia nervosa, bulimia nervosa, and binge eating. Eating disorders are dangerous behaviors that result in big health problems.

Girls with eating disorders can do major damage to their bodies. Restricting what you eat can make you sick like feeling nauseous, tired, dizzy, or irritable. If this behavior goes on too long, it can mess up your menstrual cycle, dry out your hair and skin, and might even cause early osteoporosis, a disease of the bones. The physical consequences can become life threatening.

The physical problems are only half the story. The emotional problems can be serious too. An unhealthy attitude about food and body image is the main problem. Some girls use food to make themselves feel better; others stop eating to feel like they are in control of their life. Both behaviors leave people feeling bad about what they are eating; and worst of all, the more people begin to obsess over what they are eating (or not eating), the less they care about other things like school, friends, or other activities.

About This Chapter: Information in this chapter is from "What Are Eating Disorders," "Anorexia Nervosa," "Bulimia Nervosa," and "Binge Eating Disorder," Girl Power, sponsored by the U.S. Department of Health and Human Services, December 2005.

How Do People Get Eating Disorders

Experts do not know exactly how people develop eating disorders, but it is likely the result of many factors. Many people who suffer from eating disorders—a fear of becoming fat, feelings of not measuring up to other people's expectations, or feeling helpless. Some people with eating disorders feel they have to be perfect in every way—having a perfect body, getting perfect grades, and being an excellent athlete. People who suffer from eating disorders may be depressed or feel they lack control over their lives. Sometimes, they also feel like they do not fit in or do not belong. Often, the problems begin when a person is dealing with a difficult transition, shock, or loss.

Girls often experiment with different ways to lose as much weight as possible or to keep their weight down. Here are some examples of unsafe methods girls use to control their weight:

- **Diuretics** (or water pills) make your body lose water but also important nutrients. In extreme cases, this can cause heart problems.

- **Laxatives** can cause stomachaches and cramps as well as other serious problems to your digestive system. Laxatives can become habit-forming.

- **Self-induced vomiting**, even once in a while, can pop blood vessels in your face and swell up your neck glands. Because your food is not being digested right, you may suffer stomachaches, constipation, heartburn, or diarrhea. Also, repeated vomiting can ruin your teeth and give you cavities.

- **Diet pills** can cause your heart to beat faster and make you jittery. They also are habit-forming. Once they wear off, you become hungry and want to eat, so you reach for another pill to control your appetite.

- **Serious over exercising** is another unhealthy way some people control their weight. Exercising for long periods of time when it is not part of a program (like with your school coach) is not smart. Over exercising will make you feel tired and increase your chance of injuries.

Anorexia Nervosa: The Relentless Pursuit Of Thinness

People who suffer from this disorder have an intense and irrational fear of gaining weight because they see themselves as being fat, even when everyone else does not. Anorexics feel that they are heavier than the rest of the people around them and want to do something about it. They feel the need to become thinner and thinner, and the quickest way to lose weight is to not eat at all. Food, calories, and body weight take control of the person's life. Anorexics often become isolated; they stop seeing friends and having fun.

Cindy's Story

Cindy was 12 when she developed anorexia nervosa. A rather shy, studious girl, she tried hard to please everybody. She was attractive, but just a little bit overweight. She was afraid that she was not pretty enough to get the attention of boys in her class. Her father jokingly told her that she would never get a boyfriend if she did not lose some weight. She took him seriously, though, and began to diet. "I thought that being thin was the most important thing. I thought it was the only way to get people to like me or notice me. I started worrying that if I ever gained weight I would become ugly."

Soon after the pounds started dropping off, Cindy's periods stopped. She became obsessed with dieting and food, and she developed strange eating habits. She stopped eating all fast food and anything with fat in it. Every day she weighed all the food she would eat on the kitchen scale, cutting solids into tiny pieces and measuring liquids exactly. Cindy knew the calorie and fat counts of everything. She put her daily ration in small containers lining them

> ### ♣ It's A Fact!!
> ### Signs And Symptoms Of Anorexia
>
> - Missing periods
> - Strange eating habits like restricting certain foods or drastically reducing how much food you eat
> - Feeling moody
> - Denying hunger
> - Extreme concern with body weight and shape
> - Over exercising
> - Significant or extreme weight loss
>
> Source: "Anorexia Nervosa," Girl Power.

up in neat rows. She also exercised all the time, sometimes as much as 3 hours a day to burn lots of calories. "I would inline skate, do exercise tapes, or run eight miles a day." She never took an elevator if she could walk up steps.

Cindy managed to push away her friends and was mostly alone. "Every day I counted calories and fat grams, weighed myself, and stood in front of a mirror looking for any fat." Cindy was constantly freezing, even when she wore tights and two pairs of wool socks under her jeans. She did not have much energy, and her grades started slipping. No one was able to convince Cindy that she was in danger.

Finally, her doctor insisted that she be hospitalized for treatment of her illness. While in the hospital, she secretly continued her exercise routine in the bathroom, doing lots of sit-ups and knee bends. It took several hospitalizations and a good deal of family therapy for Cindy to face and solve her problems. Now, Cindy is in therapy and is making headway. Her weight is up and her eating habits are healthier. Cindy's advice to other girls: "If you like yourself, you will not change for others, even to be thin. People who like you only because you are thin are not worth it."

Bulimia Nervosa: The Diet-Binge-Purge Disorder

People who suffer from bulimia eat large amounts of food in a quick, automatic, and helpless fashion. This is called a binge. This may numb their feelings for a little bit, but eventually people suffering from bulimia feel physical discomfort and anxiety about gaining weight. As a result, they purge the food they have eaten by making themselves vomit, using laxatives, over exercising, or limiting their diets. Some people use a combination of all these forms of purging.

Karen's Story

Karen developed bulimia nervosa at 14, and like Cindy, her strange eating behaviors began when she started to diet. Karen would diet and exercise to lose weight, but unlike Cindy, she regularly ate huge amounts of food and maintained her normal weight by forcing herself to vomit. Karen often felt angry, frightened, and depressed. "My looks were everything to me," Karen

---

♣ It's A Fact!!
Signs And Symptoms
Of Bulimia

- Sneaking food

- Making excuses to go to the bathroom after meals

- Eating large amounts of food on the spur of the moment

- Taking laxatives, vomiting, and/or over exercising to purge food

- Extreme concern with body weight and image

- Enamel on teeth begins to wear away, causing cavities

Source: "Bulimia Nervosa," Girl Power.

---

said. "I felt guilty if I ate anything with fat in it and was afraid I would gain a lot of weight, so I would make myself vomit. But at the same time, eating a lot of food was the only thing that made me feel better."

Unable to understand her own behavior, she thought no one else would either. She felt isolated and lonely. Typically, when things were not going well, she would be overcome with an uncontrollable desire for sweets. "After a bad day at school all I could think about was coming home and eating," Karen said. She would sneak the food into her room and even had hiding places for it so her family would not catch on. "I would eat pounds of candy and cake at a time and not stop until I was exhausted or in severe pain." Then, feeling really guilty and disgusted, she would make herself vomit.

Karen's eating habits embarrassed her so much that she kept them secret, until a teacher heard her vomiting in the school bathroom. The teacher referred her to a doctor where she became involved in group therapy and had regular visits with a doctor. Karen learned how to treat her illness and gained understanding from others with the same problem. "Now when I have a bad day, I call a friend instead of turning to food," Karen said. "Sometimes it is still hard, but I now have the confidence in myself to do it."

Binge Eating Disorder: Compulsive Eating

Binge eating is another type of eating disorder. Here, a person eats an amount of food larger than what others would eat in the same amount of time. When someone is bingeing, she usually does not have much control over how much she is eating. Binge eating is different from anorexia and bulimia because people do not regularly vomit, over exercise, or abuse laxatives after they have eaten.

♣ It's A Fact!!

Signs And Symptoms Of Binge Eating

- Eating large amounts of food, even when not hungry
- Eating faster than normal
- Eating alone or in secret
- Eating until uncomfortably full

Source: "Binge Eating Disorder," Girl Power.

Chapter 40

Self-Esteem

You have many possibilities and choices. You can follow your heart and plan your future. You can make goals for yourself and develop your talents. All these choices are exciting, but they can also be a little confusing. How do you make the choices that are right for you? How do you get the life you want?

It is self-respect. Self-esteem is that voice inside of you that tells you that you are special and can achieve your goals. Self-esteem does come from the inside, but there are outside things that can affect your self-esteem, too.

Your Peers

Everyone wants to have friends and feel part of a group. This is normal and part of growing up. It is good and healthy to have friends. But it is not healthy when it means giving into pressure just to fit in. Only you know what is best for you. Do not let your friends make decisions for you or tell you to do things that are unsafe, unhealthy, or unkind, and that you will later wish you had not done. Part of self-esteem is having the power to be yourself because you are such a special person.

About This Chapter: Information in this chapter is from "Self-Esteem," Girl Power, sponsored by the U.S. Department of Health and Human Services, December 2005.

Your Parents And Other Adults

Sometimes adults can get so busy that you may feel they do not even notice you exist. This is not how they really intend for you to feel. Sometimes the pressures of being an adult make it hard for parents to take the time that they would like to spend listening to and helping you. Sometimes they are so used to working and being with adults that they forget that talking to young people is different from talking to adults.

When you start to feel that your parents are too busy, remember that the situation is temporary. In the meantime, talk to an older brother or sister, teacher, or another older person that you respect and trust. Ask your parents when a good time would be to talk and make a list of things you would like to talk about. Maybe you and your parents could choose a regular time to set aside just for you—a special time each day or week. Practice what you want to say to them and speak up.

Future Goals

What do you want to be when you grow up? What would you like to become really good at? What are some hobbies you would like to learn? If you put your mind to it, you can reach your goals. By setting goals for yourself and trying to meet them, you can feel great about yourself. Try a new sport, audition for the school play, or learn about careers in which you may be interested. Your self-esteem will improve when you have a goal to work toward. So go ahead, dream and plan. Reach for the stars!

♣ It's A Fact!!
Self-esteem is the confidence or satisfaction you have in yourself.

Positive Body Image

Think about all the things your body can do. Have you ever thought about just how amazing your body really is? Take a moment and appreciate all that your body does for you—running, dancing, breathing, laughing, thinking, smiling, etc. Every day your body carries you one step closer to your goals.

Bodies come in many different shapes, sizes, and colors. Your body type is uniquely yours, but your family genes may help to determine how it will be shaped. As you grow and develop, your body will begin to take on its genetically programmed shape. This basic shape cannot be changed. It is all in your genes. Wear clothes that are comfortable and make you feel good about your body. Work with your body, not against it.

Some people are shaped like a spoon. Their upper body is smaller than their lower body. Other people are shaped like an hourglass. This shape is curvy with a larger upper and lower body, but smaller waist. Another shape is a ruler. This shape is straight with not much difference between the upper and lower body. The lower body of someone who is funnel shaped is narrower than their upper body. No category is better or worse than any other, only different. Learn to like and respect your body the way it is built, and make the most of what you have.

Chapter 41

Self-Injury

What does hurting yourself mean?

Hurting yourself, sometimes called self-injury, is when a person deliberately hurts his or her own body. Some self-injuries can leave scars that will not go away, while others leave marks or bruises that eventually will go away. These are some forms of self-injury:

- Cutting yourself (such as using a razor blade, knife, or other sharp object to cut the skin)

- Punching yourself or other objects

- Burning yourself with cigarettes, matches, or candles

- Pulling out your hair

- Poking objects through body openings

- Breaking your bones or bruising yourself

- Plucking hair for hours

About This Chapter: Information in this chapter is from "Hurting Yourself," GirlsHealth.gov, sponsored by The National Women's Health Information Center, U.S. Department of Health and Human Services, Office on Women's Health, March 2006.

Why do some teens want to hurt themselves?

Many people cut themselves because it gives them a sense of relief. Some people use cutting as a means to cope with any problem. Some teens say that when they hurt themselves, they are trying to stop feeling lonely, angry, or hopeless. Some teens who hurt themselves have low self-esteem, they may feel unloved by their family and friends, and they may have an eating disorder, an alcohol or drug problem, or may have been victims of abuse.

Teens who hurt themselves often keep their feelings bottled up inside and have a hard time letting their feelings show. Some teens who hurt themselves say that feeling the pain provides a sense of relief from intense feelings. Cutting can relieve the tension from bottled up sadness or anxiety. Others hurt themselves in order to "feel." Often people who hold back strong emotions can begin feeling numb, and cutting can be a way to cope with this because it causes them to feel something. Some teens also may hurt themselves because they want to fit in with others who do it.

Who are the people who hurt themselves?

People who hurt themselves come from all walks of life, no matter their age, gender, race, or ethnicity. About one in 100 people hurts himself or herself on purpose. More females hurt themselves than males. Teens usually hurt themselves by cutting with sharp objects.

What are the signs of self-injury?

These are some signs of self-injury:

- Cuts or scars on the arms or legs

- Hiding cuts or scars by wearing long sleeved shirts or pants, even in hot weather

- Making poor excuses about how the injuries happened

Self-injury can be dangerous. Cutting can lead to infections, scars, numbness, and

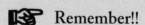 **Remember!!**

If you are hurting yourself, please get help. It is possible to overcome the urge to cut. There are other ways to find relief and cope with your emotions. Please talk to your parents, your doctor, or an adult you trust, like a teacher or religious leader.

even hospitalization and death. People who share tools to cut themselves are at risk of getting and spreading diseases like HIV and hepatitis. Teens who continue to hurt themselves are less likely to learn how to cope with negative feelings.

Are you or a friend depressed, angry, or having a hard time coping with life?

If you are thinking about hurting yourself, please ask for help. Talk with an adult you trust, like a teacher or minister or doctor. There is nothing wrong with asking for help. Everyone needs help sometimes. You have a right to be strong, safe, and happy.

Do you have a friend who hurts herself or himself?

Please try to get your friend to talk to a trusted adult. Your friend may need professional counseling and treatment. Help is available. Counselors can teach positive ways to cope with problems without turning to self-injury.

Have you been pressured to cut yourself by others who do it?

If so, think about how much you value that friendship or relationship. Do you really want a friend who wants you to hurt yourself, cause you pain, and put you in danger? Try to hang out with other friends who do not pressure you in this way.

Chapter 42

Suicide

Why do some teens think about suicide?

Thinking about suicide often goes along with stressful events and feeling sad. Some teens feel so overwhelmed and sad that they think they will never feel better. Some things that can cause these feelings include the following:

- Death of a loved one

- Seeing a lot of anger and violence at home

- Having parents get divorced

- Having a hard time in school, struggling with grades, or having problems with other teens

- Depression, alcohol, or drug problems

- Anger or heartbreak over a relationship breakup

- Feeling like you do not belong, either within the family or with friends

- Feeling left out or alone

Sometimes, teens may feel very sad for no one clear reason.

About This Chapter: Information in this chapter is from "Suicide," GirlsHealth.gov, sponsored by The National Women's Health Information Center, U.S. Department of Health and Human Services, Office on Women's Health, March 2006.

Every teen feels anxiety and confusion at some point, but it helps to get through tough times by turning to people you trust and love. If you do not think you have people like this in your life, talk to a school counselor, teacher, doctor, or another adult who can help you talk about your feelings. There are ways to help teens deal with these intense feelings and work on feeling better in the future.

How common is the problem of teen suicide?

Suicide is one of the leading causes of death for teens. Girls try to commit suicide more often than boys. The important thing for you to know is that it does not have to happen. It is also important to know that suicide is not a heroic act, even though sometimes media images can make it seem so. Often, a person who is thinking about attempting suicide is not able to see that suicide is never the answer to problems. Remember, there is always help, as well as support and love, out there for you or a friend.

How can you help a friend?

If you have a friend or friends who have talked about suicide, take it seriously. The first thing you should do is to tell an adult you trust right away. You may wonder if your friend(s) will be mad at you, but telling an adult is the right thing to do. This can be someone in your family, a coach, a school nurse, counselor, or a teacher. You can call 911 or the toll-free number of a suicide crisis line. You cannot help your friend(s) alone. They will need a good support system, including friends, family, teachers, and professional help. Suggest that they should talk with a trusted adult. Offer to listen and encourage them to talk about their feelings. Do not ignore their worries or tell them they will get better on their own. Listening shows that you take your friend(s) and their problems seriously and that you are there to help.

☞ Remember!!

If someone is in danger of hurting himself or herself, do not leave the person alone. You may need to call 911.

What about you?

If you feel suicidal, talk to an adult right away. Call 911 or 1-800-SUI-CIDE, or check in your phone book for the number of a suicide crisis center. The centers offer experts who can help callers talk through their problems and develop a plan of action. These hotlines can also tell you where to go for more help in person.

Things may seem bad at times, but those times do not last forever. Your pain right now probably feels like it is too overwhelming to cope with, and suicide may feel like the only form of relief; but remember that people do make it through suicidal thoughts. Ask for help—you can feel better. Do not use alcohol or drugs, because they cannot take your problems away. If you cannot find someone to talk with, write down your thoughts. Try to remember and write down the things you are grateful for. List the people who are your friends and family and care for you. Write about your hopes for the future. Read what you have written when you need to remind yourself that your life is important.

There is no reason that you or a friend has to continue hurting. There are ways to find help and hope.

What if someone you know attempts or dies by suicide?

If someone you know attempts or dies by suicide, it is important to remember that it is not your fault. You may feel many different emotions: anger, grief, guilt, or you may even feel numb. All of your feelings are okay; there is not a right or wrong way to feel. If you are having trouble dealing with your feelings, talk to a trusted adult. It is important that you feel strong ties with people at this time.

Chapter 43

Bullying

So what is bullying?

A lot of young people have a good idea of what bullying is because they see it every day. Bullying happens when someone hurts or scares another person on purpose, and the person being bullied has a hard time defending himself or herself. Usually, bullying happens over and over. These are some examples of bullying:

- Punching, shoving, and other acts that hurt people physically
- Spreading bad rumors about people
- Keeping certain people out of a group
- Getting certain people to gang up on others

Why do kids bully?

There are all kinds of reasons why young people bully others, either occasionally or often. Do any of these sound familiar to you?

- Because I see others doing it
- Because it's what you do if you want to hang out with the right crowd

About This Chapter: Information in this chapter is excerpted from "So what is bullying," "Why do kids bully," "Effects of bullying," and "Cyberbullying," Health Resources and Services Administration (HRSA), U.S. Department of Health and Human Services, cited March 2006.

- Because it makes me feel stronger, smarter, or better than the person I'm bullying

- Because it's one of the best ways to keep others from bullying me

Whatever the reason, bullying is something we all need to think about. Whether we have done it ourselves, or whether friends or other people we know are doing it, we all need to recognize that bullying has a terrible effect on the lives of young people. It may not be happening to you today, but it could tomorrow.

What are the effects of bullying?

If you have ever heard an adult, or anyone else, say that bullying is "just a fact of life" or "no big deal," you are not alone. Too often, people just do not take bullying seriously, or until the sad, and sometimes scary, stories are revealed. Here are some facts:

- **It happens a lot more than some people think.** Studies show that between 15–25% of U.S. students are bullied with some frequency, while 15–20% report they bully others with some frequency.

- **It can mess up a kid's future.** Young people who bully are more likely than those who do not bully to skip school and drop out of school. They are also more likely to smoke, drink alcohol, and get into fights.

- **It scares some people so much that they skip school.** As many as 160,000 students may stay home on any given day because they are afraid of being bullied.

- **It can lead to huge problems later in life.** Children who bully are more likely to get into fights, vandalize property, and drop out of school; and 60% of boys who were bullies in middle school had at least one criminal conviction by the age of 24.

What is cyberbullying?

In recent years, technology has given children and youth a new means of bullying each other.

Cyberbullying, which is sometimes referred to as online social cruelty or electronic bullying, can involve the following:

• Sending mean, vulgar, or threatening messages or images

• Posting sensitive, private information about another person

• Pretending to be someone else in order to make that person look bad

• Intentionally excluding someone from an online group

Children and youth can cyberbully each other through these methods:

• E-mails

• Instant messaging

• Text or digital imaging messages sent on cell phones

• Web pages

• Web logs (blogs)

• Chat rooms or discussion groups

• Other information communication technologies

How common is cyberbullying?

Although very little research has been conducted on cyberbullying, studies have found the following:

• 18% of students in grades 6–8 said they had been cyberbullied at least once in the last couple of months; and 6% said it had happened to them 2 or more times.

• 11% of students in grades 6–8 said they had cyberbullied another person at least once in the last couple of months, and 2% said they had done it two or more times.

• 19% of regular internet users between the ages of 10 and 17 reported being involved in online aggression; 15% had been aggressors, and 7% had been targets (3% were both aggressors and targets).

Who are the victims and perpetrators of cyberbullying?

In a recent study of students in grades 6–8 the following was found:

- Girls were about twice as likely as boys to be victims and perpetrators of cyberbullying.

- Of those students who had been cyberbullied relatively frequently (at least twice in the last couple of months) the following was found:

  - 62% said that they had been cyberbullied by another student at school, and 46% had been cyberbullied by a friend.

  - 55% did not know who had cyberbullied them.

- Of those students who admitted cyberbullying others relatively frequently the following was found:

  - 60% had cyberbullied another student at school, and 56% had cyberbullied a friend.

What are the most common methods of cyberbullying?

In a recent study of students in grades 6–8, the most common way that children and youth reported being cyberbullied was through instant messaging. Somewhat less common ways involved the use of chat rooms, e-mails, and messages posted on websites.

How does cyberbullying differ from other traditional forms of bullying?

Although there is little research yet on cyberbullying among children and youth, available research and experience suggest that cyberbullying may differ from more traditional forms of bullying in a number of ways including the following:

- Cyberbullying can occur any time of the day or night.

- Cyberbullying messages and images can be distributed quickly to a very wide audience.

- Children and youth can be anonymous when cyberbullying, which makes it difficult (and sometimes impossible) to trace them.

Chapter 44

Dating Violence

Teen life, with its fads, crushes, clashes, and breakups, seems to be a world away from abusive relationships. Yet, there is a dark side to all of the social drama. Many teens go through the same types of abuse—sexual, physical, and emotional—that we know some adults go through.

Dating violence often involves sex. More than one in four female college students say they have suffered rape, or attempted rape, at least once since age 14. At a large college, more than half of the women surveyed noted some type of unwanted sex, most often from their dates.

Such violence can start at an early age. About one in 12 eighth and ninth graders suffered sexual violence in dating.

Still, dating violence is common outside of sexual situations. Studies show that more than one in five high school students, and almost one in three college students, have been victims of dating violence that did not involve sex.

Most victims of physical dating violence are females. Seven in 10 pregnant teens report abuse by their partners. Although female high school and college students are just as likely as male students to inflict dating violence, females most often do it to defend themselves.

About This Chapter: Information in this chapter is from "Dating Violence Common Among Teens," Family Guide, 2006, Center for Substance Abuse Prevention, Substance Abuse and Mental Health Services Administration, U.S. Department of Health and Human Services.

Abuse in dating is not just about hurting a partner physically. Bullying, for example, is a form of emotional abuse. Many young people face other types of emotional abuse in the form of the following:

- Name calling

- Blame

- Threats

- Envy

- Anger

- Attempts to control a partner's dress, activities, and friendships

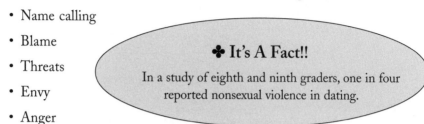

♣ It's A Fact!!

In a study of eighth and ninth graders, one in four reported nonsexual violence in dating.

Teens may be confused by a boyfriend or girlfriend who abuses them and may not know how to deal with a dating partner's mind games. Threats and rage may be followed by vows of love and pleas for forgiveness.

Teens may be afraid to break up with their partners out of fear that their partner will hurt them or will harm himself or herself. A teen may want to be there to help a boyfriend or girlfriend, may hope that things will get better, or simply may not realize what can happen. Over time, violence can escalate, and teen victims may mistakenly begin to believe that they deserve the abuse.

Signs of abuse can be both physical and emotional. Outward signs include the following:

- Bruises and injuries

- Changes in the way a person looks or dresses

- Person stops hanging out with old friends

- Giving up things a person cares about

New friends, as well as changes in attitudes, styles, hobbies, and school activities are common in young people. Still, they can be clues that a boyfriend or girlfriend is controlling a teen.

Emotional abuse is harder to see than physical abuse, since it happens over time and can take several forms. A young person suffering emotional abuse may become insecure, destructive, angry, or withdrawn. He may abuse alcohol or drugs and may even become suicidal.

Part Six

How Lifestyle Choices Can Affect Your Health

Chapter 45

The Physical Consequences Of Tobacco Use

The Health Consequences Of Smoking On The Human Body

Smoking harms your body in many different ways. It damages the immune system and increases the risk of infections. Smokers tend to be less healthy than nonsmokers.

Many illnesses in smokers last longer than in nonsmokers, and smokers are more likely to be absent from work because of illnesses, and are more likely to require longer hospitalizations than nonsmokers.

Smokers have a greater risk of complications and have a lower survival rate after surgery because of damage to the body's defenses. They are at increased risk of infections, pneumonia, and other respiratory complications.

About This Chapter: Information in this chapter is from the "The Health Consequences of Smoking on the Human Body," January 2005, "The Health Consequences of Smoking on the Human Brain," January 2005, "The Health Consequences of Smoking on the Human Eyes," January 2005, "The Health Consequences of Smoking on the Human Mouth and Throat," January 2005, "The Health Consequences of Smoking on the Human Lungs," January 2005, "The Health Consequences of Smoking on the Human Heart," January 2005, "The Health Consequences of Smoking on the Human Stomach," January 2005, "The Health Consequences of Smoking on the Human Kidneys," January 2005, "The Health Consequences of Smoking on the Human Bladder," January 2005, "The Health Consequences of Smoking on the Human Pancreas," January 2005, "The Health Consequences of Smoking on Pregnancy," July 2005, Centers for Disease Control and Prevention.

As you age, your bones become less dense, leading to a greater risk of hip fracture. The bone density of smokers tends to be lower than that of non-smokers.

Smoking causes peripheral artery disease that can affect the blood flow throughout the entire body. In peripheral artery disease, the arteries that supply blood to the legs are narrowed by atherosclerosis.

Although atherosclerosis is more commonly thought of as a heart disease, it can affect arteries anywhere in the body, including those in the legs and brain. Healthy arteries are strong, flexible and elastic, and the inner walls are smooth, allowing blood to flow freely through them to nourish tissues and organs.

Smoking causes many types of cancer, which is the second leading cause of death among Americans. It is responsible for one of every four deaths in the United States. Each year more than half a million Americans, more than 1,500 people a day, die of cancer.

Cancer was one of the first diseases linked to smoking. In 1964, the first Surgeon General's report on smoking and health concluded that smoking causes lung cancer. In later years, the list of diseases linked to smoking has grown.

The Health Consequences Of Smoking On The Human Brain

The brain is your body's center for mood and conscious thought. It controls most of your voluntary movements and makes thinking and feeling possible. It also regulates unconscious body processes, such as digestion and breathing. Arteries leading from the heart and lungs carry oxygen and other chemicals to the brain. Smoking a cigarette sends chemicals to the brain, changing its chemistry, and affecting a smoker's mood. Nicotine reaches the brain ten seconds after smoke is inhaled.

Smoking is a major cause of strokes. Strokes are the third leading cause of death in the United States. About 600,000 strokes occur in the United States each year, and about 30 percent of those strokes cause death.

The Health Consequences Of Smoking On The Human Eyes

The eyes work like cameras. Each eye has a lens. Light is focused by these lenses and projected onto a delicate membrane lining on the inner eye (retina). The retina is a collection of light-sensitive cells at the back of the eye. The light that hits these cells is changed into nerve impulses and sent to the brain where it is interpreted so people can see.

If you smoke, you have a two to three times greater risk of developing cataracts than a nonsmoker. Cataracts are a leading cause of blindness worldwide.

The Health Consequences Of Smoking On The Human Mouth And Throat

The mouth and throat (also called your pharynx) are the body's entry points for food and air. The esophagus is a muscular tube that moves food from your mouth into your stomach. The larynx allows the passage of air to and from your lungs. The larynx is sometimes called the voice box because it is used to create the sounds of speech.

Smokers have more periodontitis or gum disease than nonsmokers. Smoking causes oral or mouth cancer.

When people smoke pipes or cigars, they are also at increased risk of getting mouth cancer. Reducing the use of cigarettes, pipes, cigars, smokeless tobacco, and other tobacco products could prevent most of the estimated 30,200 new cases and 7,800 deaths from oral cavity and pharynx cancers annually in the United States.

Smoking causes throat cancer. Smoking causes cancer of the larynx. In 2003, roughly 3,800 deaths occurred from laryngeal cancer, in the United States.

Smoking causes cancer of the esophagus. Esophageal cancer is the seventh leading cause of cancer death in men in the United States. Reductions in smoking and in use of smokeless tobacco could prevent many of the approximately 12,300 new cases and 12,000 deaths from esophageal cancer that occur annually in the United States.

Smokers are more likely to have upper respiratory tract infections like colds and sore throats due to viral or bacterial infections. Smoking harms the body's ability to fight infections.

The Health Consequences Of Smoking On The Human Lungs

Lungs are located in your chest. They move air in and out of your body, taking in oxygen and pushing out carbon dioxide. The oxygen is carried through a complicated network of branching airways (called bronchi), which eventually lead to tiny air sacs (called alveoli). This network of airways looks somewhat like an upside-down tree.

♣ It's A Fact!!

Smoking among youth can hamper the rate of lung growth and the level of maximum lung function.

Source: Excerpted from "Facts on Youth Smoking, Health, and Performance," Tobacco Information and Prevention Source (TIPS), Centers for Disease Control and Prevention, January 2005.

Lung cancer is the leading cause of cancer death in the United States. Compared to nonsmokers, men who smoke are about 23 times more likely to develop lung cancer, and women who smoke are about 13 times more likely to develop lung cancer. Smoking causes about 90 percent of lung cancer deaths in men and about 80 percent in women.

In 2003, about 157,200 people died from lung cancer, and there were about 171,900 new cases in the United States.

Smoking low-tar cigarettes does not substantially reduce the risk of lung cancer.

Smoking causes injury to the airways and air sacs of your lungs, which can lead to chronic obstructive pulmonary disease (COPD), which includes emphysema. COPD is the fourth leading cause of death in the United States with more than 100,000 deaths per year. Smoking causes more than 90 percent of these deaths.

Smokers have more acute lower respiratory illnesses, such as pneumonia or acute bronchitis, than nonsmokers. These are usually diagnosed as infections of the lower respiratory tract (bronchial tubes and lung illnesses). They are caused by viral or bacterial infections.

Smoking is related to asthma among children and adolescents. Asthma is a disease that causes inflammation of the airways, causing them to become constricted, and obstruct airflow in and out of the lungs. There is currently no cure for asthma, which may recur throughout life.

Smoking is related to chronic coughing and wheezing among adults, children, and adolescents.

Smoking during childhood and adolescence retards lung growth. Lung function, which is a measure of how effectively your lungs move air in and out of the body, decreases naturally as you get older, but the decline is faster in smokers.

Smoking during pregnancy causes reduced lung function in infants.

The Health Consequences Of Smoking On The Human Heart

The heart is a fist-sized muscle that pumps blood around your body, circulating oxygen and nutrients to all your body's organs and tissues. Poisons from cigarettes are also carried everywhere the blood flows. Circulating blood also picks up waste products from the body's cells. The kidneys, liver, and lungs filter out these waste products.

Smoking causes coronary heart disease, which is the leading cause of death in the United States. More than 61 million Americans suffer from some form of cardiovascular disease, including high blood pressure, coronary heart disease, stroke, congestive heart failure, and other conditions. More than 2,600 Americans die every day because of cardiovascular diseases, about 1 death every 33 seconds. Cigarette smoking has been associated with all types of sudden cardiac death in both men and women.

Smoking-caused coronary heart disease may contribute to congestive heart failure. An estimated 4.6 million Americans have congestive heart failure, and 43,000 die from it every year.

In 2000, about 1.1 million Americans had heart attacks. Even with treatment, 25 percent of men and 38 percent of women die within one year of a heart attack.

Smoking low-tar nicotine cigarettes rather than regular cigarettes does not reduce your risk of coronary heart disease.

Smoking causes atherosclerosis, or hardening of the arteries. Poisons in the blood from smoking cigarettes contribute to the development of atherosclerosis. Most cases of coronary heart disease, stroke, and artery disease are caused by atherosclerosis.

Smoking causes abdominal aortic aneurysm, a bulge in the wall of the aorta near the stomach. Each year, about 15,000 Americans die of an abdominal aortic aneurysm. It is the 13th leading cause of death in the United States. Aneurysms are four times more common in men than women.

The Health Consequences Of Smoking On The Human Stomach

Your stomach is a muscular sac between the esophagus and small intestine. Walls of the stomach are lined with three layers of powerful muscles that grind food and mix it with gastric juices, liquefying it before passing it into your small intestine. One of these juices, hydrochloric acid, is so strong it can dissolve iron nails. The stomach's delicate tissues are protected from this powerful acid by a thick coating on the stomach lining.

Smoking causes stomach cancer. In 2003, there were an estimated 22,400 new cases of stomach cancer in the United States and an estimated 12,100 deaths.

Smokers are more likely to have peptic ulcers than nonsmokers.

The Health Consequences Of Smoking On The Human Kidneys

Kidneys are two bean-shaped organs, each about the size of a fist. They are located in the middle of the back, one on each side of the spine just below the rib cage. Kidneys are filters that purify the blood. They remove waste products and water from the blood, creating urine.

Smoking causes kidney cancer. In 2003, an estimated 31,900 new cases of kidney cancer were diagnosed in the United States, and an estimated 11,900 people died from the disease. It is the tenth leading cause of cancer death in men in the United States.

The Health Consequences Of Smoking On The Human Bladder

Your bladder is a muscular, balloon-shaped organ located in your pelvis. It stores urine that your kidneys produce during the process of filtering your blood. Like other organs in your body, cancerous cells can sometimes form in the bladder and spread throughout the body. Smoking causes bladder cancer. In 2003, an estimated 57,400 new cases of bladder cancer were diagnosed in the United States, and an estimated 12,500 people died from the disease.

The Health Consequences Of Smoking On The Human Pancreas

Your pancreas is located near the top of your small intestine. It has two very different purposes in your body. First, it helps digestion by releasing enzymes into the small intestine. Second, it regulates glucose levels in the blood. It does this by releasing hormones called insulin and glucagon into the bloodstream.

Smoking causes pancreatic cancer. In 2003, an estimated 30,700 new cases of pancreatic cancer were diagnosed in the United States, and 30,000 deaths were attributed to it.

The Health Consequences Of Smoking On Pregnancy

An estimated 6 million women become pregnant each year in the United States, and more than 11,000 give birth every day. Between 12 and 22 percent of these women will smoke during pregnancy. Smoking has a negative impact on the health of both unborn and newborn children. Only 18 to 25 percent of women quit smoking once they become pregnant.

Smoking is harmful during every part of the development of the baby and continues to be harmful after a baby is born. Smoking can cause babies to be born prematurely and to have low birth weight, respiratory diseases, and other illnesses. Low birth weight is the leading cause of infant deaths.

♣ It's A Fact!!

- Smoking hurts young people's physical fitness in terms of both performance and endurance, even among young people trained in competitive running.

- The younger people start smoking cigarettes, the more likely they are to become strongly addicted to nicotine.

- Teens who smoke are 3 times more likely than nonsmokers to use alcohol, 8 times more likely to use marijuana, and 22 times more likely to use cocaine. Smoking is associated with a host of other risky behaviors, such as fighting and engaging in unprotected sex.

- Smoking is associated with poor overall health and a variety of short-term adverse health effects in young people and may also be a marker for underlying mental health problems, such as depression, among adolescents. For high school seniors who are regular smokers and began smoking by grade nine the following is likely to be true:

  - They are 2.4 times more likely than their nonsmoking peers to report poorer overall health.

  - They are 2.4 to 2.7 times more likely to report cough with phlegm or blood, shortness of breath when not exercising, and wheezing or gasping.

  - They are 3.0 times more likely to have seen a doctor or other health professional for an emotional or psychological complaint.

Source: Excerpted from "Facts on Youth Smoking, Health, and Performance," Tobacco Information and Prevention Source (TIPS), Centers for Disease Control and Prevention, January 2005.

Smoking during pregnancy increases the risk of placenta previa and placental abruption.

Women who smoke while pregnant have a higher risk of premature rupture of membranes before labor begins. This can lead to premature birth and possibly infant death.

Secondhand smoke may have terrible effects on a newborn baby. Smoking by mothers causes sudden infant death syndrome (SIDS). Infants exposed to secondhand smoke are at twice the risk of SIDS than unexposed infants.

Chapter 46

How Alcohol Affects Your Health

Binge Drinking

- Binge drinking is generally defined as having five or more drinks on one occasion, meaning in a row or within a short period of time. However, among women, binge drinking is often defined as having four or more drinks on one occasion. This lower cut-point is used for women because women are generally of smaller stature than men and absorb and metabolize alcohol differently than men.

- In 2001, there were approximately 1.5 billion episodes of binge drinking in the U.S. Binge drinking rates were highest among those aged 18 to 25 years.

- Binge drinkers were 14 times more likely to report alcohol-impaired driving than non-binge drinkers.

- Binge drinking is associated with a number of adverse health effects, including unintentional injuries (e.g., motor vehicle crashes, falls, burns, drowning, and hypothermia); violence (homicide, suicide, child abuse, domestic violence); sudden infant death syndrome; alcohol poisoning; hypertension; myocardial infarction; gastritis; pancreatitis; sexually transmitted diseases; meningitis; and poor control of diabetes.

About This Chapter: Information in this chapter is excerpted from "General Alcohol Information," January 2005, Centers for Disease Control and Prevention.

Heavy Drinking

- Heavy drinking is consuming alcohol in excess of one drink per day on average for women and greater than two drinks per day on average for men.

- In 2002, 5.9% of U.S. adults reported heavy drinking in the past 30 days; the prevalence of heavy drinking was greater for men (7.1%) than for women (4.5%).

- Heavy drinking is associated with a number of chronic health conditions, including chronic liver disease and cirrhosis, gastrointestinal cancers, heart disease, stroke, pancreatitis, depression, and a variety of social problems.

Alcohol Dependence

- A person is defined as being dependent on alcohol if he or she reports three or more of the following symptoms in the past year: tolerance (that is, needing more alcohol to become intoxicated); withdrawal; alcohol use for longer periods than intended; desire and/or unsuccessful efforts to cut down or control alcohol use; considerable time spent obtaining or using alcohol, or recovering from its effects; important social, work, or recreational activities given up because of use; and continued use of alcohol despite knowledge of problems caused by or aggravated by use.

- In 2002, 3.7% of past-year drinkers were alcohol-dependent.

Underage Drinking

- As of 1988, all states prohibit the purchase of alcohol by youth under the age of 21 years. Consequently, underage drinking is defined as consuming alcohol prior to the minimum legal drinking age of 21 years.

- In 2003, 44.9% of 9th through 12th graders reported drinking alcohol on one or more of the past 30 days; prevalence of current drinking was higher for females (45.8%) than among males (43.8%).

- In 2003, 28.3% of 9th through 12th graders reported binge drinking (having five or more drinks of alcohol in a row or within a couple of hours) at least once during the past 30 days. The prevalence of binge drinking was higher for males (29%) than among females (27.5%).

- Zero tolerance laws, which make it illegal for youth under age 21 years to drive with any measurable amount of alcohol in their system (i.e., with a blood alcohol concentration (BAC) 0.02 g/dL or more), have reduced traffic fatalities among 18 to 20 year olds by 13% and saved an estimated 21,887 lives from 1975 through 2002.

Alcohol-Impaired Driving

- In 2002, 2.2% of U.S. adults reported alcohol-impaired driving in the past 30 days.

- In 1993, there were approximately 123 million episodes of alcohol-impaired driving in the United States.

- In 2001, there were approximately 1.4 million arrests for driving under the influence of alcohol or narcotics. This is an arrest rate of 1 of every 137 licensed drivers in the United States.

Total Deaths Due To Alcohol

- In 2000, there were approximately 85,000 deaths attributable to either excessive or risky drinking in the U.S., making alcohol the third leading actual cause of death.

- Alcohol-related deaths in the United States vary considerably by state and are directly related to the amount of alcohol consumed and the pattern of alcohol use.

♣ It's A Fact!!

Alcohol use is a leading risk factor in the three leading causes of death among youth: unintentional injuries (including motor vehicle crashes and drowning); suicides; and homicides. Other adverse consequences of underage drinking include risky sexual behavior and poor school performance.

Alcohol Motor Vehicle Crash Deaths

- In 2002, 17,419 people in the United States died in alcohol-related motor vehicle crashes, accounting for 41% of all traffic-related deaths.

- In 1995, 36% of all crash fatalities among youth aged 15 to 20 years were alcohol-related.

- From 1997 through 2002, 2,355 children died in alcohol-related motor vehicle crashes; 1,588 (68%) of these children were riding with a drinking driver.

Alcohol And Unintentional Injuries

- Alcohol-related unintentional injuries and deaths include motor vehicle crashes, drowning, falls, hypothermia, burns, suicides, and homicides.

- Approximately 31.1% of those who die from unintentional, non-traffic injuries in the United States have a blood alcohol concentration of 0.10 g/dL or greater.

- Patients treated in an emergency department (ED) for an unintentional injury are 13.5 times more likely to have consumed five or more alcohol-containing beverages within six hours of their injury compared to age and sex matched community controls.

Alcohol And Violence

- In 1997, about 40% of all crimes (violent and non-violent) were committed under the influence of alcohol, and 40% of convicted rape and sexual assault offenders said that they were drinking at the time of their crime.

- Approximately 72% of rapes reported on college campuses occur when victims are so intoxicated they are unable to consent or refuse. In addition, two-thirds of victims of intimate partner violence reported that alcohol was involved in the incident.

- Nearly one-half of the cases of child abuse and neglect are associated with parental alcohol or drug abuse.

- Approximately 23% of suicide deaths are attributable to alcohol.

Alcohol And Pregnancy

- Adverse health effects that are associated with alcohol-exposed pregnancies include miscarriage, premature delivery, low birth weight, sudden infant death syndrome (SIDS), and prenatal alcohol-related conditions (for example, fetal alcohol syndrome and alcohol-related neurodevelopmental disorders).

- Alcohol-related neurodevelopmental disorder and alcohol-related birth defects are believed to occur approximately three times as often as fetal alcohol syndrome (FAS).

- Fetal alcohol syndrome is one of the leading causes of mental retardation and is directly attributable to drinking during pregnancy. FAS is characterized by growth retardation, facial abnormalities, and central nervous system dysfunction (that is, learning disabilities and lower IQ), as well as behavioral problems.

- The incidence of FAS in the United States ranges from 0.2 to 1.5 per 1,000 live births.

- Any maternal alcohol use during the three months before pregnancy or during the first trimester is associated with a six-fold increased risk of SIDS. In addition, binge drinking (five or more drinks at a time) during a mother's first trimester of pregnancy is associated with an eight-fold increase in the odds that the infant will die of SIDS.

Alcohol And Sexually Transmitted Disease

- Among teens aged 14 to 18, 20% of those who reported drinking before age 14 also reported being sexually active compared to 7% of those who did not report drinking before this age.

- In 1998, an estimated 400,000 college students between the ages of 18 and 24 had unprotected sex after drinking, and an estimated 100,000 had sex when they were so intoxicated they were unable to consent.

♣ **It's A Fact!!**
Alcohol use by young adults is associated with earlier initiation of sexual activity, unprotected sexual intercourse, multiple partners, and an increased risk for sexually transmitted diseases.

- Among adults aged 18 to 30, binge drinkers were twice as likely as those who did not binge drink to have had two or more sex partners.

- People who abuse alcohol are more likely to engage in risky behaviors, such as having unprotected sex, having more sex partners, and using intravenous drugs. In a single act of unprotected sex with an infected partner, a teenage woman has a 1% risk of acquiring HIV, a 30% risk of getting genital herpes, and a 50% chance of contracting gonorrhea.

Hepatitis C (HCV) And Chronic Liver Disease

- Alcohol consumption can exacerbate the HCV infection and accelerate disease progression to cirrhosis. Alcohol may also exacerbate the side effects of antiviral treatment for HCV infection, impairing the body's response to the virus.

- In 2003, there were 12,207 deaths from alcohol-related chronic liver disease (CLD). Approximately 75% of those deaths occurred among men.

- Approximately 40% of the deaths from unspecified liver disease in the United States are attributable to heavy alcohol consumption.

Alcohol And Cancer

- Alcohol-related cancers include oral-pharyngeal, esophagus (squamous cell type), prostate, liver, and breast. In general, the risk of cancer increases with increasing amounts of alcohol.

- Excessive drinkers are three times more likely to develop liver cancer and four times more likely to develop esophageal cancer than nondrinkers.

- Oral cancers are six times more common in heavy alcohol users than in nonalcohol users.

- Compared to nondrinkers, women who consume an average of one alcoholic drink per day increase their risk of breast cancer by approximately 7%. Women who consume an average of two to five drinks per day increase their risk of developing breast cancer by approximately 50% compared to that of nondrinkers.

Chapter 47

Medical Consequences Of Drug Abuse

Drug addiction is a brain disease. Although initial drug use might be voluntary, drugs of abuse have been shown to alter gene expression and brain circuitry, which in turn affect human behavior. Once addiction develops, these brain changes interfere with an individual's ability to make voluntary decisions, leading to compulsive drug craving, seeking, and use.

The impact of addiction can be far reaching. Cardiovascular disease, stroke, cancer, HIV/AIDS, hepatitis, and lung disease can all be affected by drug abuse. Some of these effects occur when drugs are used at high doses or after prolonged use, however, some may occur after just one use.

HIV, Hepatitis, And Other Infectious Diseases

Drug abuse not only weakens the immune system but is also linked to risky behaviors like needle sharing and unsafe sex. The combination greatly increases the likelihood of acquiring HIV/AIDS, hepatitis, and many other infectious diseases.

About This Chapter: Information in this chapter is from "Medical Consequences of Drug Abuse," June 2005, "HIV, Hepatitis and Other Infectious Diseases," April 2005, "Cardiovascular Effects," April 2005, "Respiratory Effects," April 2005, "Gastrointestinal Effects," April 2005, "Musculoskeletal Effects," April 2005, "Kidney Damage," April 2005, "Liver Damage," April 2005, "Neurological Effects," April 2005, "Mental Health Effects," April 2005, "Hormonal Effects," April 2005, "Other Health Effects," April 2005, National Institute on Drug Abuse, National Institutes of Health.

Cardiovascular Effects

Researchers have found a connection between the abuse of most drugs and adverse cardiovascular effects, ranging from abnormal heart rate to heart attacks. Injection drug use can also lead to cardiovascular problems such as collapsed veins and bacterial infections of the blood vessels and heart valves.

Respiratory Effects

Drug abuse can lead to a variety of respiratory problems. Smoking cigarettes, for example, has been shown to cause bronchitis, emphysema, and lung cancer. Marijuana smoke may also cause respiratory problems. The use of some drugs may also cause breathing to slow, block air from entering the lungs, or exacerbate asthma symptoms.

Gastrointestinal Effects

Among other adverse effects, many drugs of abuse have been known to cause nausea and vomiting soon after use. Cocaine use can also cause abdominal pain.

Musculoskeletal Effects

Steroid use during childhood or adolescence, resulting in artificially high sex hormone levels, can signal the bones to stop growing earlier than they normally would have, leading to short stature. Other drugs may also cause severe muscle cramping and overall muscle weakness.

> **♣ It's A Fact!!**
>
> Cardiovascular disease, stroke, cancer, HIV/AIDS, hepatitis, and lung disease can all be affected by drug abuse.
>
> Source: "Medical Consequences of Drug Abuse," June 2005, National Institute on Drug Abuse.

Kidney Damage

Some drugs may cause kidney damage or failure, either directly or indirectly, from dangerous increases in body temperature and muscle breakdown.

Liver Damage

Chronic use of some drugs, such as heroin, inhalants, and steroids, may lead to significant damage to the liver.

Neurological Effects

All drugs of abuse act in the brain to produce their euphoric effects; however, some of them also have severe negative consequences in the brain such as seizures, stroke, and widespread brain damage that can impact all aspects of daily life. Drug use can also cause brain changes that lead to problems with memory, attention, and decision-making.

Mental Health Effects

Chronic use of some drugs of abuse can cause long-lasting changes in the brain, which may lead to paranoia, depression, aggression, and hallucinations.

Hormonal Effects

Steroid abuse disrupts the normal production of hormones in the body, causing both reversible and irreversible changes. These changes include infertility and testicle shrinkage in men, as well as masculinization in women.

Other Health Effects

In addition to the effects various drugs of abuse may have on specific organs of the body, many drugs produce global body changes such as dramatic changes in appetite and increases in body temperature, which may impact a variety of health conditions. Withdrawal from drug use also may lead to numerous adverse health effects, including restlessness, mood swings, fatigue, changes in appetite, muscle and bone pain, insomnia, cold flashes, diarrhea, and vomiting.

Chapter 48

Making Decisions About Sex

Many Teens Are Saying "No"

Do not be fooled into thinking most teenagers are having sex. They aren't. There is a lot to know and think about before you decide to say "yes" to have sex.

You Are More Than Just A Body

During the teen years, you may be strongly attracted to another person. Your body may send you strong messages that make you want to get closer to that person, but your body will not tell you how having sex now may harm you.

You may not know that the following is true:

- Almost 1,000,000 teens become pregnant each year. Abstinence, which is not having sex, is the only 100% sure way to protect against the risk of pregnancy.

- Teens are more likely to have problems during pregnancy.

- Babies of young, teen mothers are more likely to be born with serious health problems.

About This Chapter: Information in this chapter is from "Teen Talk #1," March 2003, U.S. Department of Health and Human Services, Office of Public Health and Science, Office of Population Affairs.

- Sexually transmitted diseases (STDs) are at epidemic levels. Absti-nence (not having sex) is the only 100% sure way to avoid herpes, syphilis, gonorrhea, chlamydia, and HIV/AIDS. One in four teens who has sex gets an STD.

You Are More Than Feelings

Sexual feelings can be pretty strong, so think before you act. Think about your future. Think about the consequences.

Think about yourself. Ask yourself, "Is it better to wait for sex with my life partner?"

♣ It's A Fact!!

Decisions about sex may be the most impor-tant decisions you will ever make, so think before you act.

Source: U.S. Department of Health and Human Services.

STDs can be painful. They can make it im-possible to have a baby. Some are incurable, and some may even cause death.

Face it! Sex for teens is pretty risky to your body, feelings, and future.

Some Questions To Ask Yourself

There is a lot to know before making your decision about whether to say "yes" or "No" to having sex. Here is a checklist to help you decide:

- When I get married, will I be glad I waited to have sex?

- Would my parents approve of me having sex now?

- If I have a child, am I responsible enough to provide for its emotional and financial support?

- If the relationship breaks up, will I be glad I had sex with this person?

- Am I sure no one is pushing me into having sex?

- Do I know how to tell my partner I do not want to have sex now?

- Am I absolutely sure my partner is not infected with an STD, includ-ing HIV/AIDS?

If any of your answers to these questions is "No," then you better wait.

Should I Have Sex Now Or Should I Wait?

It is true some teens decide to go ahead, but you will have to live with the consequences of your decision.

Ask yourself these questions before making up your mind:

- If we are fully committed as a couple, why not wait until we are married?

- Am I willing to risk STDs, including HIV/AIDS, and maybe becoming sterile so I cannot have a baby?

- Am I willing to risk getting pregnant or getting someone pregnant?

- Am I ready and able to support a child on my own?

- Can I handle the guilt and conflict I may feel?

- Will my decision hurt others such as my parents and my friends?

What Should I Know If I Decide Not To Have Sex?

Contrary to rumor, at least half of all teens decide not to have sex. Many teens are worried about hurting the other person's feelings, but it is not so hard to say "No" and still remain friends. For example, you might say the following:

- "I like you a lot, but I'm just not ready to have sex."

- "I don't believe in having sex before marriage. I want to wait."

- "I enjoy being with you, but I don't think I'm old enough to have sex."

- "I don't feel like I have to give you a reason for not having sex. It's just my decision."

Also, there are different ways to show affection for another person without having sex.

Try to avoid situations where sexual feelings become strong. "Stopping" is much harder then. Talk about your feelings and what seems right for you. Stay busy with sports and group activities.

If you and your partner cannot agree, then maybe you need to find someone else whose beliefs are closer to your own.

♣ It's A Fact!!

Homosexuality: Facts For Teens

What does it mean to be homosexual?

A person is said to be homosexual if he or she is sexually or romantically attracted to members of the same gender, or sex. This does not mean that homosexuals are sexually attracted to all members of the same gender any more than heterosexuals are sexually attracted to every person of the opposite sex. Typically, the words "gay" and "lesbian" are used to refer to homosexual men and women. The term "bisexual" refers to people who are attracted to both men and women.

Researchers who study human sexuality believe that sexual orientation develops and changes over a person's lifetime. Having feelings about, or even having a sexual experience with a person of the same sex, does not necessarily mean that a person is gay or bisexual. It is not uncommon for people to experiment with their sexuality, especially during adolescence and young adulthood.

What causes homosexuality?

No one knows why some people are homosexual. Some people who study human sexuality believe that sexuality is a result of genetics, social or individual factors, alone or in combination. A common misperception is that troubled family relationships cause people to be homosexual, but no scientifically sound research supports this myth.

Is homosexuality a disease?

No, homosexuality is not a disease. All major mental health organizations, including the American Psychological Association (APA), have stated that homosexuality is not a mental disorder. Being unsure or uncomfortable about your feelings can cause anxiety and stress, which can sometimes cause physical problems like trouble sleeping, nausea, and headache. Talking with people about how you feel, such as trusted family members and friends, can help reduce your stress and anxiety.

Can people change from gay to straight or the other way around?

Regardless of their sexual orientation, people can choose how they behave and how they cope with their feelings. However, trying to be something you are not can lead to stress, anxiety and depression.

What is homophobia?

Homophobia refers to an irrational fear, prejudice, or discrimination towards homosexuals. Homophobia can take many forms, from name-calling and teasing to serious crimes like assault and murder. Homophobia is most often based on fear and ignorance.

I think I might be gay. How will I know if I really am?

You will eventually figure it out. You may consider different options or even experiment to determine what you are happy and comfortable with. The process may take a long time, and the decisions you make may be difficult for you and other people to accept.

What does "coming out" mean?

The process of telling people about one's homosexuality is often referred to as coming out. The phrase "in the closet" is sometimes used to describe a person who is gay but who has not acknowledged it yet to friends and family members.

How do I come out, and when is it appropriate?

As with any other personal information, when and whom you tell about your sexuality is your decision. It is important and healthy for you to share your feelings with others. It is also important to realize that telling others, even people you consider supportive, may not always be a positive experience. If you feel you cannot tell your parents, talk to a friend or someone else you trust. It is possible that the people who are closest to you already know and are waiting for you to be comfortable enough to talk about it.

What Should I Know About Pressure?

Be popular. Be part of the in-crowd. Be a man/Be a woman. Everybody's doing it. Sex is fun. If it feels good, do it.

It comes from everywhere—advertising, friends, movies, TV shows, songs, and books.

But stop and think. Will having sex really make you more popular, more mature, or more desirable? Probably not. In fact, having sex may even cause your partner to lose interest. The one sure thing about having sex is that you may be in for problems you do not want to deal with.

What Should I Know About Boy/Girl Relationships?

They are great, but good relationships do not develop overnight. They take time. Sex is not what makes a relationship work.

Watch out for lines like, "If you care about me, you'll have sex with me." Remember that the following is true:

- You do not have to have sex with someone to prove you like or love him or her.

- Sex should never be used to pay someone back for something. All you have to say is "Thank you."

- Sharing time, thoughts, beliefs, feelings, and most of all, mutual respect, is what makes a relationship strong.

- Saying "No" can be the best way to say "I love you."

Where Can I Get Information That Will Help Me?

If you want more information or help, talk to someone who cares about you. Ask your parents, an older brother or sister, other family members, or an adult you feel will listen and give you good advice. There are people and organizations in your community who want to help such as your family doctor; your priest, minister, or rabbi; your school nurse or counselor; or local health-care providers.

Chapter 49

Sexually Transmitted Diseases: Understanding The Risks

What is an STD?

STD stands for "sexually transmitted disease." These infections are passed from person to person during sexual activity (vaginal, oral, or anal intercourse). Some infections are curable, while others are not. It is estimated that more than 15 million new cases of STDs occur in the U.S. each year. Approximately one quarter (3.75 million) of the new cases occur among teenagers. Anyone who engages in sexual activity can get an STD.

How do I know if I have an STD?

Since many STDs do not have any obvious symptoms, the only sure way to know is by having a medical exam and lab tests.

Do latex condoms protect you from getting an STD?

For sexually active people, the most effective strategy for reducing the risk of STDs and preventing HIV/AIDS is correct and consistent use of latex condoms. However, research shows that condoms may not provide as

About This Chapter: Information in this chapter is from "Commonly Asked Questions About Sexually Transmitted Diseases (STDs)," Teen Talk #2, March 2003, U.S. Department of Health and Human Services, Office of Public Health and Science, Office of Population Affairs.

much protection against some STDs such as HPV (genital warts). Abstinence (not having sex) is the only 100% sure way to avoid an STD.

Who can I talk to?

You can talk to a parent, teacher, school nurse, family doctor, clergyman, or other responsible adult.

What are the consequences of STDs?

- **Gonorrhea and Chlamydia:** These STDs can cause serious health problems if not diagnosed and treated early. These are some of the problems:

  - Pelvic inflammatory disease (PID) can damage fallopian tubes and make it difficult or impossible to have a baby (infertility)

  - Chronic pain in the lower abdomen

  - Tubal pregnancy (also called ectopic pregnancy), a condition where the pregnancy grows in the fallopian tube rather than the uterus. It is dangerous and requires immediate medical care.

- **HPV (genital warts):** Infection with some types of HPV has been linked to cancer of the cervix.

- **Syphilis:** This STD can cause blindness, heart disease, mental illness, joint damage, and death, if not diagnosed and treated early.

- **HIV/AIDS:** People who develop AIDS have severely weakened immune systems, which can lead to infections and death. STDs increase the risk of getting and transmitting HIV/AIDS. There is no cure for AIDS at this time.

What are the symptoms of common STDs?

Chlamydia

- ¾ of women and ½ of men infected have no symptoms

> ♣ **It's A Fact!!**
> Males who are infected with STDs can transmit the infection to their partners, who, if pregnant, can transmit the infection to their babies.

- Discharge from the genital organs

- Burning with urination

- In women, lower abdominal and/or back pain; pain during intercourse

Gonorrhea

- Discharge from the genital organs

- Burning or itching during urination

- Pelvic pain

- Frequently no symptoms in females

Syphilis

- Painless sores on genitals (10 days to 3 months after infection)

- Rash (3 to 6 weeks after sores appear)

HIV/AIDS (human immunodeficiency virus/ acquired immune deficiency syndrome)

- No symptoms may appear for years until symptoms of AIDS occur

HPV (human papillomavirus)

- Genital warts (sometimes warts are not visible)

Genital Herpes

- Itching, burning, or pain in the genital area

- Blisters or sores (sores always heal but can re-appear throughout your life)

If you experience any of these symptoms, go to a doctor or clinic as soon as possible.

♣ It's A Fact!!
Common Myths

Myth: If I do not have symptoms, that means I do not have an STD.

Fact: You can be infected with an STD and not know it. The only sure way to know if you have an STD is by having a medical exam and lab tests.

Myth: HIV/AIDS is the only STD that cannot be cured.

Fact: STDs caused by viruses—genital herpes, genital warts, and HIV/AIDS—cannot be cured, although some medications may reduce the severity and/or delay the appearance of symptoms.

STDs caused by bacteria (like chlamydia, gonorrhea, and syphilis) can usually be cured with antibiotics. If they are not treated early, serious long-term problems, like pain and infertility, can develop.

How can I prevent an STD?

Abstinence (not having vaginal, anal, or oral sex) is the best and only 100 percent effective way to prevent getting a sexually transmitted disease. Only having sex with one person who has been tested for STDs is the next best way to prevent getting HIV/AIDS and other STDs. Teens who choose to have multiple sexual partners should always use latex condoms. Latex condoms can help protect against STDs and HIV/AIDS, but they do not provide perfect protection against all STDs. To those teens involved in high-risk behaviors and relationships, and to those who may have relations with high-risk populations, the message is this: the latex condom is the only contraception method that may protect against some STDs, including HIV/AIDS.

If I am taking birth control pills, can I still get an STD?

Yes. Birth control pills only protect against pregnancy, not STDs. People who take birth control pills or use hormonal injections, implants, or patches to prevent pregnancy should also use latex condoms to reduce the risk for getting an STD, including HIV/AIDS.

What should I do if I think I have an STD?

If you think you have been exposed to an STD, you should go to a clinic or doctor as soon as possible to be tested and treated. Health departments, which diagnose and treat STDs, are located in almost every county and city. They provide confidential information and will help answer any questions you may have about STDs.

When should I have a checkup?

All sexually active teens should be seen by a health provider to be screened for STDs. Teens who have had sex with more than one person are at greater risk of getting an STD or HIV/AIDS.

Chapter 50

Birth Control Methods

What is the best method of birth control (or contraception)?

Making decisions about birth control, or contraception, is not easy; there are many things to think about. Learning about birth control methods you or your partner can use to prevent pregnancy and talking with your doctor are two good ways to get started.

There is no best method of birth control. Each method has its own pros and cons. Some methods work better than others do at preventing pregnancy.

The birth control method you choose should take into account the following:

- Your overall health
- How often you have sex
- The number of sexual partners you have
- If you want to have children at some time in the future
- How well each method works (or is effective) in preventing pregnancy
- Any potential side effects
- Your comfort level with using the method

About This Chapter: Information in this chapter is excerpted from "Birth Control Methods," The National Women's Health Information Center, U.S. Department of Health and Human Services, Office On Women's Health, July 2005.

Bear in mind that no method of birth control prevents pregnancy all of the time. Birth control methods can fail, but you can greatly increase a method's success rate by using it correctly all of the time.

What are the different birth control methods that I can use?

There are many methods of birth control that a woman can use. If you decide to have sex, talk with your doctor or nurse to help you figure out what method is best for you. You can always try one method, and if you do not like it, you can try another one.

Other than not having sex, the best protection against sexually transmitted diseases (STDs) and HIV is the male latex condom. The female condom may give some STD protection.

Do not forget that all of the methods work best if used correctly. Be sure you know the correct way to use them. Talk with your doctor or nurse and do not feel embarrassed about talking with her or him again if you forget or do not understand.

Know that learning how to use some birth control methods can take time and practice. Sometimes doctors do not explain how to use a method because they may think you already know how. For example, not everyone knows that you need to leave a reservoir, or space, at the tip of the condom for the sperm and fluid when a man ejaculates, or has an orgasm.

☞ Remember!!
Keep in mind that most birth control does not protect you from HIV or other sexually transmitted diseases (STDs) like gonorrhea, herpes, and chlamydia.

Here is a list of birth control methods with estimates of effectiveness, or how well they work in preventing pregnancy when used correctly, for each method:

Continuous Abstinence: This means not having sexual intercourse (vaginal, anal, or oral intercourse) at any time. It is the only sure way to prevent pregnancy and protect against HIV and other STDs. This method is 100% effective at preventing pregnancy and STDs.

Periodic Abstinence or Fertility Awareness Methods: Periodic abstinence means you do not have sex on the days that you may be fertile. Fertility awareness means that you can be abstinent or have sex but you use a barrier method of birth control to keep sperm from getting to the egg. Barrier methods include condoms, diaphragms, or cervical caps, used together with spermicides, which kill sperm. Keep in mind that to practice these methods, you need to learn how to predict which days you are fertile. You can ask your doctor or nurse for more information. When used correctly, these methods can help prevent pregnancy 75% (or more) of the time.

The Male Condom: Condoms are called barrier methods of birth control because they put up a block, or barrier, which keeps the sperm from reaching the egg. Only latex or polyurethane condoms are proven to help protect against STDs, including HIV. Natural or lambskin condoms are available, but they are not recommended for STD prevention because they have tiny pores that may allow for the passage of viruses like HIV, hepatitis B and herpes. Male condoms are 84 to 98% effective at preventing pregnancy. Condoms can only be used once. You can buy them at a drug store. Condoms come lubricated and non-lubricated. It is best to use lubrication with non-lubricated condoms if you use them for vaginal or anal sex. You can use KY jelly or water-based lubricants, which you can buy at a drug store. Oil-based lubricants like massage oils, baby oil, lotions, or petroleum jelly will weaken the condom, causing it to tear or break. Always keep condoms in a cool, dry place. If you keep them in a hot place (like a billfold, wallet, or glove compartment), the latex breaks down, causing the condom to tear or break. Latex or polyurethane condoms are the only method other than abstinence that can help protect against HIV and other sexually transmitted diseases (lambskin condoms do not).

Oral Contraceptives: Also called "the pill," oral contraceptives contain the hormones estrogen and progestin and are available in different hormone dosages. A pill is taken daily to block the release of eggs from the ovaries. It does not protect against STDs or HIV. The pill may add to your risk of heart disease, including high blood pressure, blood clots, and blockage of the arteries, especially if you smoke. If you have a history of blood clots or breast, liver, or endometrial cancer, your doctor may advise you not to take the pill. The pill is 95 to 99.9% effective at preventing pregnancy. Some antibiotics may reduce the effectiveness of the pill in some women. Talk to your doctor or nurse about a back-up method of birth control if she or he prescribes antibiotics. There are many different types of oral contraceptives available, and it is important to talk to your doctor or nurse about which one is best for you. You will need a prescription for oral contraceptives.

The Mini-Pill: Unlike the pill, the mini-pill only has one hormone, progestin, instead of both estrogen and progestin. Taken daily, the mini-pill thickens cervical mucus to prevent sperm from reaching the egg. It also prevents a fertilized egg from implanting in the uterus (womb). The mini-pill does not protect against STDs or HIV. Mini-pills are 92 to 99.9% effective at preventing pregnancy if used correctly. The mini-pill needs to be taken at the same time each day. A back-up method of birth control is needed if you take the pill more than three hours late. Some antibiotics may reduce the effectiveness of the pill in some women. Talk to your doctor or nurse about a back-up method of birth control if she or he prescribes antibiotics. You will need to visit you doctor for a prescription.

IUD (Intrauterine Device): An IUD is a small device that is shaped in the form of a "T." Your health care provider places it inside the uterus. There are several different types of IUDs that stop fertilization by preventing sperm from reaching the egg or, if fertilization does occur, preventing the fertilized egg from implanting in the lining of the uterus. Different types can stay in your uterus for differing lengths of time (from 1 to 12 years). IUDs do not protect against STDs or HIV. In general, they are 98–99% effective at preventing pregnancy. You will need to visit your doctor to have one inserted and to make sure you are not having any problems.

The Female Condom: Worn by the woman, this barrier method keeps sperm from getting into her body. It is made of polyurethane, is packaged with a lubricant, and may protect against STDs, including HIV. It can be inserted up to 24 hours prior to sexual intercourse. Female condoms are 79 to 95% effective at preventing pregnancy. There is only one kind of female condom, called Reality®, and it can be purchased at a drug store.

Depo-Provera®: With this method, women get injections, or shots, of the hormone progestin in the buttocks or arm every 3 months. It does not protect against STDs or HIV. Women should not use Depo-Provera® for more than 2 years in a row because it can cause a temporary loss of bone density that increases the longer this method is used. It is 97% effective at preventing pregnancy. You will need to visit your doctor for the shots and to make sure you are not having any problems.

Diaphragm, Cervical Cap or Shield: These are barrier methods of birth control, where the sperm are blocked from entering the cervix and reaching the egg. The diaphragm is shaped like a shallow latex cup. The cervical cap is a thimble-shaped latex cup. The cervical shield is a silicone cup that has a one-way valve that creates suction and helps it fit against the cervix. The diaphragm and cervical cap come in different sizes, and you need a doctor to fit you for one. The cervical shield comes in one size, and you will not need a fitting. Before sexual intercourse, you use them with spermicide (to block or kill sperm) and place them up inside your vagina to cover your cervix (the opening to your womb). You can buy spermicide gel or foam at a drug store. The diaphragm is 84 to 94% effective at preventing pregnancy. The cervical cap is 84 to 91% effective at preventing pregnancy for women who have not had a child and 68 to 74% for women who have had a child. The cervical shield is 85% effective at preventing pregnancy. Barrier methods must be left in place for 6 to 8 hours after intercourse to prevent pregnancy and removed by 24 hours for the diaphragm and 48 for cap and shield. You will need to visit your doctor for a proper fitting for the diaphragm or cervical cap and a prescription for the cervical shield.

Contraceptive Sponge: This is a barrier method of birth control that was re-approved by the Food and Drug Administration in 2005. It is a soft, disk-shaped device, with a loop for removal. It is made out of polyurethane foam and contains the spermicide nonoxynol-9. Before intercourse, you wet the sponge and place it, loop side down, up inside your vagina to cover the cervix. The sponge is 84 to 91% effective at preventing pregnancy in women who have not had a child and 68 to 80% for women who have had a child. The sponge is effective for more than one act of intercourse for up 24 hours. It needs to be left in for at least six hours after intercourse to prevent pregnancy and must be removed within 30 hours after it is inserted. There is a risk of getting toxic shock syndrome, or TSS, if the sponge is left in for more than 30 hours. The sponge does not protect against STDs or HIV. There is only one kind of contraceptive sponge for sale in the United States, called the Today® Sponge, and it can be purchased at a drug store. Women who are sensitive to the spermicide nonoxynol-9 should not use this birth control method.

The Patch (Ortho Evra®): This is a skin patch worn on the lower abdomen, buttocks, or upper body. It releases the hormones progestin and estrogen into the bloodstream. You put on a new patch once a week for three weeks, and then do not wear a patch during the fourth week in order to have a menstrual period. The patch is 98 to 99% effective at preventing pregnancy, but appears to be less effective in women who weigh more than 198 pounds. It does not protect against STDs or HIV. You will need to visit your doctor for a prescription and to make sure you are not having problems.

The Hormonal Vaginal Contraceptive Ring (NuvaRing®): The NuvaRing® is a ring that releases the hormones progestin and estrogen. You squeeze the ring between your thumb and index finger and insert it into your vagina. You wear the ring for three weeks, take it out for the week that you have your period, and then put in a new ring. The ring is 98 to 99% effective at preventing pregnancy. You will need to visit your doctor for a prescription and to make sure you are not having problems. This birth control method is not recommended while breastfeeding because the hormone estrogen may decrease breast milk production.

Surgical Sterilization (Tubal Ligation or Vasectomy): These surgical methods are meant for people who want a permanent method of birth control. In other words, they never want to have a child, or they do not want more children. Tubal ligation, or "tying tubes," is done on the woman to stop eggs from going down to her uterus where they can be fertilized. The man has a vasectomy to keep sperm from going to his penis, so his ejaculate never has any sperm in it. They are 99.9% effective at preventing pregnancy.

Non-surgical Sterilization (Essure® Permanent Birth Control System): This is the first non-surgical method of sterilizing women. A thin tube is used to thread a tiny spring-like device through the vagina and uterus into each fallopian tube. Flexible coils temporarily anchor it inside the fallopian tube. A Dacron®-like mesh material embedded in the coils irritates the fallo-pian tubes' lining to cause scar tissue to grow and eventually permanently plug the tubes. It can take about three months for the scar tissue to grow, so it is important to use another form of birth control during this time. Then you will have to return to your doctor for a test to see if scar tissue has fully blocked your tubes. After three years of follow-up studies, Essure® has been shown to be 99.8 % effective in preventing pregnancy.

Emergency Contraception: This is not a regular method of birth control and should never be used as one. Emergency contraception, or emergency birth control, is used to keep a woman from getting pregnant when she has had unprotected vaginal intercourse. Unprotected can mean that no method of birth control was used. It can also mean that a birth control method was used but did not work, like a condom breaking, or a woman may have forgot-ten to take her birth control pills or may have been abused or forced to have sex when she did not want to. Emergency contraception consists of taking two doses of hormonal pills taken 12 hours apart and started within three days after having unprotected sex. These are sometimes wrongly called the "morn-ing after pill." The pills are 75 to 89% effective at preventing pregnancy. An-other type of emergency contraception is having the Copper T IUD put into your uterus within seven days of unprotected sex. This method is 99.9% ef-fective at preventing preg-nancy. Neither method of emergency contra-ception protects against STDs or HIV. You will need to visit your doctor for either a prescription for the pills or for the insertion of the IUD and to make sure you are not having problems.

☞ **Remember!!**

The only way to be sure you never get pregnant is to not have sex (abstinence).

Are there any foams or gels that I can use to keep from getting pregnant?

You can purchase what are called spermicides in drug stores. They work by killing sperm and come in several forms—foam, gel, cream, film, supposi-tory, or tablet. They are inserted or placed in the vagina no more than one hour before intercourse. If you use a film, suppository, or tablet, wait at least 15 minutes before having intercourse so the spermicide can dissolve. Do not douche or rinse out your vagina for at least six to eight hours after intercourse. You will need to use more spermicide before each act of intercourse. You may protect yourself more against getting pregnant if you use a spermicide with a male condom, diaphragm, or cervical cap. There are spermicidal products made specifically for use with the diaphragm and cervical cap. Check the package to make sure you are buying what you want.

All spermicides have sperm-killing chemicals in them. Some spermicides also have an ingredient, called nonoxynol-9, which may increase the risk of HIV infection when used frequently because it irritates the tissue in the vagina and anus, which can cause the virus to enter the body more freely. Some women are sensitive to nonoxynol-9 and need to use spermicides without it.

> ♣ **It's A Fact!!**
> Spermicides alone are only about 74% effective at preventing pregnancy.

Medications for vaginal yeast infections may decrease effectiveness of spermicides.

How effective is withdrawal as a birth control method?

Withdrawal is not the most effective birth control method. It works much better when a male condom is used.

Withdrawal is when a man takes his penis out of a woman's vagina (or "pulls out") before he ejaculates, or has an orgasm. This stops the sperm from going to the egg. "Pulling out" can be hard for a man to do and it takes a lot of self-control. When you use withdrawal, you can also be at risk getting pregnant before the man pulls out. When a man's penis first becomes erect, there can be fluid called pre-ejaculate fluid on the tip of the penis that has sperm in it. This sperm can get a woman pregnant. Withdrawal also does not protect you from STDs or HIV.

Chapter 51

Cosmetics And Your Health

What are cosmetics? How are they different from over-the-counter (OTC) drugs?

Cosmetics are put on the body to cleanse it, make it beautiful, make it attractive, or change its appearance or the way it looks. Cosmetic products include skin creams, lotions, perfumes, lipsticks, fingernail polishes, eye and face makeup products, permanent waves, hair dyes, toothpastes, and deodorants. Unlike drugs, which are used to treat or prevent disease in the body, cosmetics do not change or affect the body's structure or functions.

What's in cosmetics?

Fragrances and preservatives are the main ingredients in cosmetics.

More than 5,000 different kinds are used in products. Products marked "fragrance-free" or "without perfume" means that no fragrances have been added to make the product smell good.

Preservatives prevent bacteria and fungus from growing in the product and protect products from damage caused by air or light; but preservatives can also cause the skin to become irritated and infected. Some examples

About This Chapter: Information in this chapter is from "Cosmetics and Your Health," The National Women's Health Information Center, U.S. Department of Health and Human Services, Office On Women's Health, November 2004.

of preservatives include paraben, imidazolidinyl urea, quaternium-15, DMDM [1,3-dimethylol-5,5-dimethyl] hydantoin, phenoxyethanol, and formaldehyde.

> ❖ **It's A Fact!!**
>
> In cosmetics, fragrances are the most common cause of skin problems. Preservatives are the second.

Some ingredients cannot be used, or their use is limited, in cosmetics because they may cause cancer or other serious health problems. Those ingredients are bithionol, mercury compounds, vinyl chloride, halogenated salicylanilides, zirconium complexes in aerosol sprays, chloroform, methylene chloride, chlorofluorocarbon propellants, and hexachlorophene.

What is the role of the Food and Drug Administration (FDA) in the cosmetic industry?

A cosmetic maker can sell products without FDA approval. FDA does not review or approve cosmetics, or their ingredients, before they are sold to the public; but FDA urges cosmetic makers to do whatever tests are needed to prove their products are safe. Cosmetics makers must put a warning statement on the front labels of products that have not been safety tested, which reads, "WARNING—The safety of this product has not been determined."

FDA does require safety testing for color additives used in cosmetics. Cosmetics may only contain approved and certified colors. You will find FD&C, D&C, or external D&C listed on cosmetic labels. Here is what they mean:

- FD&C: color that can be used only in foods, drugs, and cosmetics

- D&C: color that can be used only in drugs and cosmetics

- External D&C: color that can be used only in drugs applied to the surface of the skin and cosmetics

A cosmetic maker also does not have to report product injuries. FDA collects this information on a voluntary basis only. Cosmetic makers that want to be a part of this program send reports to the FDA. Product recalls are also voluntary actions taken by cosmetic makers. FDA cannot require cosmetics recalls, but FDA does monitor cosmetic makers that do a recall.

FDA must first prove in court that a cosmetic product is a danger or some-how breaks the law before it can be taken off the market.

Are cosmetics safe?

Yes, for the most part. Serious problems from cosmetics are rare, but some-times problems can happen.

Eye infections can result from scratching the eye with a mascara wand, if the scratches go untreated. These infections can lead to ulcers on the cornea (clear covering of the eye), loss of lashes, or even blindness. To play it safe, never try to apply mascara while riding in a car, bus, train, or plane.

Sharing makeup can also lead to serious problems. Cosmetic brushes and sponges pick up bacteria from the skin; and if you moisten brushes with saliva, the problem can be worse. Washing your hands before using makeup will help prevent this problem.

Sleeping while wearing eye makeup can cause problems too. If mascara flakes into your eyes while you sleep, you might wake up with itching, blood-shot eyes, infections, or eye scratches. So be sure to remove all makeup be-fore going to bed.

Cosmetic products that come in aerosol containers also can be a hazard. For example, it is dangerous to use aerosol hairspray near heat, fire, or while smoking. Until hairspray is fully dry, it can catch on fire and cause serious burns. Fires related to hairsprays have caused injuries and death. Aerosol sprays or powders also can cause lung damage if they are deeply inhaled into the lungs.

How can I protect myself against the dangers of cosmetics?

- Never drive and put on makeup. Not only does this make driving a danger, hitting a bump in the road and scratching your eyeball can cause serious eye injury.

- Never share makeup. Always use a new sponge when trying products at a store. Insist that salespersons clean container openings with alco-hol before applying to your skin.

- Keep makeup containers closed tight when not in use.

- Keep makeup out of the sun and heat. Light and heat can kill the preservatives that help to fight bacteria. Do not keep cosmetics in a hot car for a long time.

♣ **It's A Fact!!**
The most common injury from cosmetics is from scratching the eye with a mascara wand.

- Do not use cosmetics if you have an eye infection, such as pinkeye. Throw away any makeup you were using when you first found the problem.

- Never add liquid to a product unless the label tells you to do so.

- Throw away any makeup if the color changes, or it starts to smell.

- Never use aerosol sprays near heat or while smoking, because they can catch on fire.

- Do not deeply inhale hairsprays or powders. This can cause lung damage.

- Avoid color additives that are not approved for use in the eye area, such as permanent eyelash tints and kohl (color additive that contains lead salts and is still used in eye cosmetics in other countries). Be sure to keep kohl away from children. It may cause lead poisoning.

What are "cosmeceuticals?"

Some products can be both cosmetics and drugs. This may happen when a product has two uses. For example, a shampoo is a cosmetic because it is used to clean the hair, but an antidandruff treatment is a drug because it is used to treat dandruff. So an antidandruff shampoo is both a cosmetic and a drug. Some other examples include toothpastes that contain fluoride, deodorants that are also antiperspirants, and moisturizers and makeup that provide sun protection.

These products must meet the standards for both cosmetics (color additives) and drugs.

Some cosmetic makers use the term "cosmeceutical" to refer to products that have drug-like benefits. FDA does not recognize this term. A product can be a drug, a cosmetic, or a combination of both, but the term "cosme-ceutical" has no meaning under the law.

While drugs are reviewed and approved by FDA, FDA does not approve cosmetics. If a product acts like a drug, FDA must approve it as a drug.

How long do cosmetics last?

You may not be able to use eye makeup, such as mascara, eyeliner, and eye shadow for as long as other products. This is because of the risk of eye infection. Some experts recommend replacing mascara three months after purchase. If mascara becomes dry, throw it away. Do not add water or, even worse, saliva to moisten it. That will bring bacteria into the product.

You may also need to watch certain "all natural" products that contain substances taken from plants. These products may be more at risk for bacte-ria. Since these products contain no preservatives or have non-traditional ones, your risk of infection may be greater.

If you do not store these products as directed, they might expire before the expiration date. For example, cosmetics stored in high heat may go bad faster than the expiration date. On the other hand, products stored the way they should be can be safely used until they expire.

What are hypoallergenic cosmetics?

Hypoallergenic (hy-po-al-ler-gen-ic) cosmetics are products that makers claim cause fewer allergic reactions than other products. Women with sensi-tive skin, and even those with normal skin, may think these products will be gentler; but there are no federal standards for using the term hypoallergenic. The term can mean whatever a company wants it to mean. Cosmetic makers do not have to prove their claims to the FDA.

Some products that have natural ingredients can cause allergic reac-tions. If you have an allergy to certain plants or animals, you could have an allergic reaction to cosmetics with those things in them. For example, lanolin from sheep wool is found in many lotions, but it is a common cause of allergies too.

Can cosmetics cause acne?

Some skin and hair care products can cause acne. To help prevent and control acne flare-ups, take good care of your skin. For example, use a mild soap or cleanser to gently wash your face twice a day. Choose non-comedogenic make-up and hair care products. This means that they do not close up the pores.

Are cosmetic products with alpha hydroxy acids safe?

Alpha hydroxy acids (AHAs) come from fruit and milk sugars. They are found in many creams and lotions. Many people buy products with AHAs because they claim to reduce wrinkles, spots, sun-damaged skin, and other signs of aging. Some studies suggest they may work.

Are these products safe? FDA has received reports of reactions in people using AHA products. Their complaints include severe redness, swelling (especially in the area of the eyes), burning, blistering, bleeding, rash, itching, and skin discoloration. AHAs may also increase your skin's risk of sunburn.

To find out if a product contains an AHA, look on the list of ingredients. By law, all cosmetics have ingredients on their outer label. AHAs may be called other names, like glycolic acid and lactic acid.

What precautions should I follow when using AHA products?

If you want to use AHA products, follow these safety tips:

- Always protect your skin before going out during the day. Use a sunscreen with a SPF (sun protection factor) of at least 15. Wear a hat with a brim. Cover up with lightweight, loose-fitting clothing.

- Buy products with good label information including a list of ingredients. Buy only products with an AHA level of 10 percent or less and a pH of 3.5 or more.

- Test a small area of skin to see if it is sensitive to any AHA product before using a lot of it. Stop using the product right away if you have a reaction, such as stinging, redness, or bleeding.

- Talk with your doctor or dermatologist (a doctor that treats skin problems) if you have a problem.

Chapter 52

Hair Dyes And Relaxers: Use With Caution

According to the U.S. Food and Drug Administration's (FDA) Office of Cosmetics and Colors, hair straighteners and hair dyes are among its top consumer complaint areas. Complaints range from hair breakage to symptoms warranting an emergency room visit. Reporting such complaints is voluntary, and the reported problem is often due to incorrect use of a product rather than the product itself. FDA encourages consumers to understand the risks that come with using hair chemicals and to take a proactive approach in ensuring their proper use. The agency does not have authority under the Federal Food, Drug, and Cosmetic Act to require pre-market approval for cosmetics, but it can take action when safety issues surface.

When The Product Is The Problem

When consumers notify FDA of problems with cosmetics, the agency evaluates evidence on a case-by-case basis and determines if follow-up is needed. FDA looks for patterns of complaints or unusual or severe reactions. The agency may conduct an investigation, and if the evidence supports regulatory action, FDA may request removal of a cosmetic from the market.

About This Chapter: Information in this chapter is excerpted from "Heading Off Hair-Care Disasters: Use Caution With Relaxers and Dyes," *FDA Consumer*, by Michelle Meadows, January-February 2001, U.S. Food and Drug Administration. Reviewed July 23, 2006 by David A. Cooke, M.D., Diplomate, American Board of Internal Medicine.

Safer Straightening

FDA has received complaints about scalp irritation and hair breakage related to both lye and "no lye" relaxers. Some consumers falsely assume that compared to lye relaxers, "no lye" relaxers take all the worry out of straightening.

People may think because it says "no lye" that it is not caustic, but both types of relaxers contain ingredients that work by breaking chemical bonds of the hair, and both can burn the scalp if used incorrectly. Lye relaxers contain sodium hydroxide as the active ingredient. With "no lye" relaxers, calcium hydroxide and guanidine carbonate are mixed to produce guanidine hydroxide.

Research has shown that this combination in "no lye" relaxers results in less scalp irritation than lye relaxers, but the same safety rules apply for both. They should be used properly, left on no longer than the prescribed time, carefully washed out with neutralizing shampoo, and followed up with regular conditioning. For those who opt to straighten their own hair, it is wise to enlist help because not being able to see and reach the top and back of the head makes proper application a challenge.

Scratching, brushing, and combing can make the scalp more susceptible to chemical damage and should be avoided right before using a relaxer.

How often to relax hair is a personal decision. Relaxing at intervals of six to eight weeks is common, and the frequency depends on the rate of a person's hair growth. Relaxers can cause hair breakage in the long term, and blow drying and curling can do more damage.

Consumers should be aware that applying more than one type of chemical treatment, such as coloring hair one week and then relaxing it the next, could increase the risk of hair damage. The only color recommended for relaxed hair is semi-permanent because it has no ammonia and less peroxide compared with permanent color.

Hair Dye Reactions

As with hair relaxers, some consumers have reported hair loss, burning, redness, and irritation from hair dyes. Allergic reactions to dyes include itching, swelling of the face, and even difficulty breathing.

Coal tar hair dye ingredients are known to cause allergic reactions in some people. Synthetic organic chemicals, including hair dyes and other color additives, were originally manufactured from coal tar, but today manufacturers primarily use materials derived from petroleum. The use of the term "coal tar" continues because historically that language has been incorporated into the law and regulations.

✔ **Quick Tip**

Some stylists recommend applying a layer of petroleum jelly on the scalp before applying a relaxer because it creates a protective barrier between the chemical and the skin.

The law does not require that FDA approve coal tar hair dyes, as is required for other uses of color additives. In addition, the law does not allow FDA to take action against coal tar hair dyes that are shown to be harmful, if the product is labeled with the prescribed caution statement indicating that the product may cause irritation in certain individuals, that a patch test for skin sensitivity should be done, and that the product must not be used for dyeing the eyelashes or eyebrows. The patch test involves putting a dab of hair dye behind the ear or inside the elbow, leaving it there for two days, and looking for itching, burning, redness, or other reactions.

The problem is that people can become sensitized, that is, develop an allergy to these ingredients. They may do the patch test once and then use the product for ten years before having an allergic reaction, but you are supposed to do the patch test every time, even in salons.

What about ending up with something other than the exact shade of strawberry blonde on the shelf? Do not think the color on the box is the color you will get. There are so many variables, like what chemicals are already in your hair and what your natural color is, that go into how your hair will turn out.

When using all hair chemicals, it is critical to keep them away from children to prevent ingestion and other accidents, and to follow product directions carefully. It sounds basic, but some people do not do it. If it says leave on hair for five minutes, seven minutes does not make it better. In fact, it could do damage.

Look Out For Your Eyes

Whether applying hair chemicals at home or in a hair salon, consumers and beauticians should be careful to keep them away from the eyes. FDA has received reports of injuries from hair relaxers and hair dye accidentally getting into eyes; and while it may be tempting to match a new hair color to eyebrows and eyelashes, consumers should resist the urge. There are no color additives approved by FDA for dyeing or tinting eyelashes and eyebrows.

The law does not require that FDA approve coal tar hair dyes, as is required for other uses of color additives. In addition, the law does not allow FDA to take action against coal tar hair dyes that are shown to be harmful, if the product is labeled with the following caution statement:

"Caution—This product contains ingredients which may cause skin irritation on certain individuals, and a preliminary test according to accompanying directions should first be made. This product must not be used for dyeing the eyelashes or eyebrows; to do so may cause blindness."

♣ **It's A Fact!!**

The use of permanent eyelash and eyebrow tinting and dyeing has been known to cause serious eye injuries and even blindness.

Chapter 53

Tattoos And Permanent Makeup: What Are The Risks?

The U.S. Food and Drug Administration (FDA) considers the inks used in intradermal tattoos, including permanent makeup, to be cosmetics and considers the pigments used in the inks to be color additives requiring pre-market approval under the Federal Food, Drug, and Cosmetic Act. However, because of other public health priorities and a previous lack of evidence of safety concerns, FDA has not traditionally regulated tattoo inks or the pigments used in them. The actual practice of tattooing is regulated by local jurisdictions. FDA is aware of more than 150 reports of adverse reactions in consumers to certain permanent makeup ink shades, and it is possible that the actual number of women affected was greater. In addition, concerns raised by the scientific community regarding the pigments used in these inks have prompted FDA to investigate the safe use of tattoo inks. FDA continues to evaluate the extent and severity of adverse events associated with tattooing and is conducting research on inks. As new information is assessed, the agency will consider whether additional actions are necessary to protect public health.

In addition to the reported adverse reactions, areas of concern include tattoo removal, infections that result from tattooing, and the increasing variety

About This Chapter: Information in this chapter is from "Tattoos and Permanent Makeup," Office of Cosmetics and Colors, Center for Food Safety and Applied Nutrition, U.S. Food and Drug Administration, April 2006.

of pigments and diluents being used in tattooing. More than fifty different pigments and shades are in use, and the list continues to grow. Although a number of color additives are approved for use in cosmetics, none is approved for injection into the skin. Using an unapproved color additive in a tattoo ink makes the ink adulterated. Many pigments used in tattoo inks are not approved for skin contact at all. Some are industrial grade colors that are suitable for printers' ink or automobile paint.

Nevertheless, many individuals choose to undergo tattooing in its various forms. For some, it is an aesthetic choice or an initiation rite. Some choose permanent makeup as a time saver or because they have physical difficulty applying regular, temporary makeup. For others, tattooing is an adjunct to reconstructive surgery, particularly of the face or breast, to simulate natural pigmentation. People who have lost their eyebrows due to alopecia (a form of hair loss) may choose to have "eyebrows" tattooed on, while people with vitiligo (a lack of pigmentation in areas of the skin) may try tattooing to help camouflage the condition.

Whatever their reason, consumers should be aware of the risks involved in order to make an informed decision.

What Risks Are Involved In Tattooing?

The following are the primary complications that can result from tattooing:

- **Infection:** Unsterile tattooing equipment and needles can transmit infectious diseases, such as hepatitis. The risk of infection is the reason the American Association of Blood Banks requires a one-year wait between getting a tattoo and donating blood.

- **Removal problems:** Despite advances in laser technology, removing a tattoo is a painstaking process, usually involving several treatments and considerable expense. Complete removal without scarring may be impossible.

- **Allergic reactions:** Although FDA has received reports of numerous adverse reactions associated with certain shades of ink in permanent makeup, marketed by a particular manufacturer, reports of allergic reactions to tattoo pigments have been rare. However, when they happen, they may be particularly troublesome because the pigments can be hard to remove. Occasionally, people may develop an allergic reaction to tattoos they have had for years.

- **Granulomas:** These are nodules that may form around material that the body perceives as foreign, such as particles of tattoo pigment.

- **Keloid formation:** If you are prone to developing keloids, which are scars that grow beyond normal boundaries, you are at risk of keloid formation from a tattoo. Keloids may form any time you injure or traumatize your skin.

- **MRI complications:** There have been reports of people with tattoos or permanent makeup who experienced swelling or burning in the affected areas when they underwent magnetic resonance imaging (MRI). This seems to occur only rarely and apparently without lasting effects.

There also have been reports of tattoo pigments interfering with the quality of the image. This seems to occur mainly when a person with permanent eyeliner undergoes MRI of the eyes. Mascara may produce a similar effect. The difference is that mascara is easily removable.

The cause of these complications is uncertain. Some have theorized that they result from an interaction with the metallic components of some pigments.

However, the risks of avoiding an MRI when your doctor has recommended one are likely to be much greater than the risks of complications from an interaction between the MRI and tattoo or permanent makeup. Instead of avoiding an MRI, individuals who have tattoos or permanent makeup should inform the radiologist or technician of this fact in order to take appropriate precautions and avoid complications.

A Common Problem: Dissatisfaction

A common problem that may develop with tattoos is the desire to remove them. Removing tattoos and permanent makeup can be very difficult.

Although tattoos may be satisfactory at first, they sometimes fade. Also, if the tattooist injects the pigments too deeply into the skin, the pigments may migrate beyond the original sites, resulting in a blurred appearance.

Another cause of dissatisfaction is that the human body changes over time, and styles change with the season. The permanent makeup that may have looked flattering when first injected may later clash with changing skin tones and facial or body contours. People who plan to have facial cosmetic surgery are advised that the appearance of their permanent makeup may become distorted. The tattoo that seemed stylish at first may become dated and embarrassing, and changing tattoos or permanent makeup is not as easy as changing your mind.

Consult your healthcare provider about the best removal techniques for you.

What About Temporary Tattoos?

Temporary tattoos, such as those applied to the skin with a moistened wad of cotton, fade several days after application. Most contain color additives approved for cosmetic use on the skin; however, the agency has issued an import alert for certain foreign-made temporary tattoos.

The temporary tattoos subject to the import alert are not allowed into the United States because they do not carry the FDA-mandated ingredient labels, or they contain colors not permitted by FDA for use in cosmetics applied to the skin. FDA has received reports of allergic reactions to temporary tattoos.

In a similar action, FDA has issued an import alert for henna intended for use on the skin. Henna is approved only for use as a hair dye, not for direct application to the skin. Also, henna typically produces a reddish brown tint, raising questions about what ingredients are added to produce the varieties of colors labeled as "henna," such as "black henna" and "blue henna." FDA has also received reports of allergic reactions to products applied to the skin that contain henna.

♣ It's A Fact!!

Henna is a brown to reddish brown dye made from the leaves of the *Lawsonia* plant, a flowering shrub native to North Africa and Asia.

Source: "Focus On: Henna," *FDA & You*, Issue #3, Spring/Summer 2003, Updated May 2004, U.S. Food and Drug Administration.

Chapter 54

What You Should Know Before You Get Pierced

Many young people of today are discovering body piercing. Getting a piercing can be a statement about who you are, a form of body art that is less permanent than tattooing, yet still daring. Ears, necks, lips, nose, eyebrows, cheeks, tongues (ouch!), nipples, in between fingers and toes, navels, and genitals are among the areas of the body that people have had pierced.

History

Body piercing is not a new practice. Here are some examples:

- Earlobes have been pierced for many years in many countries.

- In many cultures people adorn their face with nostril piercing.

- Septum piercing (through the nose) takes place in traditional African and New Guinean societies.

- Lip and cheek piercing have been common in many tribal societies.

About This Chapter: Information in this chapter is from "Body Piercing," February 2006. Printed with permission, © Children, Youth and Women's Health Service, Government of South Australia.

What Can Go Wrong/Risks

Here are some things that can go wrong:

- If sterile equipment and latex gloves are not used, there are risks of passing on infections like hepatitis B and C, HIV/AIDS, and tetanus.

- There is a risk of infection after piercing. Infections can become severe and may need antibiotics and removal of the piercing.

- The piercing can be rejected, much like the body rejects a splinter.

- You can get an allergic reaction to the metal.

- You will be permanently scarred.

- There is a risk of keloid formation— a large scar even from a small wound.

> ### ♣ It's A Fact!!
>
> Body piercing can cause some problems. It's a good idea to find out as much information as you can before making a decision.

- Genital piercing increases the risk of sexually transmitted diseases because the jewelry can cause a condom to break and because the piercing can be a point for an infection to enter the body.

- Some women have reported that it is more difficult to breastfeed after getting nipples pierced, possibly due to the milk ducts being blocked by jewelry and by scar tissue. A breastfeeding woman would have to take the jewelry out until after the baby is weaned. It is not practical to take the jewelry out for each feeding, every few hours. This would be really difficult at four o'clock in the morning with a baby screaming for a feeding. The jewelry can't be left in the nipple during a feeding because it could damage the baby's soft palate (inside the mouth) and because if it comes loose, the baby could choke on the jewelry. For these reasons it may be best to avoid nipple piercing if there's a possibility you'll breastfeed later on.

- Mouth jewelry may damage teeth, especially when tongue jewelry taps on the teeth.

If there is any infection, it is important to consult your doctor quickly.

Things To Consider Before Piercing

If you are considering piercing, it's good to have a lot of knowledge first. You've already read about the possible risks. Here are some questions to ask to help you make your decision:

- Ask yourself why you want to get pierced? Is it a rebellion, a way to stand out, or is it more of a personal statement, something you feel strongly about?

- Talk to people that you know have had a piercing. What was it like for them? Would they do it again?

- Where on your body will you have the piercing? Remember that some people can be quite judgmental about piercing and about your looks, and this can lessen your chances of getting a job (especially a conservative job).

- If at a later date you decide to take the jewelry out, there will be some scarring; this will, of course, be more obvious on the more exposed parts of the body such as the face.

- What rules does your place of work or your school have about piercing?

- How will your parents feel about it? Is this going to cause conflict at home?

- If you play a sport, can you keep the jewelry in while playing, or is there a danger it can get caught and tear? If you take the jewelry out for games, the hole could close.

At What Age Can You Get Piercing?

Check the laws where you live about when you can have a body piercing. Most body piercers will not pierce a person under the age of 16 or 18 except with signed parental consent.

Although this may seem unfair to younger people who really want a piercing, these rules are in place for a number of reasons. Firstly, your body is still growing and this means that the piercing can grow out or change position. Secondly, a piercing could be seen as child abuse especially if it is in a private part of your body.

Don't get your piercing done by a friend to avoid waiting. Without proper training and equipment, this can be dangerous. Wait until a reputable piercer will do the piercing correctly.

Choosing A Reputable Piercer

If you do decide to go ahead and get a piercing, here are some important things to find out first so that you can try and avoid the piercing pitfalls already described:

- It's important to go to a reputable piercer. There are many things that have to be carefully considered by the piercer including the right size jewelry, the right type of metal for different body parts, sterilization of equipment, and correct positioning of the piercing using some knowledge of the human anatomy.

- Ask around for names of reputable piercers. There are no legal regulations for the training of body piercers. This means that some piercers may not be well trained. They have varying degrees of formal training, experience, knowledge, and skill.

- Don't get just anyone to do it. Although piercers do not have formal training, a reputable piercer still has lots more knowledge than one of your friends doing your piercing at home.

Ask the piercer the following questions:

- Is all the equipment sterile? Equipment should be in new sterile packaging and then thrown out immediately after use or properly sterilized in an autoclave. An autoclave kills germs with ultra high temperatures.

- Is a brand new sterile needle used for each customer? It should then be disposed of in a locked sharps container.

- Are fresh, disposable latex gloves used for each customer?

- Does the piercer have knowledge about the human anatomy and the location of various nerves, etc. that lie beneath the skin and must be avoided?

- Does the piercer give every customer information about proper after-care of their piercing?

- Is the piercer available to you for any questions you may have after the piercing?

- What is the piercer's knowledge about correct jewelry to be used? The jewelry must be the right gauge or thickness for the particular piercing, as well as the right type of metal.

Have a look for yourself and make sure the place is clean. The piercer should be clean, sober, helpful, knowledgeable, and give you all the information you need to guide you through the experience.

What's It Like To Get A Piercing?

It takes about 15 minutes to get a piercing. This time includes marking the area to be pierced, cleaning the area, and getting everything ready. The actual piercing itself only takes from seconds to minutes depending on the type of piercing.

Whether it hurts or not is an individual thing; we all have different levels of tolerance to pain. Piercers don't generally use any anesthetic. It can be sore for a while afterwards, especially if you bump it.

After Care

After care instructions vary depending on the type of piercing. Your piercer should give you detailed instructions to follow to take care of the piercing.

It can be a good idea to ask about the instructions before the piercing, as it can be hard to concentrate afterwards, especially if you feel a little dizzy or light headed. Ask the piercer to write down the after care instructions.

☞ Remember!!

It is your right to choose a reputable piercer and to be given quality service. If you are not happy with the attitude of the piercer or the appearance of the business, don't be afraid to walk out; there are better places to choose from.

Some general rules are as follows:

- Never touch your piercing with dirty hands.

- Follow the piercer's instructions carefully.

- Use products suggested by the piercer, as different products should be used for different areas of the body.

- If you have an oral piercing (a piercing in the mouth), avoid smoking or drinking alcohol, at least until it has fully healed.

- Use condoms or dental dams for sex, including oral sex, if you have a genital or oral piercing.

- See a health professional quickly if you have pain or an infection.

Healing Time

Healing times vary from weeks to a year. It depends on the following:

- The part of the body being pierced; e.g. earlobes heal quicker than the cartilage at the top of the ear.

- Your own body's reaction to the piercing; e.g. you can be slightly sensitive to metal.

- How well you care for the piercing

Ask the piercer about expected healing times for various body parts.

Chapter 55

Decorative Contact Lenses: Are Your Eyes At Risk?

Responsible and appropriate use is critical when it comes to contact lenses. That means getting an eye exam and a valid prescription and buying contact lenses from an eye care professional licensed to sell them. It is also essential to follow directions for cleaning and wearing the lenses and to have follow-up eye exams.

These precautions apply to all contact lenses, including non-corrective lenses intended solely to change the appearance of a normal eye in a decorative fashion, such as to turn brown eyes blue. These products present the same eye health risks as contact lenses intended for vision correction.

Fortunately, most decorative contact lenses are part of product lines that include a range of corrective powers, including non-corrective lenses, which have been authorized by the U.S. Food and Drug Administration (FDA) for marketing. But the FDA has learned that some firms are not seeking FDA authorization before marketing decorative lenses.

The FDA recently issued a warning to consumers about the risk of permanent eye injury, and even blindness, associated with decorative contact

About This Chapter: Information in this chapter is from "FDA Issues Warning on Decorative Contact Lenses," *FDA Consumer*, by Michelle Meadows, January-February 2003, U.S. Food and Drug Administration.

lenses distributed without a prescription and without proper fitting by an eye care professional. These products are being distributed through beauty salons, record stores, video stores, flea markets, convenience stores, beach shops, and other retail establishments.

Reports Of Damage, Infections

The FDA has received reports of eye problems, such as damage to the cornea and eye infections, associated with decorative contact lenses. Most of the reports involve teenagers. Victor Crosby, M.D., an ophthalmologist in Athens, Georgia, reported a case of a 16-year-old female who bought contact lenses at a flea market. "She wore them for a couple of days and ended up in the emergency room with burning, redness, and sensitivity to light in both eyes," he says. "The main problem was a poor lens fit." Contact lenses that are too tight can damage the cornea. Crosby treated her with a topical steroid antibiotic for five to six days, and she fully recovered.

Others have not been as lucky. Thomas Steinemann, M.D., director of the Metro-Health Eye Clinic in Cleveland, Ohio, treated one of the worst cases related to decorative contact lenses that have been reported to the FDA so far. In September 2001, a 14-year-old female needed treatment after wearing decorative contact lenses she bought for about $20 at a video store. "She wanted to turn brown eyes green to match an outfit," Steinemann says. "But the result was a lot of pain and suffering."

She experienced an aggressive infection caused by a *Pseudomonas* bacterium in one eye. "You can not only lose vision from this infection, but you can lose the eye," Steinemann says. The teenager had to be hospitalized and treated with antibiotic drops every 30 minutes for four days. "Though the infection was eradicated by aggressive topical therapy, the eye remained inflamed for a long time," he says. She was blind in the infected eye for two months. Soon after she began to regain some vision, scar tissue formed, causing further vision loss. In June 2002, Steinemann performed a corneal transplant, which involved removing her diseased cornea and replacing it with a donor cornea. Recovery from the corneal transplant takes about a year.

Along with informing consumers about potential dangers with decorative contact lenses, the FDA is seizing decorative contact lenses on the market that violate federal law. The agency has also issued an import alert instructing the FDA and Customs officials to detain decorative contact lenses presented at U.S. ports of entry unless the FDA has cleared them for marketing.

Proper Fit, Prescription Needed

The FDA encourages consumers to discontinue use of decorative contact lenses obtained without proper fitting and a prescription, and to notify the FDA of any complaints or problems associated with these products.

It comes down to this question, Steinemann says: "Who is the advocate for the health of your eyes? It is not someone at a video store or a gas station."

✔ Quick Tip
Contact Lens Tips

- Wear contact lenses only if they are fitted and prescribed by an eye care professional such as an ophthalmologist or an optometrist.

- Do not purchase contact lenses from gas stations, video stores, record shops, or any other vendor not authorized by law to dispense contact lenses.

- Never swim while wearing contact lenses. There is a risk of eye infection when contact lenses come into contact with bacteria in swimming pool water.

- Make sure contact lenses are properly cleaned and disinfected as instructed by your eye care professional.

- Make sure you wash your hands before handling and cleaning your contact lenses.

- Never swap or share contact lenses with anyone.

- Never sleep while wearing contact lenses unless they are extended-wear lenses specifically designed for that purpose.

Chapter 56

What You Need To Know About Tanning

Do not mistake the tan you get from hours spent by the pool or under tanning lamps for a healthy summer glow. It is actually a sign of sun damage from ultraviolet (UV) rays and can cause premature aging and skin cancer. Protecting your skin now can help prevent the side effects caused by too much sun.

Long-Term Sun Damage

Leathery, wrinkled skin, and dark spots are common earmarks of a life-long sunbather. Unfortunately, since these signs of sun damage do not usually show up until many years later, you may think you are immune to the long-term effects of tanning. Everyone, no matter his or her skin tone, is at risk for skin damage.

Skin Cancer

Experts agree that natural and artificial sunlight, particularly the UV rays, damages the skin. UV rays cause the obvious short-term damage seen in a sunburn or a tan, as well as the long-term damage that accumulates with each exposure.

About This Chapter: Information in this chapter is from "The Truth About Tanning: What You Need to Know to Protect Your Skin," *FDA & You*, Issue #7, Summer 2005, U.S. Food and Drug Administration.

When you tan you greatly increase your risk of developing skin cancer. This is especially true if you spend time tanning each year because damage to the skin accumulates over time. Unlike skin cancer, premature aging of the skin will occur in everyone who is repeatedly exposed to the sun over a long time, although the damage may be less apparent and take longer to show up in people with darker skin.

There are three main types of skin cancer: melanoma, basal cell carcinoma, and squamous cell carcinoma. Melanoma is the least common but most serious because it is responsible for most of the skin cancer deaths each year. The other two types, basal cell and squamous cell carcinomas, are often referred to as non-melanoma skin cancer. Basal cell cancer is the most common skin cancer, followed by squamous cell carcinoma, which can also become a killer.

A fourth type of growth, actinic, or solar keratosis, is also of concern because it can progress into cancer. It is the most common pre-malignant skin condition, occurring in more than 5 million Americans.

Researchers still are not sure why some people develop skin cancer and others do not, but there are some preventive measures you can take that may reduce your chances of getting skin cancer. While sunscreens protect against sunburn, they do not necessarily prevent cancer. If you use sunscreens to spend more time in the sun, your skin could still be exposed to a high dose of UV, especially the long wave rays. So it is still a good idea to stay out of the sun at midday, and to protect yourself with sunglasses, a wide-brim hat, and protective clothing like a long-sleeved shirt made of thick, light-colored fabric.

Moles or freckles that change shape, color, texture, or get crusty and bleed could be a sign of skin cancer. Early-stage melanomas often show up as a light brown to black flat mark that is usually about one-quarter inch in size. Your doctor should check out any suspect spot as soon as possible. When detected in its earliest stages, skin cancer is often curable.

Prevention

The best way to protect your skin from the dangerous effects of UV rays is to take simple precautions every day. Wearing sunscreen, shielding your face and eyes with a wide-brim hat, wearing sunglasses with a UVA/UVB rating of 99% or higher, and seeking shade when possible can help decrease your risk.

Clothing can also help protect you from harmful UV in the form of protection you do not need to reapply. Fabrics can differ greatly in their ability to shield you from UV rays, and natural fibers like cotton offer little protection when wet.

The ideal sun protective fabrics are lightweight, comfortable, and protect against exposure even when wet. Items of sun protective factor (SPF) clothing are available that have thick, tightly woven fabrics with special fibers and dyes to help shield you from the sun's rays. Remember that light-color fabrics will be cooler in the summer heat.

> ❖ **It's A Fact!!**
>
> Direct sun is not the only cause of sunburn. You can get sunburned even on a cloudy day because UV rays can filter through the water droplets that make up clouds.
>
> Source: "The Truth About Tanning: What You Need to Know to Protect Your Skin," *FDA & You*, Issue #7, Summer 2005, U.S. Food and Drug Administration.

Certain medications, such as antibiotics, can make you more sensitive to the sun and put you at greater risk for sunburn. Ask your doctor whether you are taking a medication that could affect your sensitivity to the sun and what you should do.

Sunscreen

Sunscreen does not completely protect you from harmful UV rays, but it can drastically reduce their effects if used properly. Sunscreen is available in a variety of forms for you to choose from, including sprays, lotions, gels, and wax sticks. Most sunscreens are made of chemicals that absorb UV radiation. Others create a barrier that reflects the UV radiation away from the skin.

When shopping for sunscreen, choose one that is labeled as broad-spectrum because it will help protect you from both UVA and UVB rays. Check the sunscreen label for broad-spectrum ingredients, such as benzophenones (oxybenzone), cinnamates (octylmethyl cinnamate and cinoxate), suliso-benzone, salicylates, titanium dioxide, zinc oxide, and avobenzone (Parsol® 1789).

All sunscreens are labeled with SPF numbers. The higher the SPF number, the more protection against sunburn the sunscreen provides. To get the most protection out of sunscreen choose one with an SPF of at least 15. Some sunscreens are labeled as being water-resistant. These sunscreens stay on the skin longer even if they get wet from pool water, ocean water, or sweat. But water-resistant does not mean waterproof. Water-resistant sunscreens still need to be reapplied, so check the label for reapplication times.

The effectiveness of a sunscreen is reduced if it is applied incorrectly or if it is washed off, rubbed off, or sweated off. To make sure you are getting the maximum sunscreen protection, apply an even layer of sunscreen and reapply it according to the directions.

Sunscreen usually needs about 15–30 minutes to soak in to the skin before you go outside. Read the label to see how long you should wait. If the label does not indicate how long, wait 30 minutes to be safe.

♣ **It's A Fact!!**

Protect Yourself With These Sun Safety Tips

- Avoid the sun, or seek shade, from 10 a.m. to 4 p.m. when the sun's rays are strongest.

- Apply an SPF 15 or higher sunscreen.

- Allow 30 minutes for skin to absorb sunscreen before going outside.

- Check the label and reapply sunscreen according to the instructions.

- Wear a wide-brimmed hat.

- Protect eyes with sunglasses that have a UV/UVB protection of at least 99%.

- Check with your doctor to find out if you are taking medications that will make you more sensitive to the sun.

Source: "The Truth About Tanning: What You Need to Know to Protect Your Skin," *FDA & You*, Issue #7, Summer 2005, U.S. Food and Drug Administration.

In The Salon

With the convenience offered by a tanning salon, it may be tempting to lie in a tanning bed or sit in front of a tanning lamp. Fight the urge! Tanning beds and lights are just as dangerous as tanning at the pool or on the beach. The UVA rays emitted by a tanning lamp or bed are often much more intense than those produced by the sun. The aging and cancer risks associated with outdoor tanning are the same as tanning in a salon. For these reasons, the U.S. Food and Drug Administration (FDA) does not recommend the use of indoor tanning equipment.

If you insist on using a tanning lamp or bed, follow these steps to reduce the dangers of UV exposure:

- Be sure to wear the goggles provided, making sure they fit snugly and are not cracked.

- Start slowly and use short exposure times to build up a tan over time.

- Follow manufacturer-recommended exposure times for your skin type. Check the label for exposure times.

- Stick to your time limit.

- After a tan is developed, tan no more often than twice a week.

Sunless Tanning

Sunless tanning delivers a false glow by coating your skin with the chemical dihydroxyacetone (DHA). DHA interacts with the dead surface cells in the epidermis to darken skin color and simulate a tan, and the result usually lasts for several days.

You should know that while the FDA allows DHA to be "externally applied" for skin coloring, there are restrictions on its use. DHA should not be inhaled, ingested, or used in such a way that the eyes and eye area are exposed to it because the risks, if any, are unknown.

Before using a sunless tanning booth, ask the tanning salon these questions to make sure you will be protected: Will my eyes and the area surrounding them be protected? Will my nose, mouth, and ears be protected? Will I be protected from inhaling the tanning spray through my nose or mouth? If the answer to any of these questions is "no," look for another salon. Otherwise you are putting yourself at risk for exposure to chemicals with potentially dangerous effects.

You should also take precautions if you are applying a self-tanner at home. Most self- tanners contain the same DHA used in sunless tanning salons. Self-tanners are available in many forms, including lotions, creams, and sprays that you apply and let soak in to your skin. Follow the directions on the self-tanner label carefully and take care not to get the self-tanner in your eyes, nose, or mouth.

Tanning Pills

You may have seen ads that promise to give you a golden glow just by swallowing a pill. This may sound too good to be true, because it is. These, so-called, tanning pills are unsafe and none are approved by the FDA. Some tanning pills contain the color additive canthaxanthin. When large amounts of canthaxanthin are ingested, the substance can turn the skin a range of colors from orange to brown. They can also cause serious health problems including liver damage; a severe itching condition called urticaria; and an eye disorder called canthaxanthin retinopathy, in which yellow deposits form in the retinas.

✔ Quick Tip
Do A Skin Cancer Check

No matter how much time you spend in the sun, you should protect yourself by checking for signs of skin cancer. Do a thorough body check and look for changes in the size, shape, color, or feel of birthmarks, moles, and spots. If you find any changes or find sores that are not healing, let your doctor know right away.

Use a hand mirror or full-size mirror and follow these easy steps:

1. Check the back of your neck, ears, and scalp.

2. Check your body and head—front, back, and sides.

3. Bend your elbows and check the underside of your arms.

4. Check all in-view parts like fingers, hands, and feet.

Source: "Do a Skin Cancer Check," *FDA & You*, Issue #3, Spring/Summer 2003, Updated May 2004, U.S. Food and Drug Administration.

Chapter 57

Plastic Surgery: Is It A Healthy Choice For Teens?

When you hear of plastic surgery, what do you think of? A Hollywood star trying to delay the effects of aging? Somebody's cute "new" nose that cost quite a few allowances? People who want to change the size of their stomachs, breasts, or other parts of their appearance because they see it done so easily on TV?

Those are common images of plastic surgery, but what about the 4-year-old boy who has his chin rebuilt after a dog bit him? Or the young woman who has the birthmark on her forehead lightened with a laser?

What is plastic surgery?

Just because the name includes the word "plastic" does not mean patients who have this surgery end up with a face full of fake stuff. The name is not taken from the synthetic substance but from the Greek word *plastikos*, which means to form or mold (and which gives plastic its name as well).

About This Chapter: Information in this chapter is from "Plastic Surgery." This information was provided by TeensHealth, one of the largest resources online for medically reviewed health information written for parents, kids, and teens. For more articles like this one, visit www.TeensHealth.org, or www.KidsHealth.org. © 2004 The Nemours Foundation.

Plastic surgery is a special type of surgery that involves both a person's appearance and his or her ability to function. Plastic surgeons strive to improve patients' appearance, self-image, and confidence through both reconstructive and cosmetic procedures.

Reconstructive procedures correct defects on the face or body. These include physical birth defects like cleft lips and palates and ear deformities, traumatic injuries like those from dog bites or burns, or the aftermath of disease treatments like rebuilding a woman's breast after surgery for breast cancer.

Cosmetic (also called **aesthetic**) procedures alter a part of the body that the person is not satisfied with. Common cosmetic procedures include making the breasts larger (augmentation mammoplasty) or smaller (reduction mammoplasty), reshaping the nose (rhinoplasty), and removing pockets of fat from specific spots on the body (liposuction). Some cosmetic procedures are not even surgical in the way that most people think of surgery—that is, cutting and stitching. For example, the use of special lasers to remove unwanted hair, and injections or sanding skin to improve severe scarring, are two such treatments.

Why do teens get plastic surgery?

Most teens do not, of course, but some do. Interestingly, the American Society of Plastic Surgeons reports a difference in the reasons teens give for having plastic surgery and the reasons adults do: Teens view plastic surgery as a way to fit in and look acceptable to friends and peers. Adults, on the other hand, frequently see plastic surgery as a way to stand out from the crowd.

The number of teens who choose to get plastic surgery is on the rise. According to the American Society of Plastic Surgeons, 335,000 people 18 years and younger had plastic surgery in 2003, up from about 306,000 in 2000.

Some people turn to plastic surgery to correct a physical defect or to alter a part of the body that makes them feel uncomfortable. For example, guys with a condition called gynecomastia (excess breast tissue) that does not go away with time or weight loss may opt for reduction surgery. A girl or guy with a birthmark may turn to laser treatment to lessen its appearance.

Other people decide they want a cosmetic change to feel better about the way they look. Teens who have cosmetic procedures, such as otoplasty (surgery to pin back ears that stick out) or dermabrasion (a procedure that can help smooth or camouflage severe acne scars), often say that having the surgery gives them greater confidence and boosts their self-esteem.

♣ It's A Fact!!

The most common procedures teens choose include nose reshaping, ear reshaping, acne and acne scar treatment, and breast reduction.

Is plastic surgery the right choice?

Reconstructive surgery helps repair significant defects or problems. But what about having cosmetic surgery just to change your appearance? Is it a good idea for teens? It can be. But like everything else, there are right and wrong reasons. And there are no quick fixes.

Unlike on TV, cosmetic surgery is unlikely to change your life, or even get you a date to the prom. Shows like *I Want a Famous Face* are actually far from reality. In fact, it is impossible for a surgeon to make one person look exactly like another. You and Brad Pitt probably have very different bone structures.

In reality, most board-certified plastic surgeons spend a lot of time interviewing teens who want plastic surgery to decide if they are good candidates for the surgery. Some doctors will not perform certain procedures (like rhinoplasty) on a teen until they are sure that person is old enough and has finished growing. For rhinoplasty, that means about 14 or 15 for girls and a little older for guys.

Girls who want to enlarge their breasts for cosmetic reasons usually must be at least 18 because saline implants are only approved for women 18 and older. In some cases, though, such as when there is a tremendous size difference between the breasts, or one breast has failed to grow at all, a plastic surgeon may get involved earlier.

Doctors also want to know that teens are emotionally mature enough to handle the surgery and that they are doing it for the right reasons. Many plastic surgery procedures are just that—surgery. They involve anesthesia, wound healing, and other serious risks. Doctors who perform these procedures want to know that their patients are capable of understanding and handling the stress of surgery.

Here are a few things to think about if you are considering plastic surgery:

- Almost all teens (and many adults) are self-conscious about their bodies. Almost everyone wishes there were a thing or two that could be changed. A lot of this self-consciousness goes away with time. Ask yourself if you are considering plastic surgery for only yourself or whether it is to please someone else.

- A person's body continues to change through the teen years. Body parts that might appear too large or too small now can become more proportionate over time. Sometimes, for example, what seems like a big nose looks more the right size as the rest of the person's face catches up during growth.

- Getting in good shape through appropriate weight control and exercise can do great things for a person's looks without surgery. In fact, it is never a good idea to choose plastic surgery as a first option for something like weight loss that can be corrected in a non-surgical manner. Sure, gastric bypass or liposuction may seem like quick and easy fixes compared to sticking with a diet. Both of these procedures, however, carry far greater risks than dieting, and doctors should reserve them for extreme cases when all other options have failed.

- Some people's emotions have a really big effect on how they think they look. People who are depressed, extremely self-critical, or have a

distorted view of what they really look like sometimes think that changing their looks will solve their problems. In these cases, it will not.
Working out the emotional problem with the help of a trained thera-
pist is a better bet. In fact, many doctors will not perform plastic surgery on teens who are depressed or have other mental health problems
until these problems are treated first.

What's involved?

If you are considering plastic surgery, talk it over with your parents. If you
are serious, and your parents agree, the next step is meeting with a plastic
surgeon to help you learn what to expect before, during, and after the procedure, as well as any possible complications or downsides to the surgery. Depending on the procedure, you may feel some pain as you recover, and
temporary swelling or bruising can make you look less like yourself for a
while.

Procedures and healing times vary, so you will want to do your research
into what is involved in your particular procedure and whether the surgery is
reconstructive or cosmetic. It is a good idea to choose a doctor who is certified by the American Board of Plastic Surgery.

Cost will likely be a factor, too. Elective plastic surgery procedures can be
expensive. Although medical insurance covers many reconstructive surgeries, the cost of cosmetic procedures almost always comes straight out of the
patient's pocket. Your parents can find out what your insurance plan will and

☞ Remember!!

Plastic surgery is not something to rush
into. If you are thinking about plastic surgery,
find out as much as you can about the specific procedure you are considering and talk it over with doctors and your parents. Once you have the facts,
you can decide whether the surgery is
right for you.

will not cover. For example, breast enlargement surgery is considered a purely cosmetic procedure and is rarely covered by insurance, but breast reduction surgery may be covered by some plans because large breasts can cause physical discomfort, and even pain for many girls.

Chapter 58

Teens And Breast Implants: Consider These Facts

Breast implant surgery is a growing trend among teenaged women. According to the American Society for Aesthetic Plastic Surgery (ASAPS), women 18 and under accounted for 11,326 breast implant surgeries performed in American women in 2003, compared to 3,872 in 2002.

Despite more than a decade of controversy over their safety, breast implants are more popular than ever among women who want to build upon what nature gave them or who want to restore what disease has taken away. Whatever the reason, opting for breast implants is a personal decision that should be made only after a woman fully understands and accepts the potential risks of the devices and the importance of follow-up evaluations with her doctor.

Breast implants are designed to change the size and shape of the breast (augmentation), to rebuild the breast (reconstruction), and to replace existing implants (revision). There are two primary types of breast implants: saline-filled and silicone gel-filled. Depending on the type of implant, the shell is either pre-filled with a fixed volume of solution or filled through a valve during the surgery to the desired size. Some allow for adjustments of the filler volume after surgery. Breast implants vary in shape, size, and shell texture.

About This Chapter: Information in this chapter is from "Teens and Breast Implants," *FDA & You*, Issue #4, Fall 2004, U.S. Food and Drug Administration.

At this time, there are two manufacturers with approved saline-filled
breast implants. No manufacturer
has yet received FDA approval to
market a silicone gel-filled breast
implant for augmentation.

> ♣ **It's A Fact!!**
> Because it has not been well
> studied in young people, the U.S.
> Food and Drug Administration
> (FDA) discourages the use of any
> breast implant in a patient
> younger than 18.

Health officials worry that teens and
their parents may not realize the risks asso-
ciated with breast implants. They also want to be sure that the teen's body has
finished developing, and that they are psychologically ready to handle the outcome of surgery. While every surgical procedure has potential risks, such as infection, bleeding, and scarring, there are risks that are specific to breast implants.
Learning about them is key to being properly informed about the procedure.

"I didn't know my breasts were still growing when I signed up for the
surgery," admits Kacey Long, who got saline-filled breast implants in July
2001, when she was 19. Prior to her surgery, the college student from Ennis,
Texas, was a 34B, the breast size she thought she would be for life.

Teenagers who are dissatisfied with their bodies see breast implants as
harmless and, according to Long, a fun thing to do to improve self-image.
Following implantation, Long's breast size increased to a 34D. But complications convinced her to have the implants removed a short time later. Three
years later, Long's breasts measured 36C, one size larger than before she was
implanted, suggesting that her own breasts continued to develop even after
the implants were removed.

Many of the changes to the breast that occur with an implant cannot be
undone. If a teen chooses to have her implants removed, she may experience
dimpling, puckering, wrinkling, or other cosmetic changes. "When you're
making a decision that can impact your life at 19," Long advises other young
women, "you need to research the subject like you're 50 years old."

Consider these breast implant facts:

• Breast implants will not last a lifetime. Either because of rupture or
  other complications, you will likely need to have the implants removed.

- Your breast may not be fully developed and could continue to grow larger, even after implant surgery.

- You are likely to need additional doctor visits and operations because of one or more complications over the course of your life.

- You are likely to have the implants removed, with or without replacement, because of one or more complications over the course of your life.

- Many of the changes to your breasts following implantation may be cosmetically undesirable and cannot be undone.

- If you choose to have your implants removed, you may experience unacceptable dimpling, puckering, wrinkling, loss of breast tissue, or other undesirable cosmetic changes of the breasts.

Part Seven

How To Handle Illness And Injury

Chapter 59

Talking To Your Doctor

Tips For Talking With Your Doctor

Stay Positive

It will help to go to your doctor's visits with a good attitude. It is also important to remember that your doctor and other caregivers are on your side. Think teamwork! Think positive!

Keep Track Of How You Are Feeling

Your doctor visits will be easier if you keep notes on how you are feeling. This will make it easier for you to answer questions about your symptoms and how medicines make you feel. This also makes it easier for you to bring up anything that you are worried about. Make sure to be honest about where it hurts and how long it has been hurting. Also let your doctor know how you feel about your health and treatments. Are you scared, worried, or sad? Your care will be easier if your doctor knows how you are feeling.

Your doctor can also tell you about counselors and support groups to help you talk about your feelings.

About This Chapter: Information in this chapter is from "Talking to the Doctor," GirlsHealth.gov, sponsored by The National Women's Health Information Center, U.S. Department of Health and Human Services, Office on Women's Health, May 2005.

Bring A List Of Your Current Medications To Your Appointment

You and your parents need to bring a list of all the medicines you take with you to your appointment. If you are able to take medicines you can buy at the pharmacy without a prescription (an order from the doctor), make sure to also include them in your list. This way, the doctor does not have to look through your records to see what you are taking, and you can spend more time talking about how you are feeling.

Read About Your Condition

It will help to learn as much as you can about your illness or disability by reading information from your doctor, national organizations, the library, and the Internet. You can also learn about it by talking to adults and other people who have the same illness or disability. Make sure to talk to your doctor about what you learn because not all information you will find on the Internet is good.

Ask Questions

Do not be afraid to ask your doctor any questions you have. This will help you understand your own health better. To remember all the questions you have, even when you are not in the doctor's office, write them down and bring the list with you to your appointments. You can also write down what your doctor says. Be sure to talk with your parents about the things you want to ask the doctor. This will make getting answers even easier.

Ask Special Questions About Your Treatment

While some health problems do not need treatment, most of them can be helped by medicine, surgery, changes in daily habits, such as what you eat, or a few of these together. You will get the most out of treatments when you understand what is going on and when you and your parents make choices together. In case your doctor talks about a new treatment at your next visit, here are some questions you can write down to take with you:

- How long will it take?

- What will happen? (Is it a shot, pill or operation?)

♣ It's A Fact!!

Being able to talk freely with your doctor will not only make you feel better, it will also help your doctor better know how to care for you.

• Will it hurt?

• How many treatments do I have to have?

• Will I be able to go to school?

• Are there things I won't be able to do, such as ride a bike?

• Is this treatment to try to cure my health problem or help take away some of my symptoms?

• Will these treatments make me tired or feel pain? How long will this last?

• What happens if I miss a treatment?

• What will we do if the treatments don't work?

• Is this the best treatment out there for me?

For some health problems, and depending on the patient, there is more than one treatment the doctor can give you. If the treatment you get makes you feel badly, it is okay to ask if there are others you can try. There may not be others, but you and your doctor can talk about it.

Talking About Personal Things

It is okay to be nervous about talking to your doctor about things that make you uncomfortable. Who wants to talk to a strange adult about sex, feeling sad, or what you eat? But it is easier than you think. Doctors are there to talk about everything that is going on with your body, and they will never think any less of you no matter what you ask or what your problem is. In fact, they are very used to personal issues (and they likely have had to seek help for their own). It is also very important for your health that you tell them everything that is going on with you. By not telling them about a strange smell, rash, pain, or anything else going on with your body, you could be making a health problem worse.

Talking about personal issues with your doctor can be confidential, which means that your doctor has to keep everything you say secret. Doctors might feel they have to tell your parents what you say if they think you are in danger or are not able to make choices on your own. Ask your doctor about the privacy policy before you begin.

Chapter 60

Glossary Of Medical Specialties

Which Medical Specialist For You?

Everyone knows that a medical doctor is a physician who has had years of training to understand the diagnosis, treatment, and prevention of disease. The basic training for a physician specialist includes four years of premedical education in a college or university, four years of medical school, and after receiving the M.D. degree, at least three years of specialty training under supervision (called a "residency"). Training in subspecialties can take an additional one to three years.

The process most widely used by physicians to tell whether and why you are sick is to ask you, and/or family members, questions about your health and past medical history. This process, called taking a history, is usually followed by an appropriate physical examination of your body to determine how well it is functioning and whether there are signs of disease. Doctors also use a variety of tests such as lab tests, x-rays, other imaging techniques, and additional procedures to evaluate your health and identify any diseases or other health problems, which may be present. Some of these diagnostic procedures (e.g., cardiac catheterization, CT scans, biopsy of internal tissues) are very complicated. They require many years of training in order to use them safely and accurately.

After the diagnostic process is completed, the doctor will recommend treatment if it is needed. Treatment may involve medication, surgery (there are many types of surgical specialists), or other complex procedures.

Some specialists are primary care doctors, such as family physicians, general internists, and general pediatricians. Other specialists concentrate on certain body systems, specific age groups, or complex scientific techniques developed to diagnose or treat certain types of disorders.

A subspecialist is a physician who has completed training in a general medical specialty and then takes additional training in a more specific area of that specialty called a subspecialty. This training increases the depth of knowledge and expertise of the specialist in that particular field. For example, cardiology is a subspecialty of internal medicine and pediatrics, pediatric surgery is a subspecialty of surgery, and child and adolescent psychiatry is a subspecialty of psychiatry. The training of a subspecialist within a specialty requires an additional one or more years of full-time education.

Training Of A Specialist

The training of a specialist begins after the doctor has received the M.D. degree from a medical school in what is called a residency. Resident physicians dedicate themselves for three to seven years to full-time experience in hospital and/or ambulatory care settings, caring for patients under the supervision of experienced specialists. Educational conferences and research experience are often part of that training. In years past, the first year of post-medical school training was called an internship but is now called residency.

> ### ✣ It's A Fact!!
> Specialties in medicine developed because of the rapidly expanding body of knowledge about health and illness and the constantly evolving new treatment techniques for disease.
>
> Source: © 2005 American Board of Medical Specialties. All rights reserved. Reprinted with permission.

Licensure, the legal privilege to practice medicine, is governed by state law and is not designed to recognize the knowledge and skills of a trained specialist. A physician is licensed to practice general medicine and surgery by a state board of medical examiners after passing a state or national licensure examination.

♣ **It's A Fact!!**

Each state or territory has its own procedures to license physicians and sets the general standards for all physicians in that state or territory.

Source: © 2005 American Board of Medical Specialties. All rights reserved. Reprinted with permission.

Who Credentials A Specialist And/Or Subspecialist?

Specialty boards certify physicians as having met certain published standards. There are 24 specialty boards that are recognized by the American Board of Medical Specialties (ABMS) and the American Medical Association (AMA). Remember, a subspecialist first must be trained and certified as a specialist.

In order to be certified as a medical specialist by one of these recognized boards, a physician must complete certain requirements. Generally, these include the following:

1. Completion of a course of study leading to the M.D. or D.O. (Doctor of Osteopathy) degree from a recognized school of medicine.

2. Completion of three to seven years of full-time training in an accredited residency program designed to train specialists in the field.

3. Many specialty boards require assessments and documentation of individual performance from the residency training director or from the chief of service in the hospital where the specialist has practiced.

4. All of the ABMS Member Boards require that a person seeking certification have an unrestricted license to practice medicine in order to take the certification examination.

5. Finally, each candidate for certification must pass a written examination given by the specialty board. Fifteen of the 24 specialty boards also require

an oral examination conducted by senior specialists in that field. Candidates who have passed the exams and other requirements are then given the status of "Diplomate" and are certified as specialists. A similar process is followed for specialists who want to become subspecialists.

All of the ABMS Member Boards now, or will soon, issue only time-limited certificates, which are valid for six to ten years. In order to retain certification, diplomates must become recertified and must periodically go through an additional process involving continuing education in the specialty, review of credentials, and further examination. Boards that may not yet require recertification have provided voluntary recertification with similar requirements.

How To Determine If A Physician Is A Certified Specialist

Certified specialists are listed in The Official ABMS Directory of Board Certified Medical Specialists published by Marquis Who's Who. The ABMS Directory can be found in most public libraries, hospital libraries, university libraries, medical libraries, and is also available on CD-ROM. Alternatively, you could ask for that information from your county medical society, the American Board of Medical Specialties, or one of the specialty boards.

The ABMS also arranges for the publication of lists of certified specialists/subspecialists and operates a toll free phone line (866-ASK-ABMS) to verify the certification status of individual physicians. Additionally, information about the ABMS organization and links to an electronic directory of certified specialists can be accessed through the ABMS website at www.abms.org.

Almost all board certified specialists are also members of their medical specialty societies. These societies are dedicated to furthering standards, practice, and professional and public education within individual medical specialties. Some, such as the American College of Surgeons and the American College of Obstetricians and Gynecologists, require board certification for full membership. A physician who has attained full membership is called a "Fellow" of the society and is entitled to use this designation in all formal communications, such as certificates, publications, business cards, stationery, and signage. Thus, "John Doe, M.D., F.A.C.S. (Fellow of the American

College of Surgeons)" is a board certified surgeon. Similarly, F.A.A.D. (Fellow of the American Academy of Dermatology) following the M.D. or D.O. in a physician's title would likely indicate board certification in that specialty.

The Purpose Of Certification

The intent of the certification process, as defined by the member boards of the American Board of Medical Specialties, is to provide assurance to the public that a certified medical specialist has successfully completed an approved educational program and an evaluation, including an examination process designed to assess the knowledge, experience, and skills requisite to the provision of high quality patient care in that specialty.

Glossary Of Clinical Specialties

Allergy and immunology: Concerned with the hypersensitivity to foreign substances and protection from the resultant infection or disorder.

Anesthesiology: Concerned with purposeful depression of nerve function, characterized by loss of feeling or sensation, usually by anesthetics, and induced to allow performance of surgery or other painful procedures; also concerned with treating pain associated with diseases/conditions.

Cardiology: Concerned with the study of the heart, its physiology, and its functions. Cardiovascular specialists are trained in diseases of the heart, lungs, and blood vessels.

Chiropractic: An occupational discipline based on the relationship of the spine to health and disease. X-rays and palpation analyze the spine, and vertebrae are adjusted manually to relieve pressures on the spinal cord.

Colon and rectal surgery: Concerned with the diagnosis and treatment of diseases of the intestinal tract, colon, rectum, anal canal, and perianal area by medical and surgical means. The specialty is also concerned with other organs and tissues involved with primary intestinal disease.

Critical care: Concerned with the diagnosis, treatment, and support of patients with multiple organ dysfunction (i.e., critically ill) during a medical emergency or crisis.

✎ What's It Mean?

Accreditation: A process of review and approval of medical schools and graduate medical education training programs, residency programs, conducted by credentialing bodies and certifying that the programs have met certain standards. This process does not certify or accredit individuals. The Liaison Committee on Medical Education (LCME), a joint committee of the Association of American Medical Colleges (AAMC) and the American Medical Association (AMA) conducts accreditation of medical schools. The Residency Review Committees (RRCs) of the Accreditation Council of Graduate Medical Education (ACGME) are responsible for accrediting residency programs. There are 26 RRCs, and their members come from relevant Member Boards of the ABMS, specialty societies, and the AMA. The ACGME oversees the activities of the RRCs and approves or disapproves their recommendations.

Candidate: Individual who has applied for specialty board certification.

Certification: The process of voluntary testing and evaluation of physicians who wish to become board certified in a particular medical specialty. A physician may elect to begin the certification process only after completion of an approved residency training program. Certification by a specialty board enables the public to identify those practitioners who have met a standard of training and experience set beyond the level required for licensure. Certifying boards, unlike state licensing boards, are national in scope and independent.

Diplomate: Individual who has met all specialty board requirements, including passing an examination, and is board certified in a particular medical specialty.

Fellowship: Physicians attain Fellowship status in a specialty society when they demonstrate outstanding achievement in their profession. Typical criteria for Fellowship in a specialty society include years of membership, years as a practitioner in the specialty, and professional recognition by peers.

Fellowship Training: A period of training, usually 1–2 years, which occurs after completion of a general or primary residency. Its goal is to qualify a physician as a subspecialist in an area of medical practice such as cardiology, hand surgery, etc.

Internship: The old term used to describe the first year of postgraduate training following graduation from medical school. Physicians participating in this training were formerly called interns but are now known as Postgraduate Year 1 (PGY-1) residents and the year is called the PGY-1 year. It is usually taken under the sponsorship of a single clinical department.

Licensure (Medical): Legal permission granted by a state or territorial government to a physician to take personal, unsupervised responsibility for the diagnosis and treatment of patients in the practice of medicine. Most states and territories require that physicians complete at least 1 year, and several require 3 years, of graduate medical education to qualify for licensure. In addition, applicants for licensure must pass an examination. Qualifications for medical licensure in each jurisdiction are determined by that jurisdiction. Federal, state, and territorial governments do not license physicians as specialists nor certify physicians as specialists.

Residency: A variable period of postgraduate education and training (3–7 years), based upon the specialty selected, in which a physician participates with the expectation of becoming a specialist in a field of medical practice. These educational experiences occur in a variety of settings including hospitals, clinics, offices, and other relevant medical educational centers.

Residency Matching: The process by which most medical students obtain an appointment for their postgraduate training. The matching process is performed by independent agencies such as the National Resident Matching Program (NRMP). The NRMP receives rank order preferences from students and training institutions and matches them by computer according to the highest ranked match. Residency information is available from medical schools, training programs, The *AMA Directory of Graduate Medical Education Programs*, hard copy and online, and the Fellowship and Residency Electronic Interactive Data Access (FREIDA) service of the AMA.

Specialty Boards: There are 24 approved medical specialty boards that grant certification. These boards form the umbrella organization, the American Board of Medical Specialties (ABMS). The specialty boards influence graduate medical education since they set the criteria required of physicians seeking admission to the certification examinations. Each board sets the minimum length of time for education in an accredited residency and the content of the certifying exam.

Specialty Societies: Membership organizations of physicians involved in a given field of practice. Specialty societies represent the interests of practitioners. In most specialty societies, it is necessary to be board certified to be eligible for membership.

Training: Usually refers to a period of postgraduate medical education during which a physician gains the experience necessary to assume responsibility for the care of patients.

Transitional Year Residency: A training program for physicians equivalent to the PGY-1 residency training year but organized and sponsored by several institutions or clinical departments to provide training in multiple specialties of medicine rather than in a single specialty.

Dentistry: Concerned with the teeth, oral cavity, associated structures, and the diagnosis and treatment of their diseases.

Dermatology: Concerned with the skin.

Emergency medicine: Concerned with resuscitation, transportation, and care, from the point of injury or beginning of illness.

Endocrinology: Concerned with the metabolism, physiology, and disorders of the internal (endocrine) system. This branch of medicine also deals with diabetes, metabolic and nutritional disorders, pituitary diseases, and menstrual and sexual problems.

Family practice: Concerned with the provision of continuing, comprehensive primary health care for the entire family.

Gastroenterology: Concerned with the study of the physiology and diseases of the digestive system and related structures.

Geriatrics: Concerned with the physiological and pathological aspects of the aged, including the clinical problems of senescence and senility.

Hematology: Concerned with blood and blood-forming tissues.

Infectious diseases: Concerned with illnesses caused by microorganisms.

Internal medicine: Concerned with the diagnosis and treatment of diseases of the internal organ systems in adults.

Medical genetics: Concerned with the reliable prediction of certain genetically linked disorders. The clinical areas include: clinical biochemical genetics, clinical cytogenetics, clinical genetics, clinical/medical genetics, and clinical molecular genetics.

Nephrology: Concerned with the kidney.

Neurological surgery: Concerned with disorders of the central, peripheral, and autonomic nervous systems, including supporting structures and vascular supply; the evaluation and treatment of pathological processes that modify function or activity of the nervous system, and the management of pain.

Neurology: Concerned with the nervous system.

Nuclear medicine: Concerned with diagnostic, therapeutic, and investigative use of radioactive compounds in pharmaceutical form.

Nursing: Concerned with the provision of care and services essential to the promotion, maintenance, and restoration of health by attending to a patient's needs.

Nutrition: Concerned with nutrients and other substances contained in food and their action, interaction, and balance in relation to health and disease.

Obstetrics and gynecology: Concerned with management and care of women during pregnancy, parturition, and puerperium; the physiology and disorders primarily of the female genital tract; and female endocrinology and reproductive physiology. This physician may serve as a primary care source for women.

Oncology: Concerned with the study of neoplasms (cancer).

Ophthalmology: Concerned with eye defects and diseases.

Optometry: The professional practice of primary eye and vision care that includes the correction of visual defects with lenses or glasses.

Orthopedic surgery: A surgical specialty that treats and corrects deformities, diseases, and injuries to the skeletal system and associated structures.

Otolaryngology: Concerned with disorders of the ear, nose, throat, respiratory and upper alimentary systems, and related structures of the head and neck.

Pathology: Concerned with the causes and nature of disease including diagnosis, prognosis, and treatment through knowledge gained by the laboratory application of the biological, chemical, and physical sciences.

Pediatrics: Concerned with the physical, emotional, and social health of children from birth to young adulthood. Care encompasses a broad spectrum of health services. Neonatology is also covered under this specialty.

Pharmacology: Concerned with the effectiveness and safety of medications.

Physical medicine and rehabilitation: Concerned with rehabilitating patients who are physically diseased, injured, or recovering from elective surgery. Physicians practicing this specialty are physiatrists.

Plastic surgery: Deals with the repair, reconstruction, or replacement of physical defects of form or function involving the skin, musculoskeletal system, craniomaxillofacial structures, extremities, breast and trunk, and external genitalia.

Podiatry: Concerned with the foot.

Preventive medicine: Concerned with maintaining health and well-being, and preventing disease, disability, and premature death.

Psychiatry: Concerned with mental disorders, addictive disorders, emotional disorders, mood disorders, anxiety disorders, substance-related disorders, sexual and gender identity disorders, and adjustment disorders.

Psychology: Concerned with recognizing and treating behavior disorders.

Pulmonary medicine: Concerned with the respiratory system.

Radiation oncology: Concerned with the therapeutic application of radiant energy and its modifiers, especially regarding malignant tumors.

Radiology: Concerned with the use of x-ray and other forms of radiant energy in the diagnosis and treatment of disease.

Rheumatology: Concerned with inflammatory or degenerative processes and metabolic derangement of connective tissue structures that pertain to a variety of musculoskeletal disorders (for example, arthritis).

Sleep medicine: Concerned with disturbances of sleep patterns or behaviors.

Speech-language pathology: Concerned with the study of speech/language and swallowing disorders and their diagnosis and correction.

Sports medicine: Responsible for continuous care, enhancement of health and fitness, and prevention of injury and illness to an individual engaged in physical exercise (sports).

Surgery: Concerned with manual or operative procedures used in the diagnosis and treatment of diseases, injuries, or deformities.

Thoracic surgery: Concerned with the operative, perioperative, and critical care of patients with pathologic conditions within the chest.

Urology: Concerned with the urinary tract in both sexes and the genital tract in the male.

Chapter 61

Managing The Benefits And Risks Of Medicines

Although medicines can make you feel better and help you get well, it is important to know that all medicines, both prescription and over-the-counter, have risks as well as benefits.

The benefits of medicines are the helpful effects you get when you use them, such as lowering blood pressure, curing infection, or relieving pain. The risks of medicines are the chances that something unwanted or unexpected could happen to you when you use them. Risks could be less serious, such as an upset stomach, or more serious, such as liver damage.

When a medicine's benefits outweigh its known risks, the U.S. Food and Drug Administration (FDA) considers it safe enough to approve. But before using any medicine, as with many things that you do every day, you should think through the benefits and the risks in order to make the best choice for you.

There are several types of risks from medicine use such as the following:

• The possibility of a harmful interaction between the medicine and a food, beverage, dietary supplement (including vitamins and herbals),

About This Chapter: Information in this chapter is from "Think it Through: A Guide to Managing the Benefits and Risks of Medicines," *FDA & You*, Issue #6, Spring 2005, U.S. Food and Drug Administration.

or another medicine. Combinations of any of these products could increase the chance that there may be interactions

- The chance that the medicine may not work as expected

- The possibility that the medicine may cause additional problems

For example, every time you get into a car, there are risks—the possibility that unwanted or unexpected things could happen. You could have an accident, causing costly damage to your car, or injury to yourself or a loved one. But there are also benefits to riding in a car: you can travel farther and faster than walking, bring home more groceries from the store, and travel in cold or wet weather in greater comfort.

To obtain the benefits of riding in a car, you think through the risks. You consider the condition of your car and the road, for instance, before deciding to make that trip to the store.

The same is true before using any medicine. Every choice to take a medicine involves thinking through the helpful effects as well as the possible unwanted effects.

Talk With Your Doctor, Pharmacist, Or Other Health Care Professional

- Keep an up-to-date, written list of all of the medicines (prescription and over-the-counter) and dietary supplements, including vitamins and herbals, that you use, even those you only use occasionally.

- Share this list with all of your health care professionals.

- Tell about any allergies or sensitivities you have.

- Tell about anything that could affect your ability to take medicines, such as difficulty swallowing or remembering to take them.

- Tell if you are, or might become pregnant, or if you are nursing a baby.

- Always ask questions about any concerns or thoughts you have.

Know Your Medicines—Prescription And Over-The-Counter

- The brand and generic names
- What they look like
- How to store them properly
- When, how, and how long to use them
- How and under what conditions you should stop using them
- What to do if you miss a dose
- What they are supposed to do and when to expect results
- Side effects and interactions
- Whether you need any tests or monitoring
- Written information to take with you

Read The Label And Follow Directions

- Make sure you understand the directions; ask if you have questions or concerns.
- Always double-check that you have the right medicine.
- Keep medicines in their original labeled containers, whenever possible.
- Never combine different medicines in the same bottle.
- Read and follow the directions on the label and the directions from your doctor, pharmacist, or other health care professional. If you stop the medicine, or want to use the medicine differently than directed, consult with your health care professional.

Avoid Interactions

- Ask if there are interactions with any other medicines or dietary supplements (including vitamins or herbal supplements), beverages, or foods.
- Use the same pharmacy for all of your medicine needs, whenever possible.

- Before starting any new medicine or dietary supplement (including vitamins or herbal supplements), ask again if there are possible interactions with what you are currently using.

Monitor Your Medicines' Effects And The Effects Of Other Products That You Use

- Ask if there is anything you can do to minimize side effects, such as eating before you take a medicine to reduce stomach upset.

- Pay attention to how you are feeling and note any changes. Write down the changes so that you can remember to tell your doctor, pharmacist, or other health care professional.

- Know what to do if you experience side effects and when to notify your doctor.

- Know when you should notice an improvement and when to report back.

Weighing The Risks, Making The Choice

You must decide what risks you can and will accept in order to get the benefits you want. For example, if facing a life-threatening illness, you might choose to accept more risk in the hope of getting the benefits of a cure or living a longer life. On the other hand, if you are facing a minor illness, you might decide that you want to take very little risk. In many situations, the expert advice of your doctor, pharmacist, or other health care professionals can help you make the decision.

☞ **Remember!!**
Think it through and work together with your doctor, pharmacist, or other health care professional to better manage the benefits and risks of your medicines.

Chapter 62

The Safe Use Of Over-The-Counter Drugs

Types Of Over-The-Counter Drugs

Over-the-counter (OTC) drugs should be taken with the same caution as drugs prescribed by your doctor. Special care is necessary if you use more than one of these products at the same time, or if you take an OTC product while also being treated with a prescription product; and there are some OTC drugs that should not be taken by people with certain medical problems. If possible, ask your parent, pharmacist, or physician for advice before taking any OTC product you have not used before.

Besides getting expert advice, the most important thing you can do before buying an OTC drug is to read the label. The name of the product is not always the same as the name of the drug it contains, and some products contain more than one ingredient. For example, a product for coughs and one for colds might each contain phenylpropanolamine. A person taking both products at the same time might get too much of this ingredient, which is also in some OTC diet pills.

About This Chapter: This chapter begins with "Types Of Over-The-Counter Drugs," from "The Safe Use of Over-the-Counter Drugs," *FDA & You*, Issue #3, Spring/Summer 2003, Updated May 2004, U.S. Food and Drug Administration. Text under the heading "Over-The-Counter Drug Facts Label," from "The Over-the-Counter Drug Facts Label—Take a Look," *FDA & You*, Issue #5, Winter 2005, U.S. Food and Drug Administration.

Aspirin And Other Fever Reducers

Teens (as well as children) should not take products containing aspirin (acetylsalicylic acid) or salicylates when they have chickenpox, flu, or symptoms that might be the flu (this includes most colds). Children and teenagers who take aspirin and other salicylates during these illnesses may develop a rare but life-threatening condition called Reye syndrome. (Symptoms usually occur near the end of the original illness and include severe tiredness, violent headache, disorientation, and excessive vomiting.)

Acetaminophen (sold under brand names such as Tylenol) can also reduce fever and relieve pain and has not been associated with Reye syndrome. Remember though, because fevers in most colds do not normally go above 100° Fahrenheit and do not cause much discomfort, you usually do not have to take any drug for the fever. If you think you have a cold, but your temperature is running higher, consult your doctor because you might have flu or a bacterial infection.

Sniffle And Cough Combinations

OTC drugs to relieve stuffy noses often contain more than one ingredient. Some of these products are marketed for allergy relief and others for colds. They usually contain both an antihistamine and a nasal decongestant. The decongestant ingredient "un-stuffs" nasal passages while antihistamines dry up a runny nose; but some of these products may also contain aspirin or acetaminophen, and some contain a decongestant alone. Some of these drugs are "extended-release" or "long-acting" preparations that continue to work for up to 12 hours. Others are immediate-release products and usually work for four to six hours. It is important to read the label and check with the pharmacist; to be sure you are getting the right product for your symptoms.

Most antihistamines can cause drowsiness, while many decongestants have the opposite effect. Still, it is hard to predict whether any one product will make you sleepy or keep you awake, or neither, because reactions to drugs can vary from one person to another. So it is best not to drive or operate machinery until you find out how the drug affects you. In addition, alcohol, sedatives, and tranquilizers intensify the drowsiness effect of antihistamines, so it is best not to take them at the same time unless a doctor tells you to.

As you can see, selecting a product to treat a stuffy nose can be tricky, so can choosing a product to treat a cough. In addition to one or more ingredients specifically for coughs, many cold or cough syrups contain the same ingredients that are in allergy and cold pills. This means that if you are taking acetaminophen pills or cold pills, you should read the label or consult the pharmacist to make sure you are not getting a double dose of ingredients by taking a cold or cough syrup.

There are several different types of ingredients to treat coughs, depending on the kind of cough you have. Some ingredients make it easier for you to bring up phlegm, while others suppress the cough. Before taking any kind of cough medicine, it is a good idea to first try drinking plenty of liquids and adding moisture to the air by using a vaporizer or boiling water. Sometimes just doing these things will reduce the cough enough that you will not have to take any medicine. If a cough lasts more than a few days, see your doctor.

Stomach Help

If you are constipated, drinking more water, getting more exercise, and eating high-fiber foods such as fruits and vegetables, will often solve the problem.

Though appropriate for some medical conditions, laxatives can be habit forming and can make constipation worse when overused. Not having a bowel movement every day does not necessarily mean that you are constipated, for some people it is normal.

If you have diarrhea, it is a good idea to rest, eat only small amounts of food at a time, and drink plenty of fluids to prevent dehydration. OTC products marketed to stop diarrhea may contain loperamide (Imodium AD), or attapulgite (Diasorb, Kaopectate, and others), or bismuth subsalicylate (Pepto-Bismol and others). Teens should avoid products with bismuth subsalicylate if they have flu or chickenpox symptoms because of the risk of Reye syndrome.

If you are running a fever above 100° Fahrenheit, or if your upset stomach symptoms are severe or continue for more than a day or two, consult your doctor. She may recommend one of the many OTC products available for these problems.

Skin Treatment

Rashes can be caused by many different things, including allergies, fungus, and poison oak or ivy. So it is best to get a doctor's opinion about what is causing your rash before treating it.

There are topical OTC products that you apply directly to the skin, which are available specifically to treat poison ivy and oak. Some of these products contain calamine, which protects the skin, and benzocaine, which dulls the pain or itching. Other products contain an antihistamine or hydrocortisone, which relieve itching. Antihistamine creams, such as Benadryl, and hydrocortisone products, such as Cortaid and Caldecort, can also be used for rashes from allergies and insect bites, but you should not use them for more than seven days without seeing a doctor.

Acne, another type of skin problem, can also be treated with topical OTC products. Many of these lotions (such as Clearasil products and Oxy 5 and 10) contain benzoyl peroxide in strengths of 2.5, 5, or 10 percent. It is best to try the lower dosage level first, to keep your skin from getting too dry.

Benzoyl peroxide can also increase your sensitivity to sun, causing you to burn more easily. If you use a product with benzoyl peroxide, remember to wear sunscreen during the day to protect your skin.

Expert Advice

Before buying any product you have not already used, it is best to read the labeling and, if possible, ask the pharmacist how the product works and what it should be used for. And, if still in doubt, check with your doctor.

Over-The-Counter Drug Facts Label

Always Read The Drug Facts Label

Reading the drug facts label is the most important part of taking care of yourself when using OTC medicines. This is especially true because many OTC medicines are taken without seeing a doctor. If you read the OTC drug facts label and still have questions about the product, talk to your doctor, pharmacist, or other health care professional.

What's On The Drug Facts Label

A drug facts label includes information such as the following:

- **Active Ingredient:** Therapeutic substance and amount in the product

- **Uses:** Symptoms or diseases the product will treat or prevent

- **Warnings:** Special concerns or situations related to the medication.

- **Inactive Ingredients:** Substances such as colors or flavors

---

♣ It's A Fact!!
Products Containing Salicylates

The following products do not have aspirin in their brand names, but they contain aspirin or other salicylates and should not be taken by teens who have symptoms of flu or chickenpox unless told to do so by a doctor. (Ingestion of salicylates during these illnesses can increase the risk of Reye syndrome in children and teens.)

- Alka-Seltzer Effervescent Antacid and Pain Reliever (also the extra-strength version)

- Alka-Seltzer Plus Night-Time Cold Medicine

- Anacin Maximum Strength Analgesic Coated Tablets

- Ascriptin A/D Caplets (also the regular and extra strength versions)

- Bayer Children's Cold Tablets

- Bufferin (all formulations)

- Excedrin Extra-Strength Analgesic Tablets and Caplets

- Pepto-Bismol

- Vanquish Analgesic Caplets

In addition, many products to treat arthritis contain aspirin.

This list contains many common products, but is not all-inclusive, so be sure to read the label before purchasing any OTC medication.

Source: "The Safe Use of Over-the-Counter Drugs," *FDA & You*, Issue #3, Spring/Summer 2003, Updated May 2004, U.S. Food and Drug Administration.

- **Purpose:** Product action or category

- **Directions:** How to take

- **Other Information:** How to store and other facts about the product

The drug facts labeling requirements do not apply to dietary supplements, which are regulated as food products, and are labeled with a supplement facts panel.

Reading The Drug Facts Label: The Key To Proper Medicine Use

The label tells you what a medicine is supposed to do, who should or should not take it, and how to use it, but efforts to provide good labeling cannot help unless you read and use the information. It is up to you to be informed and to use OTC drug products wisely and responsibly.

✔ Quick Tip
Protect Yourself Against Tampering

- Read the label. Be alert to the tamper-evident features on the package before you open it. These features are described on the label.

- Inspect the outer packaging for signs of tampering before you buy a product.

- Examine the medicine itself before taking it. Check for capsules or tablets that differ from the others that are enclosed. Do not use medicine from packages with tears, cuts, or other imperfections.

- Never take medicine in the dark.

- Examine the label and the medicine every time you take it or give it to someone else.

- Tell somebody if the product does not look right. Do not buy or use medicine that looks suspicious. Always tell the store manager about questionable products so that they can be removed.

- Before buying any medicine, you should stop and take a look. Before taking it, you should look again.

Source: "Protect Yourself Against Tampering," *FDA & You*, Issue #5, Winter 2005, U.S. Food and Drug Administration.

Chapter 63

Basic First Aid

Accidents happen anywhere and anytime. The first response to an accident is the most important. Oftentimes, first aid given at the scene can improve the victim's chances of survival and a good recovery. The right response is better than an incorrect quick one. Any response, even if it is wrong, is better than none at all.

Unconscious Victim

If the victim is unconscious, perform rescue breathing. (Rescue breathing is explained later on in this chapter.) If the victim's heart has stopped beating, perform cardiopulmonary resuscitation (CPR) if you have been properly trained to do so.

Shock

Shock usually accompanies severe injury or emotional upset. The signs are cold and clammy skin, pale face, chills, confusion, frequent nausea or vomiting, and shallow breathing. Until emergency help arrives, have the victim lie down with the legs elevated. Keep the victim covered to prevent chilling or loss of body heat. Give non-alcoholic fluids if the victim is able to swallow and has not sustained an abdominal injury.

About This Chapter: Reprinted with permission. Dawna L. Cyr and Steven B. Johnson, "Basic First Aid," Bulletin #2325 of the Maine Farm Safety Program (Orono, ME: University of Maine Cooperative Extension.) © 1995, 2002.

Bleeding

Until emergency help arrives, try to control bleeding. If possible, first put on rubber or latex gloves before touching any blood. If these are not available, a clean plastic bag can be used to cover your hands.

If finger or hand pressure is inadequate to control bleeding, place a thick pad of clean cloth or bandage directly over the wound, and hold in place with a belt, bandage, neckties, or cloth strips. Take care not to stop the circulation to the rest of the limb. For injuries where a tie cannot be used, such as to the groin, back, chest, head, and neck, place a thick pad of clean cloth or bandage directly over the wound and control the bleeding with finger or hand pressure. If bones are not broken, raise the bleeding part higher than the rest of the body. If the injury is extensive, the victim may go into shock and should be treated for it.

As a last resort, a tourniquet can be applied to stop bleeding. There is a risk of sacrificing a limb to save a life. A tourniquet is a wide band of cloth or other material tightly placed just above the wound to stop all flow of blood. A tourniquet crushes the tissue and can cause permanent damage to nerves and blood vessels. Once in place, a tourniquet must be left there until a physician removes it. The victim must be taken to medical help as soon as possible.

Burns And Scalds

Until medical help arrives, immerse the burned area immediately in tap or cool water, or apply clean, cool, moist towels. Do not use ice because it may cause further damage to the burned area. Maintain this treatment until the pain or burning stops. Avoid breaking any blisters that may appear. Do not use ointments, greases, or powders.

For more severe burns or chemical burns, keep the victim quiet and treat them for shock. Remove any clothing. If the clothing sticks to the burned area, leave it there. For exposure to chemicals, flush the skin with plenty of water, but only cover the exposed area with a clean bandage if the chemical has caused a burn. If the burn victim is conscious, can swallow, and does not have severe mouth burns, give plenty of water or other non-alcoholic liquids to drink. Get the victim to a physician or hospital as soon as possible.

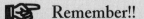

Remember!!

It is important not to come in contact with blood because of
the health risks.

Broken Bones

For fractured limbs, take the following precautions until emergency help
arrives. Place the injured part in as natural a position as possible without
causing discomfort to the patient. If the patient must be moved to a medical
facility, protect the injured part from further injury by applying splints long
enough to extend well beyond the joints above and below the fracture. Use
firm material, such as a board, pole, or metal rod, as a splint. Pad the splints
with clothing or other soft material to prevent skin injury. Fasten splints
with a bandage or cloth at the break and at points along the splint above and
below the break. Use a pressure bandage to control any bleeding.

For very serious fractures involving injuries to the body, neck, or back,
observe the following: Do not move the victim without medical supervision,
unless absolutely necessary, and then only if the proper splints have been
applied. If a victim with a suspected neck or back injury must be moved,
keep the back, head, and neck in a straight line, preventing them from being
twisted or bent during movement. Use a board or stretcher to support the
victim, if available.

Spinal Injuries

Take special care when helping a spinal injury victim. All damage to the
spinal cord is permanent, because nerve tissue cannot heal itself. The result
of nerve damage is paralysis or death.

Do not move the limbs or body of a victim with a suspected spinal injury
unless the accident scene is such that there is imminent danger of further injury
or unless it is necessary to establish breathing. The victim's body should be
stabilized to prevent any movement of the head, neck, or body. Be aware that
any movement of a victim with spinal injury may result in paralysis or death.

If the victim must be moved, keep the neck and torso of the body as straight as possible and pull in a direction that keeps the victim's spine in a straight line. Pull the body from the feet or shoulders (using both feet, both shoulders, or both arms pulled over the shoulders). It is also possible to pull the victim by the clothing. Grab the victim by the collar of the shirt and support the victim's head with your forearms while pulling. The clothing drag is preferred because the victim's head is supported while being moved. Do not pull the body sideways.

When providing patient care, it may be necessary to roll the victim over on his or her back to clear an airway or evaluate breathing. When rolling the victim over, the head, neck and torso should be moved together so that no twisting occurs.

Rescue Breathing For An Adult

When breathing movements stop, or lips, tongue, and fingernails become blue, a person needs immediate help. When in doubt, apply rescue breathing until medical help arrives. Delay in rescue breathing my cost the victim's life. Start immediately. Seconds can count.

The American Red Cross teaches the following ten steps to assist an adult who has stopped breathing:

1. Does the person respond? Tap or gently shake the victim. Shout, "Are you OK?"

2. Shout, "Help!" Call people who can phone for help.

3. Roll the person onto their back by pulling them slowly toward you. Slowly pull towards you until the victim is face up.

4. Open the airway by tilting the head back, and lift the chin. Clear the mouth and throat of any obstructions with your fingers.

5. Check for breathing. Look, listen, and feel for breathing for three to five seconds.

6. Give two full breaths. Keep the head tilted back. Pinch the nose shut, and seal your lips tight around the victim's mouth. Give two full breaths for one to one and a half seconds each.

7. Check for a pulse at the side of the neck. Feel for a pulse for five to ten seconds.

8. Phone emergency staff for help. Send someone to call for an ambulance.

9. Continue rescue breathing. Keep the head tilted back, lift the chin, and pinch the nose shut. Give one full breath every five seconds. Look, listen, and feel for breathing between breaths.

10. Recheck the pulse every minute. Keep the head tilted back, and feel for the pulse for five to ten seconds. If the victim has a pulse, but is not breathing, continue rescue breathing.

For infants and small children, follow the first five steps listed above. On the sixth step, cover the child's mouth and nose in a tight seal, and give two small breaths. Check for a pulse and call for help. Begin rescue breathing, giving one small breath every three seconds for an infant and one every four seconds for a child.

Choking

Choking occurs when food or a foreign object obstructs the throat and interferes with normal breathing. The following steps are advised if the choking victim is unable to speak or cough forcefully:

For adults and children over one year of age do the following:

1. Ask, "Are you choking?"

2. Shout, "Help!" Call for help if the victim cannot cough, speak, or breathe, is coughing weakly, or is making high-pitched noises.

3. Phone emergency staff for help. Send someone to call an ambulance.

4. Do abdominal thrusts: Wrap your arms around the victim's waist. Make a fist. Place the thumb side of the fist on the middle of the victim's abdomen just above the navel and well below the lower tip of the breastbone. Grasp the fist with the other hand. Press the fist into the abdomen with a quick upward thrust.

5. Repeat abdominal thrusts until the object is coughed up or the victim starts to breathe or cough. If the victim becomes unconscious, lower the victim onto the floor.

6. Do a finger sweep. Grasp the tongue and lower jaw and lift jaw. Slide the finger down inside of the cheek to base of tongue. Sweep the object out.

7. Open the airway. Tilt the head back and lift the chin.

8. Give two full breaths. Keep the head tilted back, pinch the nose shut, and seal your lips tight around the victim's mouth. Give two full breaths for one to one and a half seconds.

9. Give six to ten abdominal thrusts. If the air will not go in, place the heel of one hand against the middle of the victim's abdomen. Place the other hand on top of the first hand. Press into the abdomen with quick upward thrusts.

10. Repeat step six through nine until the airway is cleared or the ambulance arrives.

For infants less than one year old do the following:

1. Place the victim's head in a downward position on the rescuer's forearm with the head and neck stabilized.

2. With the heel of the rescuer's hand, administer five rapid back blows between the victim's shoulder blades.

3. If the obstruction remains, turn the victim face up, and rest on a firm surface.

4. Deliver five rapid thrusts over the breastbone using two fingers.

5. If the victim is still not breathing normally, administer mouth-to-mouth resuscitation as specified for an infant.

6. Repeat the above steps as necessary. If the obstruction cannot be removed, call for medical help immediately.

Chapter 64

Cold Weather Health Emergencies

Winter Weather

When winter temperatures drop significantly below normal, staying warm and safe can become a challenge. Extremely cold temperatures often accompany a winter storm, so you may have to cope with power failures and icy roads. Although staying indoors as much as possible can help reduce the risk of car crashes and falls on the ice, you may also face indoor hazards. Many homes will be too cold—either due to a power failure or because the heating system is not adequate for the weather. When people must use space heaters and fireplaces to stay warm, the risk of household fires increases, as well as the risk of carbon monoxide poisoning.

Exposure to cold temperatures, whether indoors or outside, can cause other serious or life-threatening health problems. Infants and the elderly are particularly at risk, but anyone can be affected. To keep yourself and your family safe, you should know how to prevent cold-related health problems and what to do if a cold weather health emergency arises.

The emergency procedures outlined in this chapter are not a substitute for training in first aid. However, these procedures will help you to know when to seek medical care and what to do until help becomes available.

About This Chapter: Information in this chapter is from "Extreme Cold: A Prevention Guide to Promote Your Personal Health and Safety," March 2005, Centers for Disease Control and Prevention.

What Is Extreme Cold?

What constitutes extreme cold and its effects can vary across different areas of the country. In regions relatively unaccustomed to winter weather, near freezing temperatures are considered "extreme cold." Whenever temperatures drop decidedly below normal, and as wind speed increases, heat can leave your body more rapidly. These weather-related conditions may lead to serious health problems. Extreme cold is a dangerous situation that can bring on health emergencies in susceptible people, such as those without shelter or who are stranded, or who live in a home that is poorly insulated or without heat.

Outdoor Safety

When the weather is extremely cold, and especially if there are high winds, try to stay indoors. Make any trips outside as brief as possible.

Dress Warmly And Stay Dry

Adults and children should wear the following:

- A hat

- A scarf or knit mask to cover face and mouth

- Sleeves that are snug at the wrist

- Mittens (they are warmer than gloves)

- Water-resistant coat and boots

- Several layers of loose-fitting clothing

> **✔ Quick Tip**
> **Eat And Drink Wisely**
>
> Eating well-balanced meals will help you stay warmer. Do not drink alcoholic or caffeinated beverages; they cause your body to lose heat more rapidly. Instead, drink warm, sweet beverages or broth to help maintain your body temperature. If you have any dietary restrictions, ask your doctor.

Be sure the outer layer of your clothing is tightly woven, preferably wind resistant, to reduce body heat loss caused by wind. Wool, silk, or polypropylene inner layers of clothing will hold more body heat than cotton. Stay dry; wet clothing chills the body rapidly. Excess perspiration will increase heat loss, so remove extra layers of clothing whenever you feel too warm. Also, avoid getting gasoline or alcohol on your skin while de-icing and fueling

✔ Quick Tip

Do not ignore shivering. It is an important first sign that the body is losing heat. Persistent shivering is a signal to return indoors.

your car or using a snow blower. These materials in contact with the skin greatly increase heat loss from the body.

Avoid Exertion

Cold weather puts an extra strain on the heart. If you have heart disease or high blood pressure, follow your doctor's advice about shoveling snow or performing other hard work in the cold. Otherwise, if you have to do heavy outdoor chores, dress warmly and work slowly. Remember, your body is already working hard just to stay warm, so do not overdo it.

Understand Wind Chill

The wind chill index is the temperature your body feels when the air temperature is combined with the wind speed. It is based on the rate of heat loss from exposed skin caused by the effects of wind and cold. As the speed of the wind increases, it can carry heat away from your body much more quickly, causing skin temperature to drop. When there are high winds, serious weather-related health problems are more likely, even when temperatures are only cool.

Avoid Ice

Walking on ice is extremely dangerous. Many cold weather injuries result from falls on ice covered sidewalks, steps, driveways, and porches. Keep your steps and walkways as free of ice as possible by using rock salt or another chemical de-icing compound. Sand may also be used on walkways to reduce the risk of slipping.

Be Safe During Recreation

Notify friends and family where you will be before you go hiking, camping, or skiing. Do not leave areas of the skin exposed to the cold. Avoid perspiring or becoming overtired. Be prepared to take emergency shelter. Pack dry clothing, a two-wave radio, waterproof matches, and paraffin fire starters with you. Do not use alcohol and other mood altering substances, and avoid caffeinated beverages. Avoid walking on ice or getting wet. Carefully watch for signs of cold weather health problems.

Cold Weather Health Emergencies

Serious health problems can result from prolonged exposure to the cold. The most common cold-related problems are hypothermia and frostbite.

Hypothermia

When exposed to cold temperatures, your body begins to lose heat faster than it can be produced. Prolonged exposure to cold will eventually use up your body's stored energy. The result is hypothermia, or abnormally low body temperature. Body temperature that is too low affects the brain, making the victim unable to think clearly or move well. This makes hypothermia particularly dangerous because a person may not know it is happening and will not be able to do anything about it.

Hypothermia is most likely at very cold temperatures, but it can occur even at cool temperatures (above 40° F) if a person becomes chilled from rain, sweat, or submersion in cold water.

Victims of hypothermia are often elderly people with inadequate food, clothing, or heating; babies sleeping in cold bedrooms; people who remain outdoors for long periods, such as the homeless, hikers, hunters, etc.; and people who drink alcohol or use illicit drugs.

Recognizing Hypothermia

The warnings signs of hypothermia in adults are shivering, exhaustion, confusion, fumbling hands, memory loss, slurred speech, and drowsiness. In infants, the warning signs of hypothermia are bright red, cold skin and very low energy.

What To Do

If you notice any of these signs, take the person's temperature. If it is below 95° Fahrenheit, the situation is an emergency, and get medical attention immediately.

If medical care is not available, begin warming the person, as follows:

- Get the victim into a warm room or shelter.

- If the victim has on any wet clothing, remove it.

- Warm the center of the body first—chest, neck, head, and groin—using an electric blanket, if available. Or use skin-to-skin contact under loose, dry layers of blankets, clothing, towels, or sheets.

- Warm beverages can help increase the body temperature, but do not give alcoholic beverages. Do not try to give beverages to an unconscious person.

- After body temperature has increased, keep the person dry and wrapped in a warm blanket, including the head and neck.

- Get medical attention as soon as possible.

A person with severe hypothermia may be unconscious and may not seem to have a pulse or to be breathing. In this case, handle the victim gently, and get emergency assistance immediately. Even if the victim appears dead, CPR should be provided. CPR should continue while the victim is being warmed, until the victim responds or medical aid becomes available. In some cases, hypothermia victims who appear to be dead can be successfully resuscitated.

Frostbite

Frostbite is an injury to the body that is caused by freezing. Frostbite causes a loss of feeling and color in affected areas. It most often affects the nose, ears, cheeks, chin, fingers, or toes. Frostbite can permanently damage the body, and severe cases can lead to amputation. The risk of frostbite is increased in people with reduced blood circulation and among people who are not dressed properly for extremely cold temperatures.

Recognizing Frostbite

At the first signs of redness or pain in any skin area, get out of the cold or protect any exposed skin; frostbite may be beginning. Any of these signs may indicate frostbite: a white or grayish-yellow skin area; skin that feels unusually firm or waxy; or numbness. A victim is often unaware of frostbite until someone else points it out because the frozen tissues are numb.

What To Do

If you detect symptoms of frostbite, seek medical care. Because frostbite and hypothermia both result from exposure, first determine whether the victim also shows signs of hypothermia, as described previously. Hypothermia is a more serious medical condition and requires emergency medical assistance.

If there is frostbite but no sign of hypothermia, and immediate medical care is not available, proceed as follows:

- Get into a warm room as soon as possible.

- Unless absolutely necessary, do not walk on frostbitten feet or toes; this increases the damage.

- Immerse the affected area in warm, not hot, water (the temperature should be comfortable to the touch for unaffected parts of the body).

- Or, warm the affected area using body heat. For example, the heat of an armpit can be used to warm frostbitten fingers.

- Do not rub the frostbitten area with snow or massage it at all. This can cause more damage.

- Do not use a heating pad, heat lamp, or the heat of a stove, fireplace, or radiator for warming. Affected areas are numb and can be easily burned.

These procedures are not substitutes for proper medical care. Hypothermia is a medical emergency, and a health care provider should evaluate frostbite. It is a good idea to take a first aid and emergency resuscitation (CPR) course to prepare for cold weather health problems. Knowing what to do is an important part of protecting your health and the health of others.

Taking preventive action is your best defense against having to deal with extreme cold weather conditions. By preparing in advance for winter emergencies, and by observing safety precautions during times of extremely cold weather, you can reduce the risk of weather-related health problems.

Chapter 65

Summer Safety

Before you pack your swimsuit or hit the hiking trail, learn how to avoid summer hazards.

Sunburn

Excessive sun exposure and frequent blistering sunburns can leave you at risk for serious health risks, like skin cancer. Everyone is at risk for skin cancer, especially people with light skin color, light hair or eye color, a family history of skin cancer, chronic sun exposure, a history of sunburns early in life, or freckles. Rays from artificial sources of light, such as tanning booths, also increase the risk of skin cancer.

What you can do: Limit sun exposure, wear protective clothing, and use sunscreen. Sunscreen should be applied 30 minutes before going outdoors and reapplied at least every two hours. Use water-resistant sunscreen with a sun protection factor (SPF) of 15 or higher. Sunscreen is formulated to protect the skin against the sun's ultraviolet light (UV), not to help the skin tan.

Wear a wide-brimmed hat, and seek shade under a beach umbrella or a tree. Sunscreens alone may not always protect you. And do not forget sunglasses, which protect the sensitive skin around the eyes, and may reduce the

About This Chapter: Information in this chapter is from "Summer Safety Savvy," *FDA & You*, Issue #6, Spring 2005, U.S. Food and Drug Administration.

long-term risk of developing cataracts. People who wear UV-absorbing contact lenses should still wear UV-absorbing sunglasses since contact lenses do not completely cover the eye.

If you do get sunburned, do not put ice or butter on it. Use a cold compress, and if you do not have that, a pack of frozen vegetables will work. Over-the-counter (OTC) pain relievers may also be helpful. Mild and moderate cases may be helped by topical corticosteroids such as hydrocortisone. Severe cases may require oral steroids prescribed by a doctor.

♣ It's A Fact!!

Some medications can increase sensitivity to the sun. Examples are tetracycline antibiotics, and non-steroidal anti-inflammatory drugs such as ibuprofen. Cosmetics that contain alpha hydroxy acids (AHAs) may also increase sun sensitivity and the possibility of sunburn. Examples are glycolic acid and lactic acid. It is important to protect your skin from the sun while using AHA-containing products and for a week after discontinuing their use.

Bites From Ticks And Mosquitoes

Ticks are usually harmless. The biggest disease threat from tick bites is Lyme disease, which is caused by the bacterium *Borrelia burgdorferi*. According to the Centers for Disease Control and Prevention (CDC), there were more than 23,000 cases of Lyme disease reported in 2002.

Lyme disease is spread by the bites of *Ixodes* ticks (the deer tick, bear tick, western black-legged tick, or black-legged tick, depending on the region of the country). These ticks are about the size of a pinhead. They can attach to any part of the body, often to moist or hairy areas such as the groin, armpits, and scalp. About 80 percent of people who get Lyme disease develop a large rash that looks like a bull's-eye. Other symptoms include muscle aches and stiff joints.

✔ Quick Tip

Watch for moles that change color or size, bleed, or have an irregular, spreading edge—all potential signs of skin cancer.

Another insect-borne illness, West Nile virus, is transmitted by infected mosquitoes and usually produces mild symptoms in healthy people; but the illness can be serious for older people and those with compromised immune systems. In 2002, there were 4,156 cases of West Nile virus in humans reported to the CDC. Less than one percent of people infected with West Nile virus develop severe illness. The symptoms are flu-like and can include fever, headache, body aches, and skin rash.

What you can do: There are no vaccines on the market for West Nile virus or Lyme disease. If you are spending time in tall grass or wooded areas, use insect repellent with DEET to ward off mosquitoes and ticks. Insect repellent should not be used on babies, and repellent used on children should contain no more than ten percent DEET.

Check yourself for ticks before bedtime. If you find a tick, remove it with tweezers, drop it in a plastic bag, and throw it away. You do not have to save the tick to show it to doctors. People who want to get a tick tested for diseases or other information could check with their local health departments, but not all of them offer tick testing. The CDC recommends cleansing the area of the tick bite with antiseptic. Early removal is important because a tick generally has to be on the skin for 36 hours or more to transmit Lyme disease.

Anti-itch cream applied to the affected area also may help.

Bee Stings

Most reactions to bees are mild, but severe allergic reactions lead to between 40 and 50 deaths each year. An allergic reaction can occur even if a person has been stung before with no complications. Symptoms of an allergic reaction are swelling in the face or an area other than where the sting occurred, hives, itching, rash, difficulty breathing, and shock.

What you can do: To keep bees away, wear light-colored clothing and avoid scented soaps and perfumes. Do not leave food, drinks, and garbage out uncovered. Treat a bee sting by scraping the stinger away in a side-to-side motion with a credit card or fingernail, and then washing the area with soap and water. Pulling the stinger or using tweezers may push more venom into the skin. For any bug bite or sting, ice or a cold compress and OTC pain-relieving creams or oral medications can help.

Because bees puncture the skin with their stingers, there is a risk of tetanus infection. After getting the regular series of childhood tetanus shots, adults should have a tetanus booster shot every ten years.

Watch for signs of allergic reaction to stings, which typically happen within the first few hours. If you have ever had an allergic reaction to a sting, experts recommend carrying epinephrine, a prescription hormone given by injection to support blood pressure, increase heart rate, and relax airways.

Heat Illness

During heat illness, the body's cooling system shuts down. Body temperature goes up, which slows down the ability to sweat. Mild symptoms of heat exhaustion include thirst, fatigue, and cramps in the legs or abdomen. Left untreated, heat exhaustion can progress to heat stroke. Serious heat-related symptoms include dizziness, headaches, nausea, rapid heartbeat, vomiting, decreased alertness, and a temperature as high as 105° Fahrenheit or more. In severe cases, the liver, kidneys, and brain may be damaged.

♣ It's A Fact!!

About 400 people die each year from heat exposure, according to the Centers for Disease Control and Prevention.

The risk of heat illness goes up during exertion and sports and with certain health conditions such as diabetes, obesity, and heart disease. Alcohol use also increases the risk, as do medications that slow sweat production, such as tricyclic antidepressants and diuretics used to treat water retention, high blood pressure, and some liver and kidney conditions.

What you can do: Air conditioning is the number one protective factor against heat illness. If you do not have air conditioning, spend time in public facilities, such as libraries and malls that have air conditioning. Reduce strenuous activities or do them during early mornings and evenings when it is cooler. If you are outside for long stretches of time, carry a water bottle, drink fluids regularly, and do not push your limits. People who play sports should wear light, loose-fitting clothes and drink water or sports drinks before, during, and after activity. If you see someone experiencing heat illness, have the person lie down in a cool place and elevate his or her legs. Use water, wet towels, and fanning to help cool the person down until emergency help comes.

Burns From Fireworks And Grills

The U.S. Consumer Product Safety Commission estimates that about 8,800 people were treated in emergency rooms in 2002 for injuries associated with fireworks. Most injuries involved the hands, head, and eyes.

Summer cookouts are fun, but open grill flames and improperly maintained propane tanks can also be a hazard.

What you can do: Stick with public firework displays handled by professionals. Children should always be closely supervised when food is being cooked indoors or outdoors. Be aware that gas leaks, blocked tubes, and overfilled propane tanks cause most gas grill fires and explosions. If you see someone's clothes catch on fire, instruct them to cover their face, stop, drop, and roll.

Generally, minor burns smaller than a person's palm can be treated at home. Larger burns, and burns on the hands, feet, face, genitals, and major joints usually require emergency treatment. To treat a minor injury, run cool water over it and cover it with a clean, dry cloth. Do not apply ice, which can worsen a burn. Do not apply petroleum jelly or butter, which can hold heat in the tissue. Consult your doctor if a minor burn does not heal in a couple of days or if there are signs of infection, such as redness and swelling.

Food Borne Illness

Typical signs of food borne illness include nausea, vomiting, cramps, and diarrhea. In serious cases, high fever, bloody stool, and prolonged vomiting may occur. Young children, pregnant women, older people, and those with compromised immune systems are hit hardest.

Bacteria, whether in food or in the air, grow faster in warmer weather. You have to be careful with all food, including melons, lettuce, potato salad, and egg dishes. Since 1996, the U.S. Food and Drug Administration (FDA) has responded to 14 outbreaks of food borne illness for which fresh lettuce or fresh tomatoes were the confirmed or suspected source. The causes included *E. coli*, salmonella, *Cyclospora*, and hepatitis A virus.

What you can do: Wash hands well, and often, with soap and water, especially after using the bathroom and before cooking or eating. Wash surfaces when cooking, keep raw food separate from cooked food, marinate food in the refrigerator, cook food thoroughly, and refrigerate or freeze food promptly. The FDA suggests never leaving food out for more than one hour when the temperature is above 90° Fahrenheit. Any other time, do not leave food out for more than two hours. Keep hot food hot and cold food cold. Wash fruits and vegetables with cool running water. Also, scrub fruits with rough surfaces like cantaloupe with a soft brush. When packing for a picnic, place cold food in a cooler with plenty of ice or commercial freezing gels. Cold food should be held at or below 40° Fahrenheit, and the cooler should be stored in shade. Hot food should be wrapped well, placed in an insulated container, and kept at or above 140° Fahrenheit.

Victims of food borne illness must stay hydrated. Try giving them ice chips to chew or clear fluid to sip after vomiting has stopped. For the next couple of days, they should only eat light foods such as bananas, rice, applesauce, toast, crackers, and soup. Seek emergency treatment if severe pain accompanies the illness, if vomiting does not stop in a couple of hours, or if bloody diarrhea is experienced.

Poison Ivy, Poison Oak, And Poison Sumac

Rashes from poison ivy, oak, or sumac are all caused by urushiol, a substance in the sap of the plants. Poison plant rashes cannot be spread from person to person, but it is possible to pick up a rash from urushiol that sticks to clothing, tools, toys, and pets.

What you can do: Learn what poison ivy looks like and avoid it. While "leaves of three, beware of me," is the old saying, "leaflets of three, beware of me" is even better because each leaf has three smaller leaflets.

Wash garden tools regularly, especially if there is the slightest chance that they have come into contact with poison ivy. If you know you will be working around poison ivy, wear long pants, long sleeves, boots, and gloves.

Hikers, emergency workers, and others who have a difficult time avoiding poison ivy may benefit from a product called Ivy Block, made by EnviroDerm Pharmaceuticals Inc., of Louisville, Kentucky. It is the only FDA-approved product for preventing rashes from poison ivy, oak, or sumac. The OTC lotion contains bentoquatam, a substance that forms a clay-like coating on the skin.

If you come into contact with poison ivy, oak, or sumac, wash the skin in cool water as soon as possible to prevent the spread of urushiol. If you get a rash, oatmeal baths and calamine lotion can dry up blisters and bring relief from itching. Talk to a health care professional about medicines that may help.

Poisoning In Children

Children may accidentally ingest sunscreens, berries, cleaning solvents, insect repellents, pesticides, plants and mushrooms, and hydrocarbons in the form of gasoline, kerosene, and charcoal fluid.

The American Academy of Pediatrics (AAP) no longer recommends that syrup of ipecac be used routinely to induce vomiting in poisoning cases. The main reason that the AAP changed its recommendation in 2003 was that, although it seems to make sense to induce vomiting to empty the stomach contents after a poisoning, research has not shown that ipecac-induced vomiting is beneficial in improving the clinical outcome of accidental poisoning cases.

Other concerns are that the continued vomiting caused by ingesting ipecac could prevent children from keeping down the activated charcoal they may be given in the emergency room. Charcoal binds to poison and keeps it out of the bloodstream. There are also some substances that you do not want coming back up because they do more damage, such as drain cleaner and other corrosives.

The FDA is considering various positions on the safety and effectiveness of ipecac syrup and whether it should still be made available OTC or switched to prescription status.

What you can do: Dangerous substances, including medication, should be kept out of reach of children. In addition, substances should be kept in their original containers to avoid confusion or mistakes. Children who have ingested poisonous substances may experience difficulty breathing, throat pain, or burns to the lips and mouth.

If you suspect that a child has ingested a poison, call the poison center immediately to relay the type of poison ingested and get advice on what to do. If you dial the nationwide poison help line, (800) 222-1222, you will be connected to your regional poison center. Convulsions, loss of breathing, or loss of consciousness, require calling 911 immediately. Take the poison with you to the emergency room, whether it is a part of a plant or the chemical's container.

Part Eight

If You Need More Information

Chapter 66

How To Find Medical Information

Searching for medical information can be confusing, especially for first-timers. However, if you are patient and stick to it, you can find a wealth of information. Today's computer technology is making it easier than ever for people to track down medical and health information. Other good sources of information include textbooks, journal articles, reference books, and health care organizations. This chapter explains how to locate these important sources of information.

Start With Your Community Library

Most people have a library in or near their community, and it is a good place to start to look for medical information. Before going to the library, you may find it helpful to make a list of topics you want information about and questions you have. Your topic list will make it easier for the librarian to direct you to the best resources.

Basic Medical References

Many community libraries have a collection of basic medical references. These references may include medical dictionaries or encyclopedias, drug

About This Chapter: Information in this chapter is from "How to Find Medical Information," NIH Publication No. 05-4745, January 2005, National Institute of Arthritis and Musculoskeletal and Skin Diseases (NIAMS), National Institutes of Health (NIH).

information handbooks, basic medical and nursing textbooks, and directories of physicians and medical specialists (listings of doctors). You may also wish to find magazine articles on a certain topic. Look in the *Reader's Guide to Periodical Literature* for articles on health and medicine that were published in consumer magazines.

Computer Databases

Infotrac, a CD-ROM computer database available at libraries or on the internet, indexes hundreds of popular magazines and newspapers, as well as some medical journals such as the *Journal of the American Medical Association* and *New England Journal of Medicine*.

Your library may also carry searchable computer databases of medical journal articles, including MEDLINE®/PubMed® (http://pubmed.gov) or the *Cumulative Index to Nursing and Allied Health Literature*. Many of the databases or indexes have abstracts that provide a summary of each journal article. Although most community libraries do not have a large collection of medical and nursing journals, your librarian may be able to get copies of the articles you want. Interlibrary loans allow your librarian to request a copy of an article from a library that carries that particular medical journal. Your library may charge a fee for this service.

Look For A Medical Library

Medical libraries can usually be found at medical, nursing, and dental schools, large medical centers, and community hospitals. Not all hospital or academic libraries are open to the public, but a librarian at your community library may be able to give you information about the closest medical library open to the public. Medical libraries may also be listed in your telephone book under "hospitals," "schools," or "universities." In addition, you can call the National Network of Libraries of Medicine (http://nnlm.gov) of the National Library of

♣ It's A Fact!!
Articles published in medical journals can be technical, but they may be the most current source of information on medical topics.

Medicine (NLM), National Institutes of Health (NIH), at (800) 338-7657 to find the location of the nearest medical library open to the public.

A medical library has a large collection of resources, including many medical and nursing textbooks, and a comprehensive collection of medical and health-related journals. Although you may not be allowed to check out materials, most libraries have photocopiers you can use to copy material you want to take home.

Use Telephone And Fax Services

Some communities have a telephone medical service that allows callers to listen to audiotapes on certain disease topics. Also, your health insurance company or health maintenance organization may have a nurse available to answer health-related questions over the telephone.

If you have access to a fax machine, you can get health information from some organizations in just a few minutes. The Centers for Disease Control and Prevention at (888) 232-3299 (toll-free) is an example of an organization that has information available by fax. Your librarian can help you locate other fax services.

Search The Internet

You can find a wealth of information on the internet—everything from the latest medical research to facts about particular conditions. The internet also offers other resources such as bulletin boards, online publications, forums for discussion of current medical issues, and online support groups.

Here are some health resources to check out on the internet:
- National Institutes of Health, http://www.nih.gov
- Combined Health Information Database, http://chid.nih.gov
- MedlinePlus®, http://medlineplus.gov
- healthfinder®, http://www.healthfinder.gov
- National Library of Medicine, http://www.nlm.nih.gov
- Agency for Healthcare Research and Quality, http://www.ahrq.gov
- American Self-Help Clearinghouse, http://www.mentalhelp.net/selfhelp

National Library Of Medicine (NLM)

MEDLINE® and MedlinePlus®: You can search the NLM's MEDLINE® database, free of charge, on the internet (http://www.nlm.nih.gov). You can conduct a search in the web-based product, PubMed®. It provides you with free access to MEDLINE® and, for a fee, allows you to use Loansome Doc Delivery Service to order copies of articles. PubMed® links you to publishers' sites for over 4,400 full-text journals; some are by subscription only. You can also access NLM databases (http://pubmedcentral.nih.gov) through the NLM Gateway®, http://gateway.nlm.nih.gov/, which searches many NLM databases simultaneously.

ClinicalTrials.gov: ClinicalTrials.gov is an information service that provides easy access to information on clinical trials for a wide range of diseases and conditions. This database provides opportunities to participate in the evaluation of new treatments. The NLM is developing the database in collaboration with all NIH institutes, other federal agencies, the pharmaceutical industry, and academic and other nonprofit organizations. You can access this database on the internet at http://clinicaltrials.gov.

Genetics Home Reference®: This is NLM's website for consumer information about genetic conditions and the genes or chromosomes responsible for those conditions. Also included are discussions of genes, gene therapy, genetic testing, and consultation. You can access the database on the internet at: http://ghr.nlm.nih.gov.

TOXNET®: This is NLM's comprehensive toxicology and environmental health database. It can be accessed at: http://toxnet.nlm.nih.gov.

✔ Quick Tip

Where To Find Medical Information

- Community library
- Federal government clearinghouses
- Associations and voluntary organizations
- Medical, hospital, or university libraries
- Personal physician
- Nurse, pharmacist, dietitian, or other health professional
- Telephone or fax services
- Computer databases
- The internet

Department Of Health And Human Services

Healthfinder®: To help people find health information on the internet, the federal government's Department of Health and Human Services has developed a website called healthfinder® (http://www.healthfinder.gov). This website serves as a gateway to the broad range of consumer health information resources produced by the government and many of its partners. It includes a searchable index and other useful tools.

Use Information Wisely

It can be hard to judge the accuracy and credibility of medical information you read in books or magazines or see on television. Even people with medical backgrounds sometimes find this task challenging. The following are some important tips to help you decide what information is believable and accurate when evaluating books, articles, and television reports:

- Compare several different resources on the same topic. Check two or three other articles or books to see whether the information or advice is similar.

- Check the author's credentials by looking up his or her affiliations, such as university and medical school attended, associations, and lists of other publications. For doctors, this information can be found in one of the physician directories at your library or on the American Medical Association's (AMA) website at http://www.ama-assn.org (click on AMA Physician Select). You can also call the American Board of Medical Specialists at (866) ASK-ABMS (275-2267) to see whether a physician is board certified in his or her specialty. Your librarian can help you find other resources to check the credentials of non-physicians.

- Ask yourself if the information or advice "rings true." That is, is it feasible, plausible, and does it make common sense, or is it wishful thinking or sensationalism?

- Look for a list of references at the end of the article or book. Information that is backed up by other medical professionals and researchers is more likely to be accurate.

- Check out your information source. Was the article published in a peer-reviewed journal? Look for a list of editorial or review board members at the beginning of a journal. In a peer-reviewed journal, other qualified members of the profession review articles for accuracy and reliability.

- Look very carefully at information published in newspapers and magazines or reported on television. Most reporters are journalists rather than medical experts. In addition, newspapers and television reporters may use sensationalism to attract more readers or viewers. Medical facts and statistics can be misrepresented or incomplete. Check to see whether the newspaper or magazine cites a source for its information and includes the credentials of the persons cited.

- Examine a magazine's list of editors. Do medical experts serve as editors and review articles? Be especially wary of personal testimonials of miracle cures. There is often no way to judge whether the story is true. Furthermore, do not trust medical product advertisements claiming miracle cures or spectacular results.

To Make Informed Decisions About Your Health Care, You Need To Understand Your Health Problem

Medical information, especially material written for health care providers, can be hard to understand, confusing, and sometimes frightening. As you read through your materials, write down any words or information you do not understand or find confusing. Make a list of your questions and concerns. During your next office visit, ask your doctor, nurse, or other health professional to review the information with you so that you understand clearly how it might be helpful to you.

If the medical information you gathered is for a personal health problem, you should share what you found with your parents. Family members and friends who understand your health problem are better able to provide needed support and care. Finally, you might want to consider joining a support group in your community. You may find it helpful to be able to talk with others who have the same health problem and share your feelings or concerns.

Chapter 67

How To Evaluate Health Information On The Internet

The growing popularity of the internet has made it easier and faster to find health information. Much of this information is valuable; however, the internet also allows rapid and widespread distribution of false and misleading information. It is important for people to carefully consider the source of information and to discuss the information they find with their health care provider. This chapter can help people decide whether the health information they find on the internet, or receive via e-mail from a website, is likely to be reliable.

Who runs the website?

Any website should make it easy for people to learn who is responsible for the site and its information.

Who pays for the website?

It costs money to run a website. The source of a website's funding should be clearly stated or readily apparent. For example, web addresses ending in ".gov" are federal government-sponsored sites, ".edu" indicates educational

About This Chapter: Information in this chapter is from "How To Evaluate Health Information on the Internet: Questions and Answers," September 2005, National Cancer Institute, U.S. National Institutes of Health.

institutions, ".org" is often used by noncommercial organizations, and ".com" denotes commercial organizations. The source of funding can affect what content is presented, how the content is presented, and what the owners want to accomplish on the site.

What is the purpose of the website?

The purpose of the website is related to who runs and pays for it. Many websites have a link to information about the site. The link, which is often called "About This Site," should clearly state the purpose of the site and help users evaluate the trustworthiness of the information on the site.

What is the original source of the information on the website?

Many health and medical websites post information collected from other websites or sources. If the person or organization in charge of the site did not write the material, the original source should be clearly identified.

How is the information on the website documented?

In addition to identifying the original source of the material, the site should identify the evidence on which the material is based. Medical facts and figures should have references (such as citations of articles in medical journals). Also, opinions or advice should be clearly set apart from information that is "evidence-based (that is, based on research results).

♣ It's A Fact!!
Health-related websites should give information about the medical credentials of the people who prepare or review the material on the website.

How current is the information on the website?

Websites should be reviewed and updated on a regular basis. It is particularly important that medical information be current and that the most recent update or review date be clearly posted. Even if the information has not changed, it is helpful to know that the site owners have reviewed it recently to ensure that the information is still valid.

How does the website choose links to other sites?

Reliable websites usually have a policy about how they establish links to other sites. Some medical websites take a conservative approach and do not link to any other sites; some link to any site that asks or pays for a link; others link only to sites that have met certain criteria.

What information about users does the website collect, and why?

Websites routinely track the path users take through their sites to determine what pages are being used. However, many health-related websites ask the user to "subscribe" or "become a member." In some cases, this may be done so they can collect a user fee or select relevant information for the user. In all cases, the subscription or membership will allow personal information about the user to be collected by the website owners.

Any website asking users for personal information should explain exactly what the site will and will not do with the information. Many commercial sites sell "aggregate" data about their users to other companies—information such as what percent of their users are women with breast cancer. In some cases, they may collect and reuse information that is "personally identifiable," such as the user's zip code, gender, and birth date. Users should be certain they read and understand any privacy policy or similar language on the site and not sign up for anything they do not fully understand.

How does the website manage interactions with users?

There should always be a way for users to contact the website owners with problems, feedback, and questions. If the site hosts a chat room or other online discussion areas, it should tell users about the terms of using the service. Is the service moderated? If so, by whom, and why? It is always a good idea to spend time reading the discussion, without joining in, to feel comfortable with the environment before becoming a participant.

How can people verify the accuracy of information they receive via e-mail?

Any e-mail messages should be carefully evaluated. The origin of the message and its purpose should be considered. Some companies or organizations use e-mail to advertise products or attract people to their websites. The accuracy of health information may be influenced by the desire to promote a product or service.

How does the federal government protect consumers from false or misleading health claims posted on the internet?

The Federal Trade Commission (FTC) enforces consumer protection laws. As part of its mission, the FTC investigates complaints about false or misleading health claims posted on the internet. The FTC's "Operation Cure-All" page, located at http://www.ftc.gov/bcp/conline/edcams/cureall/ on the internet, has information to help users evaluate health product claims.

Federal Trade Commission
Consumer Response Center
CRC–240
Washington, DC 20580
Toll Free 877-382-4357 (877-FTC-HELP)
TTY: 866-653-4261
Website: http://www.ftc.gov

The Food and Drug Administration (FDA) regulates drugs and medical devices to ensure that they are safe and effective. The FDA's "Buying Medicines and Medical Products Online" web page is located at http://www.fda.gov/buyonline/ on the internet. "Buying Prescription Medicines Online: A Consumer Safety Guide" is available at http://www.fda.gov/buyonlineguide/ on the internet.

Food and Drug Administration
5600 Fishers Lane
Rockville, MD 20857
Toll Free 888-463-6332 (888-INFO-FDA)
Website: http://www.fda.gov

Chapter 68

How To Interpret Medical Information In The News Media

Jordan was gathering information for a research project on teens and suicide. She came across a news article about how some antidepressants increase the chances of suicidal thinking and behavior in kids and teens. Jordan was confused. How could a medicine that was supposed to help kids with depression actually make them feel worse? She was also worried because her sister was taking an antidepressant. After Jordan did some of her own research and looked into the issue further, though, she discovered things that set her mind at ease.

Often, news reports on health and medicine can be confusing; and sometimes they can be downright scary. How do you know what is important and accurate?

Large newspapers, magazines, TV networks, and radio stations often have medical reporters on staff to cover developments in health and medicine. Their job is to report complicated scientific information in a way that's easy for regular people to understand. Many health stories are accurate and balanced.

About This Chapter: Information in this chapter is from "Figuring Out Health News." This information was provided by TeensHealth, one of the largest resources online for medically reviewed health information written for parents, kids, and teens. For more articles like this one, visit www.TeensHealth.org, or www.KidsHealth.org. © 2006 The Nemours Foundation.

But not all are. Sometimes, reporters try to quickly cram information into a short news story, and they may oversimplify the information. What you see may not be the whole picture.

A Study—Or Just A Story?

To catch a viewer's attention, news reports sometimes make dramatic claims. In addition, medical news reports often focus on people's personal stories, not scientific studies. Personal stories are interesting, but often they don't prove anything about health or treatments in general. It takes a well-done study to do that. And sometimes these studies just aren't dramatic or exciting enough to make the news.

When you hear about a new medical development, the first question to ask yourself is whether the news is based on a scientific study. Knowing there's a study behind the news is only the first step, though. How the study was done (and who did it) matters too. For example:

Was The Study Done In People?

A lot of medical research is done in the laboratory or in lab animals, not in people—at least, not at first. Lab studies help scientists figure out whether a drug looks promising, how it works, and whether there might be side effects. But what happens in a laboratory does not necessarily work the same in people. These studies are often a beginning, but they're usually not the end of the story.

When watching or reading a news report about a new drug or treatment, see if it tells you whether the findings involved animals or people. It might not, so you'll have to do some sleuthing on your own to get the information (see "Doing Your Own Research" later in the chapter).

Who Was In The Study?

Even if a study was done in people, it may not apply to you. For instance, findings from studies involving only adults may not be true for teens. Results of all-male studies may not apply to women. Research studies usually list who took part—their sex, age, and other characteristics. Are these people like you?

In addition to who is in a study, you'll also need to keep in mind how many people took part in it. The more people in the study, the more likely it is that the study's findings will hold true for the whole population. Sometimes a study's results are announced with a big splash and then it turns out that the study only involved a few people. When researchers do the same study using the hundreds or thousands of people necessary to get really accurate (or "significant") results, those results might be different.

It's also important for the study to follow patients long enough to be sure that a treatment really works, and that additional or more serious side effects don't develop over time.

♣ It's A Fact!!
Decoding The Numbers

A news report says that something "doubles" your risk of getting a disease. Does that mean you should be scared? Only if your chances of getting the disease are already high. News reports can make medical problems seem more common than they are. If your risk doubles from 1 in 1,000 to 2 in 1,000, that's still pretty small. And if you have a 1% chance of getting a disease, that means you have a 99% chance of not getting it.

How Was The Study Designed?

There are lots of ways researchers look into new treatments and information that can help people stay healthier. Sometimes they look back at people's medical records or ask them questions to find out what might have put them at more (or less) risk for a health condition. Those studies, called retrospective studies, can provide useful clues, but they're only as reliable as a person's memory or the accuracy of medical records.

Prospective studies are usually better. They look forward, not backward. The best of these studies follow thousands of people long enough to see whether the things they do, like diet and exercise, have a good or bad effect on their health.

For new drugs or treatments, randomized, controlled clinical trials are the best way for deciding whether a treatment works. In this kind of research, some of the participants get the drug, vitamin, or other therapy being tested. Others get what is called a placebo (a fake treatment or sugar pill that contains no medicine at all). In this type of study, the patients are "blinded"; they don't know who is getting the treatment and who is getting the placebo until the trial is over. That way, their response to the drug or placebo can't be influenced by whether they think they have been taking the real drug or not. In a double-blind study, neither the patients nor the researchers know which patients have taken the drug or the placebo until the study is over.

It's rare for one study to be the final word. Medical knowledge comes from many studies done over time, and frequently there are contradictions along the way. Often, different studies of a particular treatment or condition, all done properly, can still have different (or even completely opposite) results.

♣ **It's A Fact!!**
Who Paid For It?

A lot of medical research is funded by the government, in particular the National Institutes of Health (NIH). Foundations devoted to particular causes also pay for research, for example, the American Cancer Society funds research to help fight cancer; but some studies are funded by the companies that make the medication or device being researched. That doesn't mean the findings are false, but the organization paying for the research does have an interest in how the results turn out.

Also, the news media (and even researchers themselves) are more likely to report the findings of a study if that study shows results that are different from what is thought to be true. For example, the media are much more likely to do a story about a study that shows that eating a particular type of food may help prevent cancer, but other studies may show that eating that food doesn't really make much difference.

The scientific community can take into account all the different studies and decide that eating the food might not really help a person avoid cancer; but to the regular person who just hears about one study through the news, that food suddenly becomes a cancer-fighting miracle.

Where Do Reporters Get Their Stories?

Sometimes, reporters get their news stories by following what is published in medical journals. The best medical and scientific journals, like *The New England Journal of Medicine*, *The Journal of the American Medical Association*, *Pediatrics*, *Science*, and *Nature*, carefully review studies before publishing them so the information is trustworthy.

These publications are written for the scientific community, and the language in them can be hard for people who aren't doctors or scientists to understand. News reporters who get their information from scientific journals might do a good job of explaining the study and what it means—but not always.

Some reporters don't always wait until something is published before reporting it as news. Sometimes reporters hear information from researchers before a study has even been published, and they want to bring it to the public's attention quickly. Without a published study, though, a reporter may not have all the facts.

So how do you get closer to the truth?

Doing Your Own Research

You can get additional information about a news report on the internet. Put keywords from the news report into a search engine, and see what comes up. The results will give you lots of different perspectives, particularly if the issue is big news, so you're not relying on just one news report for the facts. You'll need to screen what you see, though. Many of the sites that show up in search results may not have the most accurate and up-to-date information.

✔ Quick Tip
News—Or Self-Promotion

It's sometimes tough to tell if you're looking at an ad or a news report. Check the fine print to see if the word "advertisement" appears on an article or website. If so, the ad may be promoting a particular treatment or point of view.

✔ Quick Tip
The Real Score On Health Quizzes

Some magazines and websites like to run quizzes on health conditions like depression, anorexia, and asthma. Quizzes like these can
get you thinking, but they are not meant for you to diagnose yourself
with a disease or medical condition. If you think you have a
problem, talk to a parent or doctor, and never stop taking a medication or change how you take it because of how you scored on a quiz.

On commercial websites (sites with URLs that end in .com), look to see
if the site has advertising. If it does, it may be biased in favor of the adver-
tiser. Of course, having advertising on a site doesn't necessarily mean it is
biased; but if you're going to be a good "information consumer," you need to
take that possibility into account.

Also check to see whether a doctor or other medical expert has reviewed
the information you're reading and whether the date on the information is
recent.

The websites of government health agencies, such as the National Institutes of Health (NIH), the Centers for Disease Control and Prevention
(CDC), and the U.S. Food and Drug Administration (FDA), usually give
accurate and unbiased information. Established medical organizations, such
as the American Academy of Pediatrics, and associations, such as the American Psychiatric Association, are other good sources.

Getting Help

The best way to get a full understanding of medical news is to ask someone like a doctor or science teacher for help in figuring out what it all means.

Jordan talked to her science teacher about the antidepressant story. She
helped Jordan understand that certain antidepressants (like the one Jordan's

sister was taking) are OK for teens. She also helped her discover that the study results didn't mean all the teens in the study committed suicide while on the medication. In fact, in this study, none of the patients on the medication committed suicide. Instead, some reported thinking about suicide more. Jordan also learned about how important it is for teens on antidepressants to see their doctors regularly so their medications can be monitored and adjusted.

Reading or watching medical news isn't a substitute for seeing a doctor. Trying to diagnose yourself or changing or stopping your medicine based on something you've read or heard can be dangerous. News reports often focus only on the positive and don't mention the downsides, or side effects, of a medication or other treatment; or they may report a dramatic or scary side effect of a medication that is really very rare, or fail to mention the large number of patients who might get very sick if they didn't take the drug. Your doctor can help you weigh the benefits and risks.

As Jordan discovered, understanding what's behind medical news can take away worry and concern; and knowing more can help you ask good questions about your own health when you see your doctor.

Chapter 69

Directory Of Health Resources

Federal Agencies

Centers for Disease Control and Prevention (CDC)
1600 Clifton Road
Atlanta, GA 30333
Toll Free: 800-311-3435
Phone: 404-639-3534
Website: http://www.cdc.gov

Health Resources and Services Administration (HRSA)
5600 Fishers Lane Rm. 9A55
Rockville, MD 20857
Phone: 301-443-0835
Website: http://www.hrsa.gov

Library of Congress
Science, Technology and
Business Division
101 Independence Avenue, S.E.
Washington, DC 20540-4750
Phone: 202-707-5000
Fax: 202-707-1925
Website: http://www.loc.gov

National Cancer Institute (NCI)
NCI Public Inquiries Office
6116 Executive Boulevard
Room 3036A
Bethesda, MD 20892-8322
Toll Free: 800-4-CANCER
(800-422-6237)
TTY: 800-332-8615
Website: http://www.cancer.gov

National Human Genome Research Institute
National Institutes of Health
Building 31, Room 4B09
31 Center Drive, MSC 2152
9000 Rockville Pike
Bethesda, MD 20892-2152
Phone: 301-402-0911
Fax: 301-402-2218
Website: http://www.genome.gov

National Institute of Allergy and Infectious Diseases (NIAID)
NIAID Office of Communications and Public Liaison
6610 Rockledge Drive, MSC 6612
Bethesda, MD 20892-6612
Phone: 301-496-5717
Fax: 301-402-3573
TDD: 800-877-8339
Website: http://www3.niaid.nih.gov

National Institute of Arthritis and Musculoskeletal and Skin Diseases (NIAMS)
Information Clearinghouse
National Institutes of Health
1 AMS Circle
Bethesda, MD 20892-3675
Toll Free: 877-22-NIAMS
Phone: 301-495-4484
Fax: 301-718-6366
TTY: 301-565-2966
Website: http://www.niams.nih.gov
E-mail: niamsinfo@mail.nih.gov

National Institute of Mental Health (NIMH)
Public Information and Communications Branch
6001 Executive Boulevard, Room 8184, MSC 9663
Bethesda, MD 20892-9663
Toll Free: 866-615-6464
Phone: 301-443-4513
Fax: 301-443-4279
TTY Toll Free: 866-415-8051
TTY: 301-443-8431
Website: http://www.nimh.nih.gov
E-mail: nimhinfo@nih.gov

National Institute on Drug Abuse (NIDA)
6001 Executive Boulevard, Rm. 5213
Bethesda, MD 20892-9561
Phone: 301-443-1124
Website: http://www.nida.nih.gov

National Institutes of Health (NIH)
9000 Rockville Pike
Bethesda, MD 20892
Phone: 301-496-4000
TTY: 301-402-9612
Website: http://www.nih.gov
E-mail: NIHinfo@od.nih.gov

National Library of Medicine (NLM)
8600 Rockville Pike
Bethesda, MD 20894
Toll Free: 888-FIND-NLM
(888-346-3656)

Phone: 301-594-5983
Fax: 301-402-1384
Website: http://www.nlm.nih.gov
E-mail: custserv@nlm.nih.gov

President's Council on Physical Fitness and Sports (PCPFS)
Department W
200 Independence Avenue, S.W.
Room 738-H
Washington, DC 20201-0004
Phone: 202-690-9000
Fax: 202-690-5211
Website: http://www.fitness.gov

Substance Abuse and Mental Health Services Administration (SAMHSA)
1 Choke Cherry Road
Rockville, MD 20857
Website: http://www.samhsa.gov

U.S. Department of Health and Human Services (HHS)
200 Independence Avenue, S.W.
Washington, DC 20201
Toll Free: 877-696-6775
Phone: 202-619-0257
Website: http://www.hhs.gov

U.S. Food and Drug Administration (FDA)
5600 Fishers Lane
Rockville, MD 20857
Toll Free: 888-INFO-FDA
(888-463-6332)
Website: http://www.fda.gov

Private Organizations

American Academy of Family Physicians
P.O. Box 11210
Shawnee Mission, KS 66207-1210
Toll Free: 800-274-2237
Phone: 913-906-6000
Website: http://www.aafp.org
E-mail: fp@aafp.org

American Board of Medical Specialties
1007 Church Street, Suite 404
Evanston, IL 60201-5913
Phone Verification: 866-ASK-ABMS
Phone: 847-491-9091
Fax: 847-328-3596
Website: http://www.abms.org

American Osteopathic Association
142 East Ontario Street
Chicago, IL 60611
Toll Free: 800-621-1773
Phone: 312-202-8000
Fax: 312-202-8200
Website: http://
www.osteopathic.org

American Society of Plastic Surgeons
444 East Algonquin Road
Arlington Heights, IL 60005
Toll Free: 888-4-PLASTIC
(888-475-2784)
Website: http://www.plasticsurgery.org

Cleveland Clinic
Department of Patient Education
and Health Information
9500 Euclid Avenue, NA31
Cleveland, OH 44195
Toll Free: 800-223-2273, ext.
43771
Phone: 216-444-3771
Website: http://
www.clevelandclinic.org
E-mail: healthl@ccf.org

Healthwise, Inc.
2601 North Bogus Basin Road
Boise, ID 83702
Toll Free: 800-706-9646
Website: http://www.healthwise.org

National Sleep Foundation (NSF)
1522 K Street, N.W., Suite 500
Washington, DC 20005
Phone: 202-347-3471
Fax: 202-347-3472
Website: http://
www.sleepfoundation.org
E-mail: nsf@sleepfoundation.org

Science News for Kids
1719 N. Street, N.W.
Washington, DC 20036
Phone: 202-785-2255
Fax: 202-659-0365
Website: http://
www.sciencenewsforkids.org
E-mail: editor@snkids.com

University of Michigan Health System
1500 E. Medical Center Drive
Ann Arbor, MI 48109
Phone: 734-936-4000
Website: http://
www.med.umich.edu

Internet Resources

Cool Nurse
http://www.coolnurse.com

FamilyDoctor.org
http://www.familydoctor.org

GirlsHealth.gov
http://www.girlshealth.gov

Girl Power
http://www.girlpower.gov

HealthAtoZ
http://www.healthatoz.com/
healthatoz/Atoz/default.jsp

KidsHealth
http://www.kidshealth.org

MayoClinic.com
http://www.mayoclinic.com

WomensHealth.gov
http://www.4woman.gov

Chapter 70

Additional Reading About Your Body And Maintaining Well-Being

Books

A Teen's Guide to Living Drug-Free
Bettie B. Youngs, Jennifer Leigh Youngs, Tina Moreno
HCI Teens, Deerfield Beach, FL
January 2003
ISBN: 0757300413

Alcohol Information for Teens:
Health Tips about Alcohol and Alcoholism
Joyce Brennfleck Shannon (Editor)
Omnigraphics, Inc., Detroit, MI
January 2005
ISBN: 0780807413

About This Chapter: This chapter includes a compilation of various resources from many sources deemed reliable. It serves as a starting point for further research and is not intended to be comprehensive. Inclusion does not constitute endorsement. Resources in this chapter are categorized by type and, under each type, they are listed alphabetically by title to make topics easier to identify.

Atlas of the Human Body
F. Netter, M.D.
Barron's Educational Series, Hauppauge, NY
November 2005
ISBN: 0764158848

Be Healthy! It's a Girl Thing: Food, Fitness, and Feeling Great
Mavis Jukes, Lilian Cheung
Crown Books for Young Readers, New York, NY
December 2003
ISBN: 0679890297

Can I Change the Way I Look: A Teen's Guide to the Health Implications of Cosmetic Surgery, Makeovers, and Beyond
Autumn Libal
Mason Crest Publishers, Broomall, PA
December 2004
ISBN: 1590848438

Cosmetic Surgery for Teens: Choices and Consequences
Kathleen Winkler
Enslow Publishers, Inc., Berkeley Heights, NJ
July 2003
ISBN: 0766019578

Diet Information for Teens: Health Tips about Diet and Nutrition
Karen Bellenir (Editor)
Omnigraphics, Inc., Detroit, MI
June 2006
ISBN: 0780808207

Drug Information for Teens: Health Tips about the Physical and Mental Effects of Substance Abuse
Sandra Augustyn Lawton (Editor)
Omnigraphics, Inc., Detroit, MI
June 2006
ISBN: 0780808622

Eating Disorders Information for Teens: Health Tips about Anorexia, Bulimia, Binge Eating, and Other Eating Disorders
Sandra Augustyn Lawton (Editor)
Omnigraphics, Inc., Detroit, MI
June 2005
ISBN: 0780807839

Fitness Information for Teens: Health Tips about Exercise, Physical Well-Being, and Health Maintenance
Karen Bellenir (Editor)
Omnigraphics, Inc., Detroit, MI
June 2004
ISBN: 0780806794

Genetics for Dummies
Tara Rodden Robinson, PhD
John Wiley and Sons, Inc., Hoboken, NJ
September 2005
ISBN: 0764595547

Good Housekeeping Family First Aid
Andy Jagoda, M.D.
Hearst, New York, NY
March 2004
ISBN: 1588162990

Human Body: A Visual Guide
Beverly McMillan
Firefly Books Ltd., Richmond Hill, Ontario
September 2006
ISBN: 1554071887

The Human Body: Uncovering Science
Chris Hawkes
Firefly Books Ltd., Richmond Hill, Ontario
May 2006
ISBN: 1554071356

Human Body Systems: Structure, Function and Environment
Daniel D. Chiras
Jones and Bartlett Publishers, Inc., Sudbury, MA
May 2003
ISBN: 0763723568

Mental Health Information for Teens: Health Tips about Mental Wellness and Mental Illness
Karen Bellenir (Editor)
Omnigraphics, Inc., Detroit, MI
July 2006
ISBN: 0780808630

Safe Sex 101: An Overview for Teens
Margaret O. Hyde, Elizabeth H. Forsyth, M.D.
Twenty-First Century Books,
Breckenridge, CO
February 2006
ISBN: 0822534398

Sexual Health Information for Teens: Health Tips about Sexual Development, Human Reproduction, and Sexually Transmitted Diseases
Deborah A. Stanley (Editor)
Omnigraphics, Inc., Detroit, MI
October 2003
ISBN: 0780804457

Teens Health and Obesity
Peter Owens
Mason Crest Publishers, Broomall, PA
July 2005
ISBN: 1590848721

Tobacco Information for Teens:
Health Tips about the Hazards of Using
Cigarettes, Smokeless Tobacco, and Other
Nicotine Products
Karen Bellenir (Editor)
Omnigraphics, Inc., Detroit, MI
December 2006
ISBN: 0780809769

Articles

"A Burning Issue: Indoor Tanning Debate Heats Up," *Current Events*, a *Weekly Reader* publication, May 6, 2005, p. 3(2).

"Brain Strain Brings Teen Turmoil," *Current Science*, a *Weekly Reader* publication, January 3, 2003, p. 13(1).

"Bulimic Teens Also Likely to Suffer from Depression," *Life Science Weekly*, December 28, 2004, p. 498.

"Clean Teens: What Do You Call a Teen Who Doesn't Drink Or Do Drugs? One of the Crowd," by Melissa Daly, *Current Health 2*, a *Weekly Reader* publication, April-May 2005, p. 20(3).

"Dark Moods: Countless Teens Are Drowning in Clinical Depression. Are You One of Them," by Pippa Wysong, *Current Health 2*, a *Weekly Reader* publication, December 2005, p. 14(5).

"Drug Problem: Two Young Men Are Campaigning Against Antidepressant Use by Teens and Children," by Kirsten Weir, *Current Science*, a *Weekly Reader* publication, November 21, 2003, p. 8(4).

"Eating Troubles," by Emily Sohn, *Science News for Kids*, February 8, 2006, p. NA.

"Empty Inside: Eating Disorders Involve Much More Than Wanting to Be Thin," by Polly Sparling, *Current Health 2*, a *Weekly Reader* publication, January 2005, p. 19(2).

"Feeling Frazzled? Today's Teens' Jam-Packed Schedules Are Causing an Excess of Stress," by Mary Lou Hurley, *Current Health 2*, a *Weekly Reader* publication, October 2004, p. 12(4).

"FDA Issues Warning on Decorative Contact Lenses," by Michelle Meadows, *FDA Consumer*, January-February 2003, p. 18(2).

"Getting Help: Two Teens in Treatment Get Real about What It's Like to Smoke Pot," *Current Health 2*, a *Weekly Reader* publication, March 2005, p. 13(1).

"Indoor Tanning: Unexpected Dangers," *Consumer Reports*, February 2005, p. 30(4).

"Modified: Are Piercings and Tattoos Safe," by Pippa Wysong, *Current Health 2*, a *Weekly Reader* publication, March 2006, p. 26(5).

"No Bones about It: Test Your Skeletal Knowledge," *Current Health 2*, a *Weekly Reader* publication, March 2006, p. 13(1).

"Teen Tanning Hazards," by Carol Rados, *FDA Consumer*, March-April 2005, p. NA.

"Tips for Teen Drivers," *Current Health 2*, a *Weekly Reader* publication, January 2004, p. 2(1).

"What Is Self-Esteem and How Can I Get It," by Edgar T. Ossolotch, *Current Science*, a *Weekly Reader* publication, March 3, 2006, p. 15(1).

"Why Teens Need More Sleep: Find out How You Can Fit More Sleep into Your Overscheduled Life (and We Don't Mean Sleeping on the Bus)," by Jan Farrington, *Current* Health 2, a *Weekly Reader* publication, November 2003, p. 6(1).

Index

Index

Page numbers that appear in *Italics* refer to illustrations. Page numbers that have a small 'n' after the page number refer to information shown as Notes at the beginning of each chapter. Page numbers that appear in **Bold** refer to information contained in boxes on that page (except Notes information at the beginning of each chapter).

$65.00   4/08

LONGWOOD PUBLIC LIBRARY
Middle Country Road
Middle Island, NY 11953
(631) 924-6400
LIBRARY HOURS

Monday-Friday	9:30 a.m. - 9:00 p.m.
Saturday	9:30 a.m. - 5:00 p.m.
Sunday (Sept-June)	1:00 p.m. - 5:00 p.m.